Immunology of HIV Infection

IMMUNOLOGY AND MEDICINE SERIES

Immunology of Endocrine Diseases
Editor: A. M. McGregor

Clinical Transplantation: Current Practice and Future Prospects
Editor: G. R. D. Catto

Complement in Health and Disease
Editor: K. Whaley

Immunological Aspects of Oral Diseases
Editor: L. Ivanyi

Immunoglobulins in Health and Disease
Editor: M. A. H. French

Immunology of Malignant Diseases
Editors: V. S. Byers and R. W. Baldwin

Lymphoproliferative Diseases
Editors: D. B. Jones and D. H. Wright

Phagocytes and Disease
Editors: M. S. Klempner, B. Styrt and J. Ho

Immunology of Sexually Transmitted Diseases
Editor: D. J. M. Wright

Mast Cells, Mediators and Disease
Editor: S. T. Holgate

Immunodeficiency and Disease
Editor: A. D. B. Webster

Immunology of Pregnancy and its Disorders
Editor: C. M. M. Stern

Immunotherapy of Disease
Editor: T. J. Hamblin

Immunology of Prophylactic Immunization
Editor: A. J. Zuckerman

Immunology of Eye Disease
Editor: S. Lightman

Lymphoproliferative Diseases
Editors: D. B. Jones and D. H. Wright

Immunology of Renal Diseases
Editor: C. D. Pusey

Biochemistry of Inflammation
Editors: J. T. Whicher and S. W. Evans

Immunology of ENT Disorders
Editor: G. Scadding

Immunology of Infection
Editors: J. G. P. Sissons, J. Cohen and L. K. Borysiewicz

Immunology of HIV Infection
Editor: A. G. Bird

Immunology of Gastrointestinal Diseases
Editor: T. T. MacDonald

IMMUNOLOGY
SERIES · SERIES · SERIES · SERIES AND SERIES · SERIES · SERIES · SERIES
MEDICINE

Volume 17

Immunology of HIV Infection

Edited by
A. G. Bird
HIV Immunology Unit
Department of Medicine
University of Edinburgh, Scotland

Series Editor: K. Whaley

SPRINGER-SCIENCE+BUSINESS MEDIA, B.V.

British Library Cataloguing in Publication Data

Immunology of HIV infection/edited by A. G. Bird.
p. cm. — (Immunology and medicine series; v. 17)
Includes bibliographical references and index.
ISBN 978-94-010-5324-2 ISBN 978-94-011-2980-0 (eBook)
DOI 10.1007/978-94-011-2980-0
1. HIV infections — Immunological aspects. 2. HIV Infections — immunology.
I. Bird, Angus Graham. II. Series.
[DNLM: W1 IM53BI v. 17 / WD 308 I345]
QR201.A37155 1991
616.97'92079 — dc20
DNLM/DLC
for Library of Congress 91-20890
CIP

Typeset by Technical Keying Services, Manchester.

Contents

Series Editor's Note

The interface between clinical immunology and other branches of medical practice is frequently blurred and the general physician is often faced with clinical problems with an immunological basis and is expected to diagnose and manage such patients. The rapid expansion of basic and clinical immunology over the past two decades has resulted in the appearance of increasing numbers of immunology journals and it is impossible for a non-specialist to keep apace with this information overload. The *Immunology and Medicine* series is designed to present individual topics of immunology in a condensed package of information which can be readily assimilated by the busy clinician or pathologist.

K. Whaley, Glasgow
August 1991

Preface

It is now 10 years since the first AIDS cases were reported in the USA. In that relatively short period of time, study of the disease has moved from the level of early clinical description to exhaustive and extensive laboratory characterization of the human immunodeficiency virus (HIV), the immune responses directed towards it and reasons for their failure.

This volume provides contributions from clinical and basic scientists who are actively involved in research in a number of areas of current interest and controversy. Further progress in the clinical management of the HIV-infected patient will undoubtedly build on the basic knowledge about HIV and its modes of pathogenesis. The intimate relationship between HIV and the human immune system provides observations and questions that are relevant to viral immunopathogenesis in general.

In the first chapter the clinical features of HIV immunodeficiency are reviewed, and aspects of its changing face are discussed. Dr Tersmette then presents evidence for changing viral characteristics at different stages of the disease. This view of close competition for ascendancy between HIV and the host immune response raises questions about current approaches to therapy.

Dr Knight and co-authors then review the interrelationships between HIV and antigen-presenting cells. These cells are essential for the initiation of specific immune responses and also form direct targets for both viral infection and consequent cytotoxic T cell action. This latter mechanism, the principal immune response responsible for inhibiting or clearing primary infection, is reviewed by Dr D. Nixon. Current evidence suggests that partially effective cellular immune responses are established against HIV in the early stages of infection, and the relevance of such responses and reasons for their eventual failure are discussed.

Improvements in the assessment of immunological competence will play an increasing role in the clinical management of individual patients with HIV infection, and in the trial assessment of new therapies. The next two chapters examine the methodologies available and review their applications and future potential.

The increasing prevalence of cellular immunodeficiency that results from HIV infection is focusing attention on the range of opportunistic infections associated with the later stages of disease. In some examples, previously rare infections are being researched closely for the first time, in others a re-examination using more powerful techniques has resulted. In some countries, especially the more socioeconomically deprived, an old infection *Mycobacterium tuberculosis* is returning as a new and virulent pathogen as a consequence of HIV infection. In Chapter 7 Dr Kumararatne and colleagues review recent new insights from investigation of the immune responses against this organism.

Finally Dr Mills reviews the prospects for vaccination against HIV infection. In the past 12 years the attitude of many immunologists towards HIV vaccine prospects has shifted from profound scepticism to cautious long-term optimism. This change has been the result of the recently published primate studies which Dr Mills discusses. However, as he points out, many problems remain and the ethical and practical problems of launching and assessing the necessary human trials are formidable. Vaccines remain a prospect for the twenty-first rather than the twentieth century, and are unlikely to substantially help the many who have already sustained infection.

Most clinicians and many immunologists find the pace and breadth of developments in the molecular virology and immunology of HIV infection daunting. Sound progress in the clinical management of this new challenge to medicine will require a working knowledge of these areas. This volume casts a spotlight on some of the more rapidly developing areas, and the series editor hopes that these reviews will encourage readers to dig more deeply into the published literature cited at the end of each contribution.

List of Contributors

R. BARTLETT
Department of Immunology
The Medical School
Birmingham B15 2TJ
UK

E. O. E. BASSI
Department of Immunology
The Medical School
Birmingham B15 2TJ
UK

A. G. BIRD
HIV Immunology Unit
Department of Medicine
University of Edinburgh
Royal Infirmary
Edinburgh EH3 9HB
UK

R. P. BRETTLE
Consultant Physician
City Hospital
Greenbank Drive
Edinburgh EH10 5SB
UK

R. A. GRUTERS
UMR 103 CNRS/Biomerieux
Ecole Normale Supérieure de Lyon
46 allée d'Italie
69463 Lyon Cedex 07
France

S. C. KNIGHT
Antigen Presentation Research Group
Clinical Research Centre
Watford Road
Harrow, Middx HA1 3UJ
UK

D. S. KUMARARATNE
Department of Immunology
The Medical School
Birmingham B15 2TJ
UK

C. L. S. LEEN
Consultant Physician
City Hospital
Greenbank Drive
Edinburgh EH10 5SB
UK

S. E. MACATONIA
Antigen Presentation Research Group
Clinical Research Centre
Watford Road
Harrow, Middx HA1 3UJ
UK

F. MIEDEMA
Department of Clinical Viro-immunology
Central Laboratory of the Netherlands
Blood Transfusion Service
PO Box 9406
1006 AK Amsterdam
The Netherlands

K. H. G. MILLS
Division of Immunology
NIBSC
Blanche Lane
South Mimms
Potters Bar, Herts EN6 3QJ
UK

D. F. NIXON
Molecular Immunology Group
Institute of Molecular Medicine
John Radcliffe Hospital
Headington, Oxford OX3 9DU
UK

LIST OF CONTRIBUTORS

S. PATTERSON
Antigen Presentation Research Group
Clinical Research Centre
Watford Road
Harrow, Middx HA1 3UJ
UK

A. PITHIE
Department of Communicable and Tropical Diseases
East Birmingham Hospital
Bordesely Green East
Birmingham B9 5ST
UK

M. TERSMETTE
Department of Clinical Viro-immunology
Central Laboratory of the Netherlands Blood Transfusion Service
PO Box 9406
1006 AK Amsterdam
The Netherlands

1
Natural history of HIV infection

C. L. S. LEEN and R. P. BRETTLE

INTRODUCTION

The original description of AIDS, or the acquired immune deficiency syndrome, appeared in 1981. It described 26 patients with Kaposi's sarcoma, a skin tumour which until then was seen only in elderly men, in African races, and in those with considerable iatrogenic immunosuppression, and in five men with oral thrush and pneumocystis pneumonia which, again, was usually associated with iatrogenic immunosuppression. The connection between the two groups was that the men were all young male homosexuals with a mean age of 32 years[1,2]. The first nine cases of AIDS amongst injection drug users were diagnosed retrospectively to have occurred in 1980, and four of these were also homosexuals[3]. The first case of tranfusion-associated AIDS occurred in a young child who had a platelet transfusion[4]. Between 1978 and 1983 in the United States the risk of acquiring HIV via blood transfusion was estimated at 0.6 cases of AIDS per 100 000 adults transfused, and 2.8 cases of AIDS per 100 000 children transfused[5]. The risk was increased by a factor of 32 for adults given more than 10 units of blood and by a factor of 27 for children given more than 10 units of blood[6]. The risk with whole blood, packed cells, platelets or frozen plasma and the mean incubation period from transfusion to the development of AIDS was 21 months for children and 31 months for adults[7]. The risk of acquiring HIV from an infected blood product appeared to be about 66% and infection was more likely the closer the donor was to developing AIDS[8]. This does rather suggest that infectivity in donors rises as they develop symptoms. Other 'high-risk groups' were also soon recognized, including haemophiliacs, the heterosexual partners of patients with AIDS and children[9–18].

The epidemiology or distribution of cases is characteristic of a blood-associated virus transmission via blood contact, via sexual intercourse and perinatally. Consequently, the patients likely to be affected are: homosexuals/bisexuals, injection drug users, the recipients of blood products (either coagulation products or blood itself, especially prior to 1985 when testing became available in the United Kingdom and the United States), the children of infected females, and heterosexual contacts of infected patients. Whilst this latter group is currently small this may change in the future. In Africa, although reporting is difficult, there appears no doubt that the disease is now heterosexually spread in the majority of cases.

At any one time approximately 50% of the cumulative number of cases have died[19]. The mortality depends upon the index condition at presentation. Those presenting with an opportunistic infection have a current case mortality rate of over 50%, whereas those with Kaposi's sarcoma have a case mortality rate of only 33%. Those patients presenting with both an opportunistic infection and Kaposi's sarcoma have a current case mortality rate of 63%[19]. The survival time also varies with the type of presentation in AIDS; the medium survival time for those patients with Kaposi's sarcoma in the absence of opportunistic infections varies between 20 and 30 months, whereas the median survival time for patients with opportunistic infections varies between 4 and 11 months[20,21].

The Centers for Disease Control (CDC) in Atlanta introduced a definition to help collate accurate information about the condition. This definition of AIDS initially required the clinical diagnosis of conditions that were moderately predictive of cellular immunodeficiency without an underlying cause. The definition was revised in 1987 to take into account serological evidence of HIV infection[22].

THE CENTERS FOR DISEASE CONTROL CLINICAL STAGING SYSTEM

It was soon recognized that, in addition to AIDS, there were a number of other conditions related to HIV infection. The exact interrelationship and natural history of HIV is as yet not known, but in an attempt to ease the problem of definition the CDC developed a classification system which is descriptive and does not attempt to define any interconnections[23]; it essentially details four mutually exclusive categories or groups of HIV infection as shown in Table 1.1.

This classification system for HIV is not meant to suggest that every individual has to progress through all stages, but it is hierarchical, i.e. having reached a particular stage patients do not revert to earlier stages if the signs or symptoms settle.

CDC stage IV is, however, further divided into five subsections which are not exclusive, and patients in this group may be included in one or more of the subgroups. The conditions detailed in stage IV contain all those conditions currently used for the definition of AIDS, as well as others that indicate clinically significant HIV infection. A similar staging system was also developed for children, but this will not be described in detail.

Table 1.1 Classification of effects of HIV infection

I	Acute infection with seroconversion		
II	Asymptomatic infection		
III	Persistent generalized lymphadenopathy		
IV	A	Constitutional disease	
	B	Neurological disease	
	C	Immunodeficiency	
		C1	CDC definition of AIDS
		C2	Infections outwith definition
	D	Tumours in CDC definitions of AIDS	
	E	Other, e.g. Hodgkin's, carcinoma, lymphoid, interstitial pneumonia	

Primary HIV infection

CDC stage I describes those individuals that undergo a self-limiting illness whilst seroconverting for HIV. Primary infection with human immunodeficiency virus may be associated with acute clinical manifestations, for example a 'glandular fever'-like illness[24–31], or less commonly an acute neurological illness, e.g. meningoencephalitis[25,32,33] and peripheral neuropathy[34].

Patients with the glandular fever-like illness complain of sore throat, non-specific flu-like symptoms and gastrointestinal disturbances. An erythematous macular rash is present in around 50% of patients; it is initially prominent in the trunk and later involves the extremities. Other skin manifestations include urticaria, loss of hair, and desquamation of palms and soles[24–26,30,35]. Generalized lymphadenopathy is a feature in around 75% of patients, and in some patients may be associated with splenomegaly and tender hepatomegaly[24,35,36].

Patients may present with symptoms of acute aseptic meningitis, e.g. headache, fever, photophobia and neck stiffness. Cerebrospinal fluid findings are typical of a viral aetiology[24,25]. HIV has been isolated from the cerebrospinal fluid in certain cases[33], and also from peripheral blood. The clinical features of HIV encephalopathy during primary infection consist of mood changes, confusion, convulsion and incontinence. Abnormalities on neurological examination include altered conscious level, extensor plantar responses and sensorimotor peripheral neuropathy including facial palsy[32,34]. Other neurological manifestations have been reported: myelopathy[37], Guillain–Barré syndrome[38], and radiculopathy[39].

The incubation period, defined as the time from exposure to clinical symptoms of acute HIV infection, has been variable, ranging from a few days[24] to up to a few months[34]. It is felt that the incubation period may be longer in sexually transmitted HIV infection possibly because of a smaller dose of inoculum and the non-parenteral route of transmission[25,40]. However, incubation periods of up to 6 months have been documented via the parenteral route[41,42].

Seroconversion, defined as time from infection to the detection of specific antibodies, has occurred from 8 days[24] to 10 weeks[25,43] after the onset of acute illness. IgM antibodies are inconsistently first detected by immunofluorescence assay (IFA), and IgG IFA has been found to be more sensitive than ELISA and Western blotting in primary HIV infection. The characteristic pattern of specific antibody responses to the various viral proteins has been described by Cooper *et al*[44]. However, in a study of sexually transmitted HIV infection, antibodies to recombinant structural proteins and p24 antigen can occasionally be detected in serum 7–14 months before seroconversion, and rarely more than 7–34 months in serum samples of high-risk patients who have not seroconverted[40].

Severe immunodepression may occur during acute HIV infection[45]. Oesophageal candidiasis has been reported in a number of patients during acute HIV infection[46–48], and other opportunistic infection, e.g. tuberculous meningitis, has been reported 8 weeks after acute HIV infection[49].

Early manifestations of HIV infection

CDC stage II describes those individuals who are essentially well or asymptomatic but have antibodies for HIV. They may be further subdivided after laboratory investigations into those with immunological abnormalities and those without; however, this stage has no prognostic value since at present the natural history of CDC stage II is incompletely understood.

CDC stage III describes those individuals with enlarged lymph nodes (greater than 1 cm) at two or more non-adjacent sites for longer than 3 months in the absence of any other illness to explain the findings. This condition is also known as persistent generalized lymphadenopathy (PGL). Commonly the enlarged nodes are found down the front and/or back of the neck, under the jaw or in the axillae, and may not be noticed by the patient. Massive enlargement can occasionally occur. Unusual sites for lymph node enlargement do occur, for instance at the elbow, behind the knee, down the front of the thigh, down the side of the chest wall, in the abdominal wall, or behind the nipples. This lymph node enlargement may be accompanied by other troublesome symptoms such as tiredness, lethargy, excessive sweating, aches and pains in muscles or joints.

Late manifestations of HIV infection

CDC stage IV is divided into five further subsections labelled A to E, and this stage has to be regarded as being more serious, although some individuals may be relatively well. AIDS-related complex or ARC is a term which is commonly used, has a number of definitions but is anyway covered within CDC stage IV.

Stage IVA describes those individuals complaining of the vague constitutional symptoms of stage III but with the addition of more serious problems such as unexplained diarrhoea, fever (greater than 38°C) for longer than 1 month or unexplained weight loss of more than 10% body weight.

Stage IVB consists of neurological problems associated with HIV other than those occurring during CDC stage I. Examples are neuropathy and myelopathy. Disabling cognitive and/or motor dysfunction interfering with occupation or the activities of daily living can also occur. Patients or relatives may notice loss of memory and loss of skills such as mental arithmetic or decision-making. Relatives may notice changes in personality which early on seem like eccentricities. Frank mental illness, dementia or loss of consciousness in the absence of other pathogens is called HIV encephalopathy, and is one criterion for the diagnosis of established AIDS.

Stage IVC describes a number of infections which occur as a result of immunodeficiency secondary to HIV infection, and is divided into two subgroups, IVC1 and IVC2. CDC stage IVC1 includes individuals suffering from one or more of 12 opportunistic infections which formed the basis of the original CDC definition of AIDS. Stage IVC2 contains those infections which are commonly associated with serious HIV infection but were not in the original description of AIDS. Examples of infections in stage IVC2 are recurrent and invasive salmonella, extensive herpes zoster or shingles, recurrent oral candidiasis, a condition almost unique to HIV called oral hairy leukoplakia, and recurrent bacterial sepsis in adults.

CDC stage IVD groups together all those malignancies specifically associated with HIV infection and, as with CDC stage IVC1, some of these conditions also fulfil the CDC definition of AIDS. Examples are the skin tumour Kaposi's sarcoma and lymphoid tumours such as non-Hodgkin's lymphoma or primary lymphoma of the brain.

Lastly, CDC stage IVE is designed to cover those conditions not yet described or those not yet fully understood, such as chronic lymphoid interstitial pneumonitis.

CLINICAL AND LABORATORY FEATURES OF HIV INFECTION

AIDS is characterized by a marked depletion of CD4 T-lymphocytes in the peripheral blood. Exactly how this depletion takes place is as yet unknown, but a number of possible mechanisms have been suggested, including a direct cytopathic effect of HIV, syncytia or giant cell formation with subsequent cell death and a form of autoimmunity against lymphocytes using either cytotoxic T cells or other antilymphocytic factors.

The major effect of HIV infection appears to be damage to the cell-mediated immune mechanism resulting in characteristic susceptibility to opportunistic infections. This susceptibility is usually to intracellular organisms such as latent viruses, fungi or protozoa. Such organisms require the presence of an intact cell-mediated immune system which relies on T lymphocytes and macrophages. This susceptibility is associated with a marked depletion of peripheral blood CD4 lymphocytes which play a key role in initiating and promoting immune responses, including the initiation of a *de novo* humoral response. Most adults with HIV infection seem to have B cell memory, although recurrent bacterial infections can occur in HIV infection. This humoral defect is worst in children where B cell memory is limited and the patient may be rendered functionally hypogammaglobulinaemic. The humoral defect also limits the usefulness of serology in the diagnosis of many disorders; for instance latent viruses may exhibit persistent and stable levels of antibodies and other organisms produce little in the way of an antibody response[50].

The marked loss of T cell immunity results in a susceptibility to reactivation of latent or controlled infections such as cytomegalovirus (CMV), toxoplasmosis or tuberculosis, or to attack by relatively non-pathogenic organisms which may be endogenous or common in the patient's environment. Examples of this type of infection are *Pneumocystis carinii* pneumonia (PCP), candidiasis or atypical mycobacteria.

The loss of T cell function also limits macrophage activity. Infection in these patients often produces little in the way of an inflammatory response and consequently little in the way of clinical signs. A number of immunological abnormalities have been described, including:

1. leucopenia and lymphopenia;
2. loss of CD4 T lymphocytes from the peripheral blood;
3. hypergammaglobulinaemia;
4. skin anergy;
5. decreased *in vitro* lymphocyte proliferation, cytotoxic T cell responses and antibody production to new antigens;
6. elevated levels of immune complexes, interferon and β_2-microglobulin[50].

The haematological abnormalities associated with HIV infection vary with the clinical state of the patient, but are commoner as HIV infection progresses. For instance 12% of AIDS/AIDS-related complex (ARC) patients were leucopenic, 20% were neutropenic, 75% were lymphopenic and 93% were anaemic[51,52]. The reasons for these abnormalities are multifactorial and involve the effects of HIV infection, drug effects, chronic infection and the effects of opportunistic infections. In a series of patients who underwent bone marrow examination a number of abnormalities were noted, including:

1. reticuloendothelial iron blockade;
2. dyserythropoiesis and megaloblastic change;
3. erythroid hypoplasia;
4. excess histiocytes and viral-associated haemophagocytosis[51].

Despite the peripheral lymphopenia, bone marrow lymphopenia is uncommon, perhaps because T cells predominate in the peripheral blood whereas B cells predominate in the bone marrow.

Idiopathic immune thrombocytopenia (ITP) is usually associated with children and middle-aged women. An ITP syndrome was noted early on to be an AIDS-related condition in homosexuals, injection drug misusers, and haemophiliacs[53–56]. In patients with AIDS about 30% have a depressed platelet count, and this often falls further with treatment for PCP[53,57]. The platelet count is generally depressed in HIV infection and ITP has been noted to occur in HIV infection before the advent of AIDS[53–55]. In Edinburgh 23% of patients had a platelet count $< 150 \times 10^9/l$, but only 4% had symptoms of excessive bruising or bleeding with counts of $< 20 \times 10^9/l$. In other studies about 5–10% of PGL patients have mildly depressed platelet counts[57]. Our experience that this is a relatively benign condition supports the USA experience. The commonest symptoms are excessive bruising, epistaxis, menorrhagia, gingival and rectal bleeding. Major life-threatening haemorrhage is rare. Platelet-associated immunoglobulin has been demonstrated in the majority of patients studied[57].

There is little variation between the risk groups with regard to presentation. In the USA, figures are available on the 30 632 cases of AIDS notified to the Centers for Disease Control by 9 February 1987[58]. These show that conditions such as KS are unusual in the absence of homo/bisexuality. Recent epidemiological studies suggest that whereas the risk of Kaposi's sarcoma is increased in patients who acquired HIV by sexual, and particularly homosexual, contact (suggesting the possibility of a second infectious cofactor)[59], no such association is evident for non-Hodgkin's lymphoma[60]. In injection drug users (IDU), KS, cytomegalovirus and chronic cryptosporidiosis are all significantly less common than for all other risk groups notified with AIDS; while PCP, tuberculosis, oesophageal candidiasis and extrapulmonary cryptococcosis are more common.

Drug use has been identified as a risk factor for tuberculosis prior to the advent of AIDS[61]; nonetheless, the incidence of tuberculosis is much higher in HIV-infected drug users than in other risk groups outside the tropics or in HIV negative drug users. In the USA most patients with AIDS and tuberculosis have been drug users[62,63]. The latter of these studies showed a prevalence of 15.1% in drug users with AIDS but only 4.4% in other risk groups within a New York hospital. A similar pattern has been shown in San Francisco[64]. In New York the rate of tuberculosis was 4% amongst HIV positive drug users compared to 0% in HIV negative drug users and the 36% increase in reported cases of tuberculosis between 1984 and 1986 has been largely ascribed to infection amongst HIV positive drug users[65,66].

Encapsulated bacteria such as *Streptococcus pneumoniae* and *Haemophilus influenzae* are frequent respiratory pathogens and causes of bacteraemia in HIV seropositive individuals[67]. IDU-related HIV patients have a higher incidence of recurrent bacterial infections such as pneumonia, 12% with a mortality of 2.2% compared to 3% with a mortality of 0% in HIV negative drug users[68]. The annual incidence of pneumonia was 9.7% for HIV seropositive drug users compared to under 2% for a population of mainly homosexual males with AIDS[69,70]. There is a rising mortality from pneumonia in young adults in New York City, primarily as a consequence of IDU-related HIV, and other cities in the USA are showing similar trends[71]. In a study of bacteraemia in Nairobi HIV seropositive individuals were five times more likely to suffer a bacteraemia (26% versus 6%) particularly with *Streptococcus pneumoniae* and *Salmonella typhimurium*[72].

The morbidity and mortality of bacterial endocarditis in HIV seropositive individuals is greater than for seronegative individuals; for instance the mortality was 24% in seropositives compared with 4% in the seronegatives. The poorer outcome was related to more frequent embolization, a greater diversity of organisms, more prolonged fever, persistent bacteraemia and greater immunological dysfunction. It was not related to recognized opportunistic infections[73,74].

This susceptibility to bacterial infection has also been noted in other contexts; for instance in a study from Uganda an increase in complications during pregnancy such as urinary tract infections or fever in HIV positive patients was noted[75].

The reasons for the increase in bacterial infections are not yet clear. Antibody production is impaired in HIV-infected patients, and low levels of IgG_2 have been associated with bacterial infection[76]. However, in another study levels of IgG2 were no different in controls, HIV-infected homosexuals or drug users, or HIV-infected patients with recurrent bacterial infections[77]. This suggests that the problem may be either a failure of production of specific antibodies or a neutrophil defect. This is not specific for injection drug users, however, and the fact that they make less or later use of medical services may be of importance. Additional factors may be that opiates themselves depress the cough reflex as well as the immune system, and unsterile IDU exposes the individual to recurrent episodes of bacterial infection.

Hepatitis B is a frequent infection amongst IDU. For instance in our population of HIV seropositives 91% have markers of infection as opposed to 51% in HIV seronegative drug users, reflecting the frequency of drug use and the extent of equipment sharing[78]. A recently described event is the reactivation of hepatitis B infection amongst drug users during the course of HIV infection[79].

Progression from HIV to AIDS

Currently the exact explanation for progression from early HIV infection to AIDS is unknown. A number of factors could be involved, including genetic susceptibility, gender, pregnancy, risk activity, coinfection with other viruses, and age. Additional immunosuppressive factors might also be important, such as the use of opiates, stimulation of the immune system via soluble antigens and DNA viruses and the acquisition of differing strains of HIV[80–84]. A number of markers of this progression have been noted, including age of the patient, low numbers of CD4 lymphocytes (a figure of less than 200/mm^3 suggests that 50% will progress in 2 years), immune thrombocytopenic purpura, the presence of HIV antigen in serum and rising levels of β_2-microglobulin[85–90].

The time from initial exposure to HIV to the onset of clinical AIDS is variable. It is possible that the vast majority of HIV-1-infected patients will eventually develop AIDS[91–95]. Currently few cofactors for progression to AIDS among HIV-infected individuals have been identified.

An extensive review of progression from HIV to AIDS in cohorts of various risk groups with known seroconversion dates revealed the following rates of progression; 0–2% at 2 years, 5–10% at 4 years, 10–25% at 6 years, 30–40% at 8 years and 48% at 10 years[96]. Updated data on the San Francisco City cohort, published recently, showed a progression rate of 51% by 10 years[97,98]. The median time for progression to AIDS was initially around 7–10 years but has now risen to 11 years[98]. There are not yet reliable assessments of progression rates in injection drug users.

Several studies have tried to assess the rate of progression to AIDS amongst drug users. However, most of these reports relate the onset of symptoms of AIDS to the length of follow-up and not to the duration of HIV infection.

Hence, these figures must be interpreted cautiously, as differing results may merely reflect differing intervals between infection and the start of the assessment period.

A study of 288 HIV positive drug users from the Bronx in New York showed that 16% had progressed to AIDS over 31 months, and in another series 25% of 25 drug users developed AIDS over a 3-year period[66,92]. Results obtained in European studies show a slower rate of progression. In a large Spanish survey of 646 IDU, the actuarial incidence of AIDS was 15% at 6 years, with a similar incidence being found amongst homosexuals[99]. Other smaller-scale studies show AIDS incidences of 6% after 14 months, 6.5% after 18 months, and 7.4% after 3 years follow-up[100–102]. In one Italian study in which seroconversion dates were estimated, there was a 17.8% progression to AIDS after 4 years of HIV infection[103].

There is increasing evidence that, amongst drug users, data collected on AIDS cases greatly underrepresent serious IDU-related HIV disease. In New York, Stoneburner and co-workers reported that there has been a rapid increase in both AIDS and non-AIDS narcotic-related deaths[104]. There were 276 narcotic-related deaths in 1978, 1607 in 1985 and nearly 2000 in 1986. Thus by 1986, for every AIDS-related death in a drug user, there was one other as a consequence of such conditions as tuberculosis, endocarditis and bacterial pneumonia. Similar data have been reported from Milan[105].

Genetic factors

There is some evidence to suggest that genetic susceptibility may affect the rate of progression to AIDS. In a study of 102 HIV seropositive men with a mean follow-up time of 43 months, AIDS developed more frequently in HLA-DR1 positive men than in those with other HLA-DR phenotypes[106]; however, with longer follow-up times the difference diminished[107]. A subsequent study of seropositive homosexual men from the Multicentre AIDS cohort study did not show any association between rapid decline in CD4 cells with the presence of HLA-DR1, but individuals with HLA-A1, Cw7, B8 combination were about 10 times more likely to suffer an accelerated progress than those without this combination[108]. In another study of HIV seropositive haemophiliacs the rapid decline in the number of CD4 lymphocytes and the development of HIV-related symptoms within 4 years of acquisition of infection was associated with HLA-A1, B8, DR3 positivity[109]. DR3 and Cw7 antigens have also been found in a high proportion of AIDS patients with opportunistic infections[110,111]. Finally, there is a reported association between HLA-DR5 and Kaposi's sarcoma[112]. However, some of these findings have not been confirmed in other studies[113,114].

Concurrent infections

Rapid progression to AIDS may be influenced by biological properties of the virus strain; for example HIV variants with rapid replication, increased syncytium-forming ability, and a broad host-cell range[115–118] (see Chapter 2). Presumably these variants will give rise to high virus loads in individuals; hence the link between high virus load and rapid progression[119].

In addition to biological variants of HIV other infectious agents have been suggested as cofactors for AIDS progression. It is possible that infectious agents and foreign antigens may stimulate T cells and hence enhance HIV replication. Coinfection of cell lines with both cytomegalovirus and HIV, and HIV superinfection of herpes simplex-infected cells have been shown to enhance HIV replication[120,121], presumably because herpes viruses may transactivate HIV long-terminal repeat sequences. In two studies, one in homosexual men and one in haemophiliac patients, CMV infection was associated with a more rapid progression to HIV disease[85,122]. However, in transfusion-transmitted HIV patients, Drew *et al.* found no evidence for CMV as a cofactor in the progression to AIDS, but the follow-up time was short at around 30 months[123]. Another study failed to find any influence of acute or chronic infection with hepatitis B or even vaccination with plasma-derived hepatitis B vaccine on progression to AIDS[124].

Coinfection with other human lymphotropic viruses is a marker for rapid progression in intravenous drug users[125], but the faster progression to AIDS in HTLV-I coinfected homosexual men, which had previously been observed in the first 3 years of a study in Trinidad, was not maintained at 72 months[126].

HIV can be activated by exogenous or endogenous signals such as lectins and cytokines, e.g. tumour necrosis factor[127]. Mycoplasmas can induce the production of tumour necrosis factor in lymphocytes and macrophages, and killed mycoplasma can stimulate HIV-1 p24 antigen production in T cell lines[128]. Tetracycline analogues have been shown to inhibit virus-induced cytopathic effects when added to chronically HIV-infected cells; an antibody directed at the binding site of *Mycoplasma genitalium* has been found to inhibit HIV replication in cell cultures[129]. Mycoplasmas have therefore been proposed as a cofactor for progression to AIDS[130]. However, introduction of mycoplasma to T cell line cultures depresses HIV-1 replication as measured by reverse transcriptase activity[131]. This issue is complex, and it is possible that the effect of mycoplasma on HIV replication is dependent on the mycoplasma species. The effect of mycoplasma on HIV progression is still unclear.

Age

There is now increasing evidence that age at the time of HIV infection is an important factor for rapid progression to AIDS. Studies among individuals infected through blood transfusion[132,133], intravenous drug users[134], and haemophiliacs[135] all suggest an adverse effect of increased age. In the Swedish transfusion study progression to AIDS at 5.5 years after infection was 47.5% in those over 60 compared to only 27.5% between 15 and 60 years of age[133]. For instance, in an Italian haemophiliac study after 5.5 years of infection 37.7% of those over 35 years of age had progressed to AIDS compared to only 18.5% of those under 35 years of age ($p < 0.02$)[136]. There was no difference in the rate of progression, however, for those above and below 18 years of age with the exception of children infected neonatally.

Drug use

Kaslow *et al.*[137] found no evidence for a role of alcohol or other psychoactive drugs in accelerating the progression of immunodeficiency in HIV seropositive homosexual and bisexual men, and no relationship between opiate use and disease progression. There is a suggestion that continued IDU may accelerate progression of HIV to AIDS; one study reported a relationship between the frequency of IDU and the loss of CD4 lymphocytes whilst another study noted a similar increased rate of decline of CD4 lymphocytes amongst a group of injectors compared to a group of non-injectors[138,139]. There was also a lower probability of disease progression amongst methadone users or ex-users compared to those that continued IDU, reported from Switzerland. Progression values from CDC stage II or III to stage IV after 2 and 3 years of follow-up were 11% (95% confidence interval 3–19%), 29% (15–43%) in the methadone group, 21% (10–32%), 29% (14–43%) in the ex-users but 36% (24–48%), 60% (45–76%) in the persistent IDU group. The progression rate in the persistent IDU group was significantly higher than that in the methadone-treated ($p<0.01$) and former drug misuser groups ($p<0.05$). Multivariate analysis showed a relative risk of 1.78 for persistent users, 0.48 in the methadone-treated group, and 0.66 in former drug misusers[140]. However, other groups have not found an increased risk for continued IDU[134,141,142]. The incidence of AIDS in the Bronx was reported to be lower (11.4 v. 33 per 1000 patient-years) for entrance to the Montefiore methadone maintenance treatment programme (MMTP) before and after 1983[143]. Similarly the proportion of drug users attending MMTP in Italy was inversely related to the cumulative incidence of AIDS. The highest AIDS incidence rates were seen in the regions with the lowest proportions of IDU attending MMTP. Nearly 40% of the variability of AIDS incidence was attributed to attendance in MMTP[144]. The reasons why continued drug use might predispose to accelerated immune decline are unknown, but one suggestion is that the drift in molecular composition demonstrated in different HIV isolates could result in an individual acquiring more infection with differing strains of HIV, which might hasten disease progression[84].

Another possible explanation is that IDU itself significantly affects the immune system, for instance frequent IDU was associated with depressed lymphocyte function irrespective of HIV serostatus. IDU has been associated with higher levels of β_2-microglobulin and activated T cells, and IDU-related HIV is associated with more immune stimulation[146–148].

One study noted that the relative hazard for smokers of cigarettes was 1.63 compared to non-smokers[149]. As yet there is no explanation of this increased risk.

Gender

As with IDU there are unfortunately few cohort studies of progression in women. There is no evidence that there is any major difference between the sexes in the rate of progression from HIV to AIDS. Gender was not reported as a significant factor in a study of progression in 58 male and 18 female

Spanish IDU[150]. The Swedish transfusion study noted shorter progression times for men, but this was not statistically significant[133]. Our own study has not to date shown gender to be predictive of progression to AIDS or CDC stage IV[151].

Pregnancy

The clinical data concerning the effect of pregnancy on the natural history of HIV are inconclusive. In one series published by Scott *et al.*[152] in 1985, of 16 mothers identified by the birth of a child with AIDS, only four (25%) of the mothers had remained well at a mean time of 2.5 years after delivery of the child. In addition 11 of the 16 women had a subsequent pregnancy during this time, and we know nothing of their total parity. Of more concern was the fact that in five of these 11 subsequent pregnancies the women developed AIDS or ARC during that subsequent pregnancy.

In a second study by Minkoff[153] from New York 34 mothers, again identified by the birth of an affected child, were followed for a mean of 27.8 months. At that time 15 out of the 34 mothers, or 44%, had become symptomatic with AIDS or ARC. Again 14 of the mothers had gone on to further pregnancies, and the authors concluded that there was a significant chance of maternal ill-health with AIDS or ARC after delivery of a child.

These original studies suggested that pregnancy, or possibly a second pregnancy, accelerated progression from asymptomatic HIV to AIDS. These findings may well have been affected by selection, since the women were identified by the development of AIDS in an affected child. In addition there were no infected but non-pregnant controls, and the length of infection with HIV was not known. However, two further studies have again suggested that pregnancy accelerates progression of HIV. In the study by Delfraissey *et al.*[154], three groups of patients were studied: those going through a pregnancy, those undergoing a spontaneous abortion and those without a pregancy. Progression to CDC stage IV was greatest for the pregnant group, 15% versus 3.6% and 5.7% in the other groups. In addition development of high-risk status, as defined by a CD4 count of below 150/mm^3, p24 antigenaemia and loss of p24 antibody was greatest in the pregnant group, 10.7% versus 13.4% and 12.4%. In the 21-month follow-up study by Deschamps *et al.*[155], progression to HIV-related ill-health or AIDS was greatest for patients having a pregnancy, 47% compared to 26%. In addition the cumulative number with symptoms at 5 years was 84% for the pregnant group compared to 53% for the non-pregnant group.

By comparison there have been five studies[156–160] reported which have shown pregnancy to have no effect on the progression of HIV. For instance Bledsoe *et al.*[159] showed that progression to AIDS for a pregnant group was only 1.8% compared to 7.8% for the non-pregnant group. Similarly Schoenbaum *et al.* compared the incidence of ill-health and AIDS in women according to the number of pregnancies, and found no differences[157].

Before leaving pregnancy we should consider the effect, if any, of HIV on an individual pregnancy. There are at least three reports[161–163] of no increase in obstetric complications, and two reports of an increase of obstetric complications such as an increase in the spontaneous abortion rate for HIV positive women[164,165]. Recent work from Edinburgh has not confirmed the increased spontaneous abortion rate, but has shown that HIV is associated with lower birth weight over and above an effect of IDU[165].

Clinical features

Persistent generalized lymphadenopathy has not been shown to be predictive of progression to AIDS[166,167]. To date, the current clinical predictors of progression to AIDS that have been identified, e.g. herpes zoster[168], oral candidiasis[168–170], and hairy oral leukoplakia[168,169,171] are unfortunately manifestations of HIV-related immunodeficiency and are therefore relatively late in the natural history of HIV infection. The 2-year progression rates in the San Francisco General Hospital cohort for men with persistent generalized lymphadenopathy, zoster, candidiasis, hairy leukoplakia and constitutional symptoms were 22%, 25%, 39%, 42%, and 100% respectively, compared with 16% in men with none of the above[169]. We therefore have to depend on laboratory markers to predict progression from asymptomatic HIV infection.

LABORATORY MARKERS OF DISEASE PROGRESSION

Laboratory and clinical markers which are predictive of rapid progression to AIDS may appear very early in HIV infection[172]. In one study, patients who had an acute seroconversion illness lasting longer than 14 days had a progression rate of 78% in 3 years compared to those who were symptom-free or who had minor symptoms[173]. Primary humoral responses to HIV proteins may also be associated with clinical outcome of infection; patients with high p24 antibody response seem to progress to AIDS more slowly[174].

Lymphocyte subsets estimations

The CD4 lymphocyte is the main target cell for HIV and the primary immunological defect in patients with AIDS is the severe depletion of CD4 lymphocytes[56,175–177]. As HIV infection progresses, there is a progressive decline in the percentage and number of CD4 cells[178]. An absolute CD4 count of 150/mm^3, or a falling CD4 count, correlates with progression, while CD4 counts higher than 500 have a much lower probability of rapid progression. This correlation between a low and declining CD4 count and disease progression is well established in the various risk groups[85,86,95,169,179–186].

CD8 cells decline shortly before the development of AIDS. In some studies high numbers of CD8 cells was found to be predictive of a rapid decline in CD4 cells[187] and it is possible that CD4/CD8 ratio may be a better predictor of rapid progression to AIDS than the absolute number of CD4 cells[178].

HIV serological markers

Low levels or absence of p24 antibodies correlate strongly with rapid disease progression[188–195], loss of p17 antibodies could be an earlier serological marker of progression than loss of p24 antibodies[196–198]. Conversely, patients with high levels of p24 antibodies progress more slowly[174].

p24 antigen can be detected when levels of p24 antibodies are low or declining[190,199,200]. A high level or an increase in p24 antigen correlates strongly with AIDS progression[169,190–195,199,201] and p24 antigenaemia has the highest predictive value for short-term prognosis[169,193]. However, p24 antigen can be detected in only up to 50% of patients with AIDS in whom plasma viraemia can be readily detected[202,203]. p24 antigen is generally not detectable in 85% or more of asymptomatic HIV-seropositive men, and it is not surprising that its usefulness as an early marker for HIV progression is not universally accepted[204].

Other immunological markers

A variety of functional immunological parameters have been associated with HIV disease progression, but most of them are impractical for everyday clinical practice and are also expensive. Indirect markers such as elevated serum IgA levels have been independently shown to be predictive[169,184,205,206].

β_2-Microglobulin

β_2-Microglobulin is the short polypeptide chain that is located in the human histocompatibility complex (HLA-A, B and C) present on the surface of most somatic cells[207–209]. Conditions giving rise to increased lymphoid cell turnover lead to increased levels of β_2-microglobulin, e.g. infection with Epstein–Barr virus[210] and cytomegalovirus[211], but not in patients with intravenous drug use[212]. Increased levels of β_2-microglobulin in the serum and cerebrospinal fluid have been described during acute HIV-1 infection[213–215]. High levels have been described in patients progressing to AIDS[214,216–218]. In the San Francisco cohort of seropositive homosexual men the 3-year actuarial progression rate to AIDS was 69% in men with serum β_2-microglobulin levels >5.0 mg/l and 12% in those with levels <3.0 mg/l. In this study, elevated serum β_2-microglobulin was the most powerful predictor of progression to AIDS[169]. Results from the MACS cohort suggest that the pattern of disease reflected by β_2-microglobulin is established in the first year of infection and persists through the following 2 years; β_2-microglobulin levels appeared to be a good indicator of HIV activity and of the rate of CD4 cell decline; β_2-microglobulin and CD4 cells had equal predictive power[96,206], and the combination of β_2-microglobulin and CD4 cells was prognostically better than either alone[219,220].

Neopterin

Neopterin, a pyrazino-pyrimidine compound derived from guanosine triphosphate, is produced by macrophages after stimulation with γ-interferon during activation of the cell-mediated immune response[221]. Blood and urine neopterin levels are raised in HIV-1-infected individuals[222–224] and are inversely correlated to absolute CD4 counts and CD4/CD8 cell ratios[223]. Changes in neopterin occur early in the course of HIV infection and high levels in asymptomatic HIV-1-infected individuals are associated with a poor prognosis[225,226]. Furthermore, the combination of neopterin levels and CD4 cell count is a better indicator of prognosis than either alone[227].

Soluble interleukin-2 receptor levels

Soluble IL-2 receptor levels have been shown to be increased in HIV infection[228,229]. It is believed that the increased levels result from activated monocytes and possibly B lymphocytes[230,231]. Elevation of soluble interleukin-2 receptor appears to have a strong correlation with serum β_2-microglobulin and neopterin levels[232,233], and seem to be inversely correlated with CD4 cell counts[234].

SURVIVAL AFTER THE DEVELOPMENT OF AIDS

In one study around 50% of patients with AIDS survived 1 year but only 20% survived 3 years[235]. Whilst it is generally assumed that survival for drug users with AIDS is shorter, a report on 5833 cases of AIDS from New York which adjusted for various factors found no difference between homosexuals and drug users in terms of survival. Injection drug use itself may be an adverse factor, however, since the combination of IDU and homosexuality did lead to a shorter survival. Also a proportional-hazards model showed a significant interaction between IDU and *Pneumocystis carinii* pneumonia (PCP) as factors shortening survival[235].

The apparent poor survival for drug users may be connected with the poor survival of women. This is possibly related to a delay in diagnosis as seen by the fact that 16.3% of women die at diagnosis of AIDS compared to 10.9% of men[235]. A greater risk of respiratory failure was observed for women with PCP, as well as a two-fold increase in the mortality compared to a matched group of men[236]. In New Jersey amongst 345 women, 95% of whom were Black and 63% drug users, the mean survival was only 14.5 weeks[237]. By comparison one series of 24 all-white women from Rhode Island suggested improved survival since the mean length of survival was 19 months and only five had PCP[238]. Overall, however, the prognosis seems to be poorer for women since in the New York series the cumulative probability of survival at 1 year was 75.4% for white males with Kaposi's sarcoma (KS) but only 37% for Black, female drug users with PCP[235].

The poor outcome for women in the USA seems to be more related to access to care than an effect of HIV. For instance there are other studies demonstrating that US women present late for care. Thirty-nine per cent of women had a CD4 count of less than 200/mm^3 at presentation[239]. In Minnesota two-thirds of women with HIV were detected by neonatal screening rather than being in medical care[240], and another study looking at survival showed that patients attending an outpatient clinic had a better survival, 70.4 weeks compared to 27.5 weeks for non-attenders[237]. Our own experience is that there is no great difference in the medical problems of women infected with HIV. In a retrospective survey of 612 HIV-related admissions there was no excess of female admissions except for detoxification, investigation of episodes of loss of consciousness and urinary tract infections[241]. The other problem faced by women, however, is cervical cancer. Increasing cervical dysplasia and more severe dysplasia occurs with increasing immunosuppression[242]. This seems to be connected with human papilloma virus (HPV), since it did not occur if women were HPV negative[243].

A Spanish study of 289 patients with AIDS revealed a median survival of just over 1 year, or 385 days[244]. The authors were able to identify a number of factors influencing survival which included age; median survival for those over 45 years 135 days and those under 45 years 625 days ($p<0.0001$); gender with a median survival of 436 days for women and 366 days for men ($p<0.05$); risk group with a median survival of 744 days for drug users and 253 days for male homosexuals ($p<0.004$); year of diagnosis with a median survival of only 72 days for those diagnosed before 1986 and 512 days for those diagnosed in 1986 or later years ($p<0.0001$); index diagnosis with a median survival of 625 for extrapulmonary tuberculosis, 339 days for other opportunistic infections, 179 days for Kaposi's sarcoma and only 75 days for lymphoma ($p<0.003$ to $p<0.0001$). In this study some 53% of the patients were IDU and 33% of the AIDS cases presented with extrapulmonary tuberculosis.

There is now good evidence showing a marked improvement in survival of patients with AIDS, particularly for those with PCP as their index diagnosis for AIDS[245,246]. For these patients the estimated 1-year survival increased from 42.7% for those diagnosed in 1984 and 1985 (95% confidence interval, 41.5–44.3%) to 54.5% for those diagnosed in 1986 and 1987 (95% confidence interval, 53.7–55.7%). The gain in survival was observed in homosexual men and in IDU of both sexes, in all age and racial groups in the United States. In this study no gain in survival was seen for patients in whom *Pneumocystis carinii* pneumonia was not an initial manifestation of AIDS[246]. Better diagnosis and treatment, particularly the introduction of zidovudine in 1986, may have contributed to the decline in mortality.

Effect of zidovudine on survival

The course of HIV infection is changing as a result of therapeutic advances and of changes in behaviour. For example, the incidence of Kaposi's sarcoma among homosexual men in the United States has decreased from 40% in the early 1980s to below 20% from 1986 onwards, reflecting a decrease in the number of sexual partners and reinforcing the possibility that Kaposi's sarcoma may be a sexually transmitted infection[58,247–249].

The life-expectancy of patients with HIV infection is presently increasing because of improved treatment for both HIV-associated infectious complications and HIV infection itself. In 1986, zidovudine was shown in a placebo-controlled study to decrease the frequency and severity of opportunistic infections and to reduce mortality in individuals with AIDS-related PCP, or symptomatic advanced ARC, and further studies of the original cohort confirmed long-term survival compared with historical controls[249,250]. In a study of 4805 patients receiving zidovudine on compassionate-use basis, Creagh-Kirk *et al.* found that zidovudine therapy is associated with increased survival of post-PCP patients[251]. In addition, patients with AIDS-related dementia have also shown improved cognitive function after receiving therapy with zidovudine[252–254]. Similar survival benefit has been observed in Europe[255], and the improved survival is not contingent on the use of aerosolized pentamidine[256]. One recent UK study suggested that survival doubled in those treated with zidovudine[257]. In an analysis of 90 patients receiving zidovudine during clinical trials, increases in β_2-microglobulin concentrations and absolute CD4 cell counts at weeks 8–12 correlated with survival[258]. If these preliminary results are confirmed it would then be theoretically possible to predict good responders to antiretroviral therapy.

The cause of death in patients with AIDS has also changed over the past decade. In one study the overall proportion of patients who developed PCP fell from 56% (20/36) in 1984 to 24% (46/194) in 1989, although it remained the index diagnosis in around half of the new patients. PCP accounted for 46% (16/35) of known causes of death in 1986 but only 3% (1/31) in 1989, and Kaposi's sarcoma was the commonest cause of death in 1989. There was also an increase in deaths due to lymphoma, and this is attributed by the authors to increased survival, and duration of immunosuppression. They also argue that malignancies may appear as a consequence of more prolonged immunosuppression[259].

Patients with symptomatic HIV infection who survive for up to 3 years on antiretroviral activity appear to have an increased likelihood of developing non-Hodgkin's lymphoma. In a study of 55 HIV seropositive men with AIDS or severe ARC on long-term anti-HIV therapy, eight developed non-Hodgkin's lymphoma after receiving antiretroviral treatment for a median of 23.8 months before the onset of lymphoma[260]. Although zidovudine can act as a mutagen, and vaginal malignancies have been reported in mice and rats receiving lifelong high-dose zidovudine[261,262], it is unlikely that this is the direct cause of the lymphoma which is more likely to be related to immunosuppression[59]. Furthermore, in the US, the incidence of non-Hodgkin's lymphoma has increased by more than 50%, and while the factors contributing to this rise are not known, the rise was observed before the AIDS epidemic and AIDS-related non-Hodgkin's lymphoma seems to account for a small percentage of this increase[263]. It is more likely that prolonged survival in the setting of profound immunosuppression with substantial CD4 cell depletion is an important factor in the developmentof these lymphomas. The patients who developed the lymphoma had less than 100 CD4 cells/mm^3 for a median of 17.8 months (range 7–35 months), and less than 50 CD4 cells/mm^3 for a median of 15.3 months (range 5.5–35 months) before the diagnosis[260].

However, the immunological improvement obtained with zidovudine is often transient[249], especially in patients with advanced disease. This may be related to a reduction in zidovudine sensitivity which has been observed in patients on long-term zidovudine therapy[264,265]. The development of resistance may have been more rapid in those who progressed to AIDS[265], but at present it is difficult to be certain whether the reduced sensitivity is the cause or effect of more rapid progression.

AZT in asymptomatic individuals

Two recent studies in HIV seropositive individuals (one in mildly symptomatic individuals[266] and one in asymptomatics[267]) have shown that individuals with CD4 cell counts of up to 500/mm^3 benefit from therapy with zidovudine. No early benefit was seen in individuals with higher than 500 CD4 positive cells per cubic millimetre. Individuals on the zidovudine trial arms had fewer progressions to AIDS and AIDS-related complex. Furthermore, low-dose zidovudine 100 mg every 4 h during waking hours was as effective as, and less toxic than, high-dose 1500 mg daily. Similar results were obtained in a small phase II study, when 300 mg zidovudine daily had clinical and virological effects similar to those of higher daily doses (600 and 1500 mg)[268]. The optimal dose of zidovudine for treatment of asymptomatic HIV seropositive individuals has therefore not yet been established.

CONCLUSIONS

While considerable progress has been made in detailing the natural history of infection with HIV there is still much to be defined. Infection with HIV exhibits marked variations, all of which may not yet have been described. HIV infection is chronic but with development in antiretroviral therapy it becomes treatable. Currently, however, treatment slows but does not reverse the progress of disease, and unless immunocompetence can be restored, mortality will remain high. The natural history of untreated HIV will then give way to the natural history of treated HIV, which will provide even more clinical variety.

References

1. Centers for Disease Control (1982). Update on Kaposi's sarcoma and opportunistic infections in previously healthy persons – United States. *Morbid. Mortal. Weekly Rep.*, **31**, 294
2. Centers for Disease Control (1981). Kaposi's sarcoma and *pneumocystis* pneumonia among homosexual men – New York and California, *Morbid. Mortal. Weekly Rep.*, **30**, 305
3. Des Jarlais, D. C., Freidman, S. and Hopkins, W. (1985). Risk reduction for the Acquired Immunodeficiency Syndrome among intravenous drug users. *Ann. Intern. Med.*, **103**, 755–9
4. Centers for Disease Control (1982). Possible transfusion-associated acquired immune deficiency syndrome (AIDS): California. *Morbid. Mortal. Weekly Rep.*, **31**, 652–4
5. Curran, J., Morgan, W., Hardy, A. *et al.* (1985). The epidemiology of AIDS: current status and future prospects. *Science*, **299**, 1352–7
6. Hardy, A., Allen, J., Morgan, W. and Curran, J. (1985). The incidence rate of acquired immunodeficiency syndrome in selected populations. *J. Am. Med. Assoc.*, **253**, 215–20
7. Peterman, T., Jaffe, H., Feorino, P. *et al.* (1985). Transfusion associated acquired immunodeficiency syndrome in the United States. *J. Am. Med. Assoc.*, **254**, 2913–17
8. Yanagi, Y., Yoshikai, Y., Leggett, K., Clark, S. P., Aleksander, I. and Mak, T. W. (1984). A human T cell-specific cDNA clone encodes a protein having extensive homology to immunoglobulin chains. *Nature*, **308**, 145–9
9. Zinkernagel, R. M. and Doherty, P. C. (1975). H-2 compatibility requirement for T-cell-mediated lysis of target cells infected with lymphocytic choriomeningitis virus:

different cytotoxic T-cell specificities are associated with structures coded for in H-2K or H-2D. *J. Exp. Med.*, **141**, 1427–36
10. Meuer, S. C., Acuto, O., Hussey, R. E. *et al.* (1983). Evidence for the T3-associated 90K heterodimer as the T-cell antigen receptor. *Nature*, **303**, 808–10
11. David, K. C., Horsburgh, C. R., Jr, Hasiba, U., Schocket, A. L. and Kirkpatrick, C. H. (1983). Acquired immunodeficiency syndrome in a patient with hemophilia. *Ann. Intern. Med.*, **98**, 284–6
12. Elliott, J. L., Hoppes, W. L., Platt, M. S., Thomas , J. G., Patel, I. P. and Gansar, A. (1983). The acquired immunodeficiency syndrome and *Mycobacterium avium–intracellulare* bacteremia in a patient with hemophilia. *Ann. Intern. Med.*, **98**, 290–3
13. Poon, M. C., Landay, A., Prasthofer, E. F. and Stagno, S. (1983) Acquired immunodeficiency syndrome with Pneumocystis carinii pneumonia and *Mycobacterium avium–intracellulare* infection in a previously healthy patient with classic hemophilia: clinical, immunologic, and virologic findings. *Ann. Intern. Med.*, **98**, 287–90
14. Ragni, M. V., Spero, J. A., Lewis, J. H. and Bontempo, F. A. (1983). Acquired immunodeficiency-like syndrome in two haemophiliacs. *Lancet*, **1**, 213–14
15. Samelson, L. E., Harford, J. B. and Klausner, R. D. (1985). Identification of the components of the murine T cell antigen receptor complex. *Cell*, **43**, 223–31
16. Reinherz, E. L., Meuer, S., Fitzgerald, K. A., Hussey, R. E., Levine, H. and Schlossman, S. F. (1982). Antigen recognition by human T lymphocytes is linked to surface expression of the T3 molecular complex. *Cell*, **30**, 735–43
17. Harris, C., Small, C. B., Klein, R. S. *et al.* (1983). Immunodeficiency in female sexual partners of men with the acquired immunodeficiency syndrome. *N. Engl. J. Med.*, **308**, 1181–4
18. Oleske, J., Minnefor, A., Cooper, R. *et al.* (1983). Immune deficiency syndrome in children. *J. Am. Med. Assoc.*, **249**, 2345–9
19. Statistics from the World Health Organization and the Centers for Disease Control (1988). *AIDS*, **2**, 145–9
20. Moss, A., McCallum, G., Volberding, P., Bacchetti, P. and Dritz, S. (1984). Mortality associated with mode of presentation in AIDS. *J. Nat. Cancer Inst.*, **73**, 1281–4
21. Rivin, B., Monroe, J., Hubschuman, B. and Thomas, P. (1984). AIDS outcome: a first follow-up. *N. Engl. J. Med.*, **311**, 857
22. Revision of the CDC Surveillance Case Definition for Acquired Immunodeficiency Syndrome (1987). *Morbid. Mortal. Weekly Rep.*, **36**(15)
23. Centers for Disease Control (1986). Classification system for HTLV-III/LAV infections. *Ann. Intern. Med.*, **105**, 234–7
24. Cooper, D. A., Gold, J., Maclean, P., Donovan, B., Finlayson, R., Barnes, T. G., Michelmore, H. M., Brooke, P. and Penny, R. (1985). Acute AIDS retrovirus infection: definition of a clinical illness associated with seroconversion. *Lancet*, **1**, 537–40
25. Ho, D. D., Sarngadharan, M. G., Resnick, L., Dimarzo-Veronese, F., Rota, T. R. and Hirsch, M. S. (1985). Primary human T-lymphotropic virus type III infection. *Ann. Intern. Med.*, **103**, 880–3
26. *Lancet* (Editorial) (1984). Needlestick transmission of HTLV-III from a patient infected in Africa. *Lancet*, **2**, 1376–7
27. Boiteux, F., Vilmer, E., Girot, R., Muller, J-Y., Rouzioux, C., Chamaret, S. and Montagnier, L. (1985). Lymphadenopathy syndrome in two thalassemic patients after LAV contamination by blood transfusion. *N. Engl. J. Med.*, **312**, 648–9
28. Tucker, J., Ludlam, C. A., Craig, A., Philip, I., Steel, C. M., Tedder, R. S., Cheingsong-Popov, R., Macnicol, M. F., McClelland, D. B. L. and Boulton, F. E. (1985). HTLV-III infection associated with glandular fever-like illness in a haemophiliac. *Lancet*, **1**, 585
29. L'Age-Stehr, J., Schwarz, A., Offerman, G., Langmaack, H., Bennhold, I., Niedrig, M. and Koch, M. A. (1985). HTLV-III infection in kidney transplant recipients. *Lancet*, **2**, 1361–2
30. Lindskov, R., Lindhardt, B. O., Weismann, K., Thomsen, K., Bang, F., Ulrich, K. and Wnatzin, G. (1986). Acute HTLV-III infection with roseola-like rash. *Lancet*, **1**, 447
31. McCray, E. (1986). The Cooperative Needlestick Surveillance Group. Occupational risk of the acquired immunodeficiency syndrome among health care workers. *N. Engl. J. Med.*, **314**, 1127–32
32. Carne, C. A., Tedder, R. S., Smith, A., Sutherland, S., Elkington, S. G., Daly, H. M., Preston, F. E. and Craske, J. (1985). Acute encephalopathy coincident with seroconversion for

anti-HTLV-III. *Lancet*, **2**, 1206–8
33. Ho, D. D., Rota, T. R., Schooley, R. T., Kaplan, J. C., Allan, J. D., Groopman, J. E., Resnick, L., Felsenstein, D., Andrews, C. A. and Hirsh, M. S. (1985). Isolation of HTLV-III from cerebospinal fluid and neural tissues of patients with neurologic syndromes related to the acquired immunodeficiency syndrome. *N. Engl. J. Med.*, **313**, 1493–7
34. Piette, A. M., Tusseau, F., Vignon, D., Chapman, A., Parrot, G., Leibowitch, J. and Montagnier, L. (1986). Acute neuropathy coincident with seroconversion for anti-LAV//HTLV-III. *Lancet*, **1**, 852
35. Romeril, K. R. (1985). Acute HTLV-III infection. *N. Z. Med. J.*, **98**, 401
36. Biggs, B. and Newton-John, H. (1986). Acute HTLV-III infection. A case followed from onset to seroconversion. *Med. J. Aust.*, **144**, 545–6
37. Denning, D. W., Anderson, J., Rudge, P. *et al.* (1987). Acute myelopathy associated with primary infection with human immunodeficiency virus infection. *Br. Med. J.*, **294**, 143–4
38. Hagberg, L., Malmvall, B-E., Svennerholm, L. *et al.* (1986). Guillain–Barré syndrome as an early manifestation of HIV central nervous system infection. *Scand. J. Infect. Dis.*, **18**, 591–2
39. Przedborski, S., Liesnard, C. and Hildebard, J. (1986). HTLV-III and vacuolar myelopathy. *N. Engl. J. Med.*, **315**, 63
40. Ranki, A., Valle, S-L., Krohn, M. *et al.* (1987). Long latency precedes overt seroconversion in sexually transmitted human-immunodeficiency-virus infection. *Lancet*, **2**, 589–93
41. Matheron, S., Dormont, D., Rey, M. A. *et al.* (1987). Kinetics of HIV infection after IV exposure to blood from an AIDS patient. Washington DC: *Proceedings, III International Conference on AIDS*, 67 (abstract)
42. Pristeria, R., Seebacher, C., Casini, M. *et al.* (1987). Acute infection by HIV in drug addicts. Washington DC: *Proceedings, III International Conference on AIDS*, p. 178 (abstract)
43. Esteban, J. I., Shih, J.W-K., Tai, C-C., Bodner, A. J., Kay, J. W. D. and Alter, H. J. (1985). Importance of Western Blot analysis in predicting infectivity of anti-HTLV-III/LAV positive blood. *Lancet*, **2**, 1083–6
44. Cooper, D. A., Imrie, A. A. and Penny, R. (1987). Antibody response to human immunodeficiency virus after primary infection. *J. Infect. Dis.*, **155**, 1113–18
45. Cooper, D. A., Tindall, B., Wilson, E. J., Imrie, A. A. and Penny, R. (1988). Characterisation of T lymphocyte responses during primary infection with human immunodeficiency virus infection. *J. Infect.*, **157**, 889–96
46. Cilla, G., Trallero, E. P., Furundarena, J. R., Cuadrado, E., Iribarren, J. A. and Neira, F. (1988). Esophageal candidiasis and immunodeficiency associated with acute HIV infection. *AIDS*, **2**, 399–400
47. Pedersen, C., Gerstoft, J., Lindhardt, B. O. and Sindrup, J. (1987). Candida oesophagitis associated with acute human immunodeficiency virus infection. *J. Infect.*, **156**, 529–30
48. Tindall, B., Hing, M., Edwards, P., Barnes, T., Mackie, A. and Cooper, D. A. (1989). Short communication; severe clinical manifestations of primary HIV infection. *AIDS*, **3**, 747–9
49. Isaksson, B., Albert, J., Chiodi, F., Furucrona, A., Krook, A. and Putkonen, P. (1988). AIDS two months after primary human immunodeficiency virus infection. *J. Infect. Dis.*, **158**, 866–8
50. Eales, L. J. and Parkin, J. M. (1988). Current concepts in the immunopathogenesis of AIDS and HIV infection. *Br. Med. Bull.*, **144**, 38–55
51. Treacy, M., Lai, L., Costello, C. and Clark, A. (1987). Peripheral blood and bone marrow abnormalities in patients with HIV related disease. *Br. J. Haematol.*, **65**, 289–94
52. Murphy, M. F., Metcalfe, P., Waters, A. H. *et al.* (1987). Incidence and mechanism of neutropenia and thrombocytopenia in patients with human immunodeficiency virus infection. *Br. J. Haematol.*, **66**, 337–40
53. Jaffe, H. S., Abrams, D. I., Anmann, A. J., Lewis, B. J. and Golden, J. A. (1983). Complications of co-trimoxazole in treatment of AIDS associated *Pneumocystis carinii* pneumonia in homosexual men. *Lancet*, **2**, 1109–11
54. Morris, L., Distenfeld, A., Amorosi, E. and Karpatkin, S. (1982). Autoimmune thrombocytopenic purpura in homosexual men. *Ann. Intern. Med.*, **96**, 714–17
55. Savona, S., Nardi, M., Lennette, E. T. and Karpatkin, S. (1985). Thrombocytopenic purpura in narcotic addicts. *Ann. Intern. Med.*, **102**, 737–41
56. Ratnoff, O. D., Menitove, J. E., Aster, R. H. and Lederman, M. M. (1983). Coincident classic hemophilia and 'idiopathic' thrombocytopenic purpura in patients under treatment

with concentrates of antihemophillic factor (factor VIII). *N. Engl. J. Med.*, **308**, 439–42
57. Abrams, D. (1986). AIDS related conditions. *Clin. Immunol. Allergy*, **6**, 581–99
58. Selik, R. M., Starcher, E. T. and Curran, J. W. (1987). Opportunistic diseases reported in AIDS patients: frequencies, associations, and trends. *AIDS*, **1**, 175–82
59. Beral, V., Peterman, T. A., Berkelman, R. L. and Jaffe, H. W. (1990) Kaposi's sarcoma among persons with AIDS: a sexually transmitted infection? *Lancet*, **335**, 123–8
60. Beral, V., Peterman, T., Berkelman, R. and Jaffe, H. (1991). AIDS-associated non-Hodgkin's lymphoma. *Lancet*, **337**, 805–9
61. Reichman, L. B., Felton, C. P. and Edsall, J. R. (1979) Drug dependence, a possible new risk factor for tuberculosis disease. *Arch. Intern. Med.*, **139**, 337–9
62. Sunderam, G., McDonald, J., Maniatis, T., Oleske, J., Kapila, R. and Reichman, L. B. (1986). Tuberculosis as a manifestation of the acquired immune deficiency syndrome (AIDS). *J. Am. Med. Assoc.*, **256**, 362–6
63. Handwerger, S., Mildvan, D., Senie, R. and McKinley, F. W. (1987). Tuberculosis and the acquired immunodeficiency syndrome at a New York City Hospital. *Chest*, **91**, 176–80
64. Chaisson, R. E., Schechter, G. F., Theuer, C. P., Rutherford, G. W., Echenberg, D. F. and Hopewell, P. C. (1987). Tuberculosis in patients with the acquired immunodeficiency syndrome. Clinical features, response to therapy, and survival. *Am. Rev. Resp. Dis.*, **136**, 570–4
65. Centers for Disease Control (Editorial) (1987). Tuberculosis and acquired immunodeficiency syndrome – New York. *Morbid. Mortal. Weekly Rep.*, **36**(48), 785–90, 795
66. Selwyn, P. A., Hartel, D., Lewis, V. A. *et al.* (1989). A prospective study of the risk of tuberculosis among intravenous drug users with human immunodeficiency virus infection. *N. Engl. J. Med.*, **320**(9), 545–50
67. Simberkoff, M. S., El-Sadr, W., Schiffman, G. and Rahal, J. J. Jr (1984). *Streptococcus pneumoniae* infections and bacteremia in patients with acquired immune deficiency syndrome, with report of a pneumococcal vaccine failure. *Am. Rev. Resp. Dis.*, **130**(6), 1174–6
68. Selwyn, P. A., Schoenbaum, E. E., Hartel, D. *et al.* (1988). AIDS and HIV-related mortality in intravenous drug users (IVDUs) (Abstract). IV International Conference on AIDS, Stockholm, Sweden, 13–16 June; Abstract 4526
69. Polsky, B., Gold, J. W., Whimbey, E. *et al.* (1986). Bacterial pneumonia in patients with the acquired immunodeficiency syndrome. *Ann. Intern. Med.*, **104**(1), 38–41
70. Selwyn, P. A., Feingold, A. R., Hartel, D., Schoenbaum, E. E. *et al.* (1988). Increased risk of bacterial pneumonia in HIV-infected intravenous drug users without AIDS. *AIDS*, **2**, 267–72
71. Centers for Disease Control (Editorial) (1988). Increase in pneumonia mortality among young adults and the HIV epidemic – New York City, United States. *Morbid. Mortal. Weekly Rep.*, **37**(38), 593–6
72. Gilks, G. F., Brindle, R. J., Otieno, L. S., Simani, P. M., Newham, R. S., Bhatt, S. M., Lule, G. N., Okelo, G. B. A., Watkins, W. M., Waiyaki, P. G., Were, J. B. O. and Warrell, D. A. (1990). Life-threatening bacteraemia in HIV-1 seropositive adults admitted to hospital in Nairobi, Kenya. *Lancet*, **336**, 545–9
73. Slim, J., Boghossian, J., Perez, G. and Johnson, E. (1988). Comparative analysis of bacterial endocarditis in HIV(+) and HIV(−) intravenous drug users (Abstract). IV International Conference on AIDS, Stockholm, Sweden, 13–16 June: Abstract 8027
74. Ruggeri, P., Sathe, S. S. and Kapila, R. (1988). Changing patterns of infectious endocarditis (IE) in parenteral drug abusers (PDA) with human immunodeficiency virus (HIV) infections (Abstract). IV International Conference on AIDS, Stockholm, Sweden, 13–16 June: Abstract 8028
75. Guay, L., Mmiro, F., Ndugwa, C., Kataha, P., Migisha, K., Goldfarb, J., Hom, D., Friesen, H., Toltzis, P., Coulter, B. and Olness, K. (1990). Perinatal outcome in HIV infected women in Uganda. VIth International Conference on AIDS: San Francisco, USA: Abstract ThC 42
76. Parkin, J. M., Helbert, M., Hughes, C. L. and Pinching, A. J. (1989). Immunoglobulin G subclass deficiency and susceptibility to pyogenic infections in patients with AIDS-related complex and AIDS. *AIDS*, **3**, 37–9
77. Jones, G., Brettle, R. P., Bird, A. G. and Leen, C. L. S. (1991). Immunoglobulin subclass responses to bacterial infection in HIV positive injection drug users. VIIth International Conference on AIDS, Florence, Italy: Abstract
78. Burns, S. M., Collacott, I. A., Hargreaves, F. D. and Inglis, J. M. (1987). Incidence of hepatitis B markers in HIV seropositive and seronegative drug misusers in the Edinburgh

area. *Commun. Dis. Scotland* (*Weekly Rep.*), **87**(08), 7–8
79. Vento, S., Di Perri, G., Luzzati, R. *et al.* (1989). Clinical reactivation of hepatitis in anti-HBs-positive patients with AIDS. *Lancet*, **1**, 332–3
80. Fauci, A. (1987). Immunopathogenesis of HIV. III International Conference on AIDS, Washington DC, 1–5 June.
81. Rivin, B., Monroe, J., Hubschuman, B. and Thomas, P. (1984). AIDS outcome: a first follow-up. *N. Engl. J. Med.*, **311**, 857
82. Tubaro, E., Borelli, G., Croce, C., Cavallo, G. and Santiangeli, C. (1983). Effect of morphine on resistance to infection. *J. Infect. Dis.*, **148**, 656–6
83. Editorial (1984). Opiates, opioid peptides, and immunity. *Lancet*, **1**, 774–5
84. Hahn, B. H., Shaw, G. M., Taylor, M. E. *et al.* (1986). Genetic variation in HTLV-III/LAV over time in patients with AIDS or at risk for AIDS. *Science*, **232**, 1548–53
85. Polk, B. F., Fox, R., Brookmeyer, R. *et al.* (1987). Predictors of the acquired immunodeficiency syndrome developing in a cohort of seropositive homosexual men. *N. Engl. J. Med.*, **316**, 61–6
86. Eyster, M. E., Gail, M. H., Ballard, J. O., Al-Mondhiry, N. and Goedert, J. J. (1987). Natural history of human immunodeficiency virus infection in haemophiliacs: effects of T-cell subsets, platelet counts and age. *Ann. Intern. Med.*, **107**, 1–6
87. Lacey, C. J. N., Forbes, M. A., Waugh, M. A., Cooper, E. H., Cooper, J. and Hambling, M. H. (1988). Serum β_2-microglobulin and HIV infection. IV International Conference on AIDS, Stockholm, Sweden, 12–16 June
88. Winkelstein, W. (1988). Beta-2 microglobulin level predicts AIDS. IV International Conference on AIDS, Stockholm, Sweden, 12–16 June
89. Gold, J., Morlet, A., Nicolas, T., Guinan, J. J. and Stevens, M. (1988). Elevation of serum Beta-2 microglobulin associated with decreased CD4 lymphocyte count in HIV infection. IV International Conference on AIDS, Stockholm, Sweden, 12–16 June
90. Lambin, P., Lefrère, J. J., Doinel, C., Fine, J. M. and Salmon, C. (1988). Neopterin and beta-2 microglobulin in sera of HIV seropositive subjects during a two year follow-up. IV International Conference on AIDS, Stockholm, Sweden, 12–16 June
91. Marthur-Wagh, U., Mildvan, D. and Senie, R. T. (1985). Follow-up at 4.5 years on homosexual men with generalised lymphadenopathy. *N. Engl. J. Med.*, **313**, 1542–5
92. Goedert, J. J., Biggar, R. J., Weiss, S. H. *et al.* (1986). Three years incidence of AIDS in five cohorts of HTLV-III infected risk group members. *Science*, **231**, 992–5
93. Melbye, M., Biggar, R. J., Ebbesen, P. *et al.* (1986). Long-term seropositivity for human T-lymphotropic virus type III in homosexual men without the acquired immune deficiency syndrome: development of immunologic and clinical abnormalities. *Ann. Intern. Med.*, **104**, 497–500
94. Taylor, J. G. M., Schwartz, K. and Detels, R. (1986). The time from infection with human immunodeficiency virus (HIV) to the onset of AIDS. *J. Infect. Dis.*, **154**, 694–7
95. Kaplan, J. E., Spira, T. J., Fishbein, D. B., Pinsky, P. F. and Schoenberger, L. B. (1987). Lymphadenopathy syndrome in homosexual men; evidence for continuing risk of developing the acquired immune deficiency syndrome. *J. Am. Med. Assoc.*, **257**, 335 –7
96. Moss, A. R. and Bacchetti, P. (1989). Natural history of HIV infection. *AIDS*, **3**, 55–61
97. Lifson, A. R., Hessol, N., Rutherford, G., O'Malley, P., Barnhart, L., Buchbinder, S., Cannon, L., Bodecker, T., Holmberg, S., Harrison, J. and Doli, L. (1990). Natural history of HIV infection in a cohort of homosexual and bisexual men: clinical and immunological outcome. VIth International Conference on AIDS, San Francisco: Abstract ThC 33
98. Rutherford, G. W., Lifson, A. R., Hessol, N. A. *et al.* (1990). Course of HIV-1 infection in a cohort of homosexual and bisexual men: an 11 year follow up study. *Br. Med. J.*, **301**, 1183–8
99. Gatell, J. M., Podzamczer, D., Clotet, B., Ocana, I., Estamy, C., Miro, J. M. and Barcelona AIDS Study Group (1989). Incidence of AIDS in Spanish HIV infected Patients (Abstract). V International Conference on AIDS, Montreal, Canada, 5–9 June: Abstract WAP 55
100. Vaccher, E., Saracchini, S., Errante, D. *et al.* (1988). Progression of HIV disease among intravenous drug abusers (IVDA): a three-year prospective study (Abstract). IV International Conference on AIDS, Stockholm, Sweden, 13–16 June: Abstract 4529
101. Zulaica, D., Arrizabalaga, J., Iribarren, J. A. *et al.* (1988). Follow-up of 100 HIV infected intravenous drug abusers (Abstract). IV International Conference on AIDS, Stockholm, Sweden, 13–16 June: Abstract 4532
102. Crovari, P., Penco, G., Valente, A. *et al.* (1988). HIV infection in two cohorts of drug

addicts prospectively studied. Association of serological markers with clinical progression (Abstract). IV International Conference on AIDS, Stockholm, Sweden, 13–16 June: Abstract 4527

103. Rezza, G., Lazzarin, A., Angarano, G. *et al.* (1989). The natural history of HIV infection in intravenous drug users: risk of disease progression in a cohort of seroconverters. *AIDS*, **3**, 87–90
104. Stoneburner, R. L., Des Jarlais, D. C., Benezra, D. *et al.* (1989). A larger spectrum of severe HIV-1 related disease in intravenous drug users in New York City. *Science*, **242**, 916–18
105. Galli, M., Carito, M., Craccu, V. *et al.* (1988). Cause of death in IV drug abusers – a retrospective survey on 4883 subjects (Abstract). IV International Conference on AIDS; Stockholm, Sweden, 13–16 June: Abstract 4520
106. Mann, D. L., Murray, C., Yarchoan, R., Blattner, W. A. and Goedert, J. J. (1988). HLA antigen frequencies in HIV-1 seropositive disease-free individuals and patients with AIDS. *J. AIDS*, **1**, 13–17
107. Mann, D., Tabor, Y., Lubet, M. and Goedert, J. (1988). Influence of MHC phenotype on cellular cytotoxicity to HIV infected cells. IV International Conference on AIDS, Stockholm, Sweden, 12–16 June: Abstract 2003
108. Kaslow, R. A., Duquesnoy, R., VanRaden, M., Kingsley, L. *et al.* (1990). A1, Cw7, B8, DR3 HLA antigen combination associated with rapid decline of T-helper lymphocytes in HIV-1 infection. A report from the Multicentre AIDS cohort study. *Lancet*, **335**, 927–30
109. Steel, C. M., Ludlam, C. A., Beatson, D. *et al.* (1988). HLA haplotype A1, B8, DR3 as a risk factor for HIV related disease. *Lancet*, **1**, 1185–8
110. Raffoux, C., David, V., Couderc, L. D. *et al.* (1987). HLA-A, B, DR antigen frequencies in patients with AIDS related persistent generalised lymphadenopathy (PGL) and thrombocytopenia. *Tissue Antigens*, **29**, 60–2
111. Scorza Smeraldi, R., Fabio, G., Lazzarin, A. *et al.* (1988). HLA-associated susceptibility to AIDS: HLA B35 is a major risk factor for Italian HIV infected intravenous drug addicts. *Hum. Immunol.*, **22**, 73–9
112. Pollack, M. S., Safai, B. and Dupont, B. (1983). HLA-DR5 and DR2 are susceptibility factors for acquired immunodeficiency syndrome with Kaposi's sarcoma in different ethnic subpopulations. *Dis. Markers*, **1**, 135–9
113. Halle, L., Castellano, F., Kaplan, C., Lefrere, J-J., Salmon, D. and Salmon C. (1988). HLA haplotype and HIV infection. *Lancet*, **2**, 342
114. Pabinger, I., Lechner, K., Kyrie, P. A., Rosenmayer, A. H. and Kirnbauer, M. (1988). HLA haplotype and HIV infection. *Lancet*, **2**, 342–3
115. Cheng-Mayer, C., Seto, D., Tateno, M. and Levy, J. A. (1988). Biological features of HIV-1 that correlate virulence in the host. *Science*, **240**, 80–2
116. Tersmette, M., Gruters, R. A., de Wolf, F. *et al.* (1989). Evidence for a role of virulent HIV strains in the pathogenesis of AIDS obtained from studies on a panel of sequential HIV isolates. *J. Virol.*, **63**, 2118–25
117. Tersmette, M., Lange, J. M. A., de Goede, R. E. Y. *et al.* (1989). Association between biological properties of human immunodeficiency virus variants and risk for AIDS and AIDS mortality. *Lancet*, **1**, 983–9
118. Fenyo, E. M., Albert, J., Morfeldt-Manson, L. and Asjo, B. (1989). Replicative capacity of sequential virus isolates from HIV-1 infected subjects and relationship to clinical progression. V International Conference on AIDS, Montreal, June: Abstract MCO 9
119. Nicholson, J. K. A., Spira, T. J., Aloisio, C. H. *et al.* (1989). Serial determinations of HIV-1 titers in HIV-infected homosexual men: association of rising titers with CD4 T cell depletion and progression to AIDS. *AIDS Res. Hum. Retrovirus*, **5**, 502–15
120. Skolnik, P. R., Kosloff, B. R. and Hirsh, M. S. (1985). Bidirectional interaction between human immunodeficiency virus type 1 and cytomegalovirus. *J. Infect. Dis.*, **157**, 508–14
121. Albrecht, M. A., Gillis, J. M., Andrea, N. T. and Hammer, S. M. (1987). Human immunodeficiency virus (HIV) – herpes simplex virus (HSV) interactions *in vitro*. Program and Abstracts of the 27th Interscience Conference on Antimicrobial Agents and Chemotherapy. Washington, DC: American Society for Microbiology: Abstract 839
122. Webster, A., Lee, C. A., Cook, D. G., Grundy, J. E., Emery, V. C., Kernoff, P. B. A. and Griffiths, P. D. (1989). Cytomegalovirus infection and progression towards AIDS in haemophiliacs with human immunodeficiency virus infection. *Lancet*, **2**, 63–6

123. Drew, W. L., Perkins, H., Garner, J. and Miner, R. (1990). CMV is not a cofactor in progression of HIV infection. VIth International Conference on AIDS, San Francisco, June: Abstract ThC680
124. Buchbinder, S., Hessol, N., Lifson, A., O'Malley, P., Barnhart, L., Bodecker, T., Cannon, L., Rutherford, G. and Hadler, S. (1990). Does infection with hepatitis B virus or vaccination with plasma derived hepatitis B vaccine accelerate progression to AIDS? VIth International Conference on AIDS, San Francisco, June: Abstract ThC 679
125. Weiss, S. H., French, J., Holland, B. *et al.* (1989). HTLV-I/II coinfection is strongly associated with risk for progression to AIDS among HIV positive intravenous drug abusers. In V International Conference on AIDS, Montreal, June: Abstract THAO 23
126. Bartholomew, C., Cleghorn, F., Hull, B., Battoo, K., Diaz, C. and Blattner, W. (1990). Update on coinfection with HIV and HTLV-I in Trinidad. VIth International Conference on AIDS, San Francisco, June: Abstract ThC 681
127. Matsuyama, T., Hamamoto, Y., Soma, G., Mizuno, D., Yamamoto, N. and Kobayashi, N. (1989). Cytocidal effect of tumour necrosis factor on cells chronically infected with human immunodeficiency virus (HIV): enhancement of viral replication. *J. Virol.*, **63**, 2504–9
128. Chowdhury, M. I. H., Koyanagi, Y., Kobayashi, S. *et al.* (1990). Mycoplasma and AIDS. *Lancet*, **336**, 247–8
129. Montagnier, L., Berneman, D., Guetard, D. *et al.* (1990). Inhibition de l'infectuosite de souches prototypes du VIH par des anticorps diriges contre une sequence peptidique de mycoplasme. *C.R. Acad. Sci. Paris*, **311**, 425–30
130. Lemaitre, M., Guetard, D., Henin, Y., Montagnier, L. and Zerial, A. (1990). Protective activity of tetracycline analogs against the cytopathic effect of human immunodeficiency virus in CEM cells. *Res. Virol.*, **141**, 5–16
131. Vasudevachari, M. B., Mast, T. C. and Salzman, N. P. (1990). Suppression of HIV-1 reverse transcriptase activity by mycoplasma contamination of cell cultures. *AIDS Res. Hum. Retrovirus*, **6**, 411–16
132. Medley, G. F., Anderson, R. M., Cox, D. R. and Billard, L. (1987). Incubation period of AIDS in patients infected via blood transfusion. *Nature*, **328**, 719–23
133. Blaxhult, A., Granath, F., Lidman, K. and Giesecke, J. (1990). The influence of age on the latency period to AIDS in people infected by HIV through blood transfusion. *AIDS*, **4**, 125–9
134. Robertson, R. J., Skidmore, C. A., Roberts, J. J. K. and Elton, R. A. (1990). Progression to AIDS in intravenous drug users, cofactors and survival. VIth International Conference on AIDS, San Francisco, June: Abstract ThC649
135. Lee, C. A., Phillips, A. N., Elford, J., Janossy, G., Griffiths, P. D. and Kernoff, P. B. A. (1990). Ten year follow-up of a cohort of 111 anti-HIV seropositive haemophiliacs. VIth International Conference on AIDS, San Francisco, June: Abstract ThC 641
136. Schinaia, N. and Chiarotti, F. (1990). The progression to AIDS in the Italian hemophilia population over a six year period. VIth International Conference on AIDS, San Francisco, June: Abstract ThC 38
137. Kaslow, A. R., Blackwelder, W. C., Ostrow, D. G. *et al.* (1989). No accelerating immunodeficiency in HIV-1 seropositive individuals. *J. Am. Med. Assoc.*, **261**, 3424–9
138. Des Jarlais, D. C., Friedman, S. R., Marmor, M. *et al.* (1987). Development of AIDS, HIV seroconversion, and potential co-factors for T4 cell loss in a cohort of intravenous drug users. *AIDS*, **1**, 105–11
139. Flegg, P. J., Jones, M. E., MacCallum, L. R., Bird, A. G., Whitelaw, J. M. and Brettle, R. P. (1989). Continued injecting drug use as a cofactor for progression of HIV. V International Conference on AIDS, 4–9 June 1989, Montreal, Canada: Abstract MAP 92
140. Weber, R., Ledergerber, B., Opravil, M., Siegenthaler, W., Luthy, R. (1990). Progression of HIV infection in misusers of injected drugs who stop injecting or follow a programme of maintenace treatment with methadone. *Br. Med. J.*, **301**, 1362–5
141. Selwyn, P. A., Hartel, D., Schoenbaum, E. E., Klein, R. S. and Friedland, G. H. (1990). Clinical progression of HIV related diseases in intravenous drug users (IVDU) in a prospective cohort study: 1985–1989. Vth International Conference on AIDS, San Francisco, June: Abstract ThC 649
142. Selwyn, P. A., Hartel, D., Schoenbaum, E. E., Davenny, K., Budner, N., Klein, R. S. and Friedman, G. H. (1990). Rates and predictors of progression to HIV disease and AIDS in a cohort of intravenous drug users (IVDUs), 1985–1990. VIth International Conference

on AIDS, San Francisco, June: Abstract FC 111
143. Hartel, D., Selwyn, P. A., Schoenbaum, E. E., Klein, R. S., Friedland, G. H. (1988). Methadone maintenance treatment (MMTP) and reduced risk of AIDS and AIDS-specific mortality in intravenous drug users (IVDUs) (Abstract). IV International Conference on AIDS, Stockholm, Sweden, 13–16 June: Abstract 8546
144. Diego, S. and Franceschi, S. (1990). Methadone maintenance programmes and AIDS in North Italy. VIth International Conference on AIDS, San Francisco, June: Abstract SD 125
145. Mientjes, G., van den Hoek, J. A. R., van Ameijden, E., Schellekens, P. T. A., Roos, M. and Coutinho, R. A. (1990). The impact of frequent injecting on the immune status of intravenous drug users (IDU). VIth International Conference on AIDS, San Francisco, June: Abstract ThC 648
146. Davenny, K., Buono, D., Schoenbaum, E. and Friedland, G. H. (1990). Baseline health status of intravenous drug users with and without HIV infection. VIth International Conference on AIDS, San Francisco, June: Abstract FB 430
147. Clarkson, R. C., Flegg, P. J., Bird, A. G., Brettle, R. P. and Robertson, J. R. (1990). Beta-2-microglobulin levels in Edinburgh drug users. VIth International Conference on AIDS, San Francisco, June: Abstract ThC 650
148. Gorter, R. W., Vranizan, K., Moss, A. R., Brodie, B. and Wolfe, H. (1990). Progression of HIV disease in intravenous drug users. VIth International Conference on AIDS, San Francisco, June: Abstract ThC 644
149. Royce, R., Winkelstein, W. and Bacchetti, P. (1990). Cigarette smoking and incidence of AIDS. VIth International Conference on AIDS, San Francisco, June: Abstract ThC 39
150. Fernandez-Cruz, E., Desco, M., Montes, M. G., Longo, N., Gonzalez, B. and Zabay, J. M. (1990). Immunological and serological markers predictive of progression to AIDS in a cohort of HIV infected drug users. *AIDS*, **4**, 987–94
151. McNeil, A., Gore, S. M., Bird, A. G. and Brettle, R. P. (1991). Progression to AIDS or ARC in the Edinburgh City Hospital cohort. VIIth International Conference on AIDS, Florence, Italy: Abstract MC 3142
152. Scott, G. B., Fischl, M. A., Klimas, N. *et al.* (1985). Mother of infants with the acquired immune deficiency syndrome. *J. Am. Med. Assoc.*, **253**, 363–6
153. Minkoff, H., Nanda, D., Menez, R. and Fikeig, S. (1987). Pregnancies resulting in infants with AIDS or AIDS related complex. *Obstet. Gynecol.*, **69**, 285–7
154. Delfraissey, J. F., Pons, J. C., Sereni, D., Chambrin, V., Meyer, D., Emgelman, Ph., Papiernik, E. and Henrion, R. (1989). Does pregnancy influence disease progression in HIV positive women? Vth International Conference on AIDS, Montreal, Canada: Abstract MBP 34
155. Deschamps, M-M., Pape, J. W., Madhavan, S. and Johnson, W. D. Jr (1989). Pregnancy and acceleration of HIV related illness. Vth International Conference on AIDS, Montreal, Canada: Abstract MBP 6
156. Nachman, S. (1987). HIV infection during pregnancy: a longitudinal study. IIIrd International Conference on AIDS, Washington, DC: Abstract TP 55
157. Schoenbaum, E. E., Daverny, K., Selwyn, P. A., Hartel, D. and Rogers, M. (1989). The effect of pregnancy on progression of HIV related disease. Vth International Conference on AIDS, Montreal, Canada: Abstract MBP 8
158. Berribi, A., Puel, J., Tricoire, J., Herne, H. and Pontonnier, G. (1990). Influence of gestation on HIV infection. VIth International Conference on AIDS, San Francisco: Abstract ThC 651
159. Bledsoe, K., Olopoenia, L., Barnes, S., Delapenha, R., Saxinger, C. and Frederick, W. (1990). Effect of pregnancy on progression of HIV infection. VIth International Conference on AIDS, San Francisco: Abstract ThC 652
160. Johnstone, F. D., MacCallum, L. and Brettle, R. (1988). Does infection with HIV affect the outcome of pregnancy? *Br. Med. J.*, **296**, 467
161. Di Lenardo, L., Truscia, D., Giaquinto, C. and Grella, P. V. (1989). A prospective study of HIV in pregnant women. Vth International Conference on AIDS, Montreal, Canada: Abstract MBP 14
162. Berribi, A., Kobuch, W. E., Puel, J., Tricoire, J., Herne, P. and Fournie, A. (1989). Effects of HIV Infection on pregnancy. Vth International Conference on AIDS, Montreal, Canada: Abstract MBP 26
163. Lopita, M. I., Temmerman, M., Sinei, S. K. F., Plummer, F., Wamola, I. and Piot, P. (1990). HIV infection as a risk factor for spontaneous first trimester abortion. VIth

International Conference on AIDS, San Francisco: Abstract ThC 653
164. Lasley-Bibbs, V., Renzzullo, P., Goldenbaum, M., Horton, J. and McNeil (1990). Patterns of pregnancy and reproductive morbidity among HIV infected women in the United States Army; a retrospective cohort study. VIth International Conference on AIDS, San Francisco: Abstract ThC 655
165. Johnstone, F. D., MacCallum, L. R., Brettle, R. P., Hamilton, B. A., Peutherer, J., Burns, S. M. and Gore, S. M. (1991). Population based, controlled study; effects of HIV infection on pregnancy. VIIth International Conference on AIDS, Florence, Italy: Abstract WC 3239
166. Edison, R., Feigal, D. W., Kirn, D. and Abrams, D. (1988). Progression of laboratory values. AIDS morbidity and AIDS mortality in a 6-year cohort with PGL. IV International Conference on AIDS, Stockholm, June: Abstract 5145
167. Kaplan, J. E., Spira, T. J., Fishbein, D. B., Bozeman, L. H., Pinsky, P. F. and Schonberger, L. B. (1988). A six year follow-up of HIV infected homosexual men with lymphadenopathy. *J. Am. Med. Assoc.*, **260**, 2694–7
168. Melbye, M., Grossman, R. J., Goedert, J. J., Eyster, M. E. and Biggar, R. J. (1987). Risk of AIDS after herpes zoster. *Lancet*, **i**, 728–31
169. Moss, A. R., Bacchetti, P., Osmond, D. *et al.* (1988). Seropositivity for HIV and the development of AIDS or AIDS related condition: three year follow-up of the San Francisco General Hospital cohort. *Br. Med. J.*, **296**, 725–50
170. Klein, R. S., Harris, C. A., Butkus Small, C., Moll, B., Lesser, M. and Friedland, G. H. (1984). Oral candidiasis in high risk patients as the initial manifestation of the acquired immunodeficiency syndrome. *N. Engl. J. Med.*, **311**, 354–8
171. Greenspan, D., Greenspan, J. S., Jearst, N. G. *et al.* (1987). Relation of oral hairy leukoplakia to infection with the human immunodeficiency virus and the risk of developing AIDS. *J. Infect. Dis.*, **155**, 475–81
172. Schechter, M. T., Craib, K. J. P., Le, T. N., Montaner, S. G., Douglas, B., Sestak, P., Willoughby, B. and O'Shaughnessy, M. V. (1990). Susceptibility to AIDS progression appears early in HIV infection. *AIDS*, **4**, 185–90
173. Pedersen, C., Lindhart, B. O., Jensen, B. L., Lauritzen, E., Gerstoft, J. and Dickmeiss, E. (1989). V International Conference on AIDS, Montreal, Canada, June: Abstract TAO 30
174. Cheingsong-Popov, R., Panagiotidi, C., Bowcock, S., Aronstam, A., Wadsworth, J. and Weber, J. (1991). Relation between humoral responses to HIV gag and env proteins at seroconversion and clinical outcome of HIV infection. *Br. Med. J.*, **302**, 23–6
175. Gottlieb, M. S., Schroff, R., Schanker, H. M. *et al.* (1981). *Pneumocystis carinii* pneumonia and mucosal candidiasis in previously healthy homosexual men. *N. Engl. J. Med.*, **305**, 1425–31
176. Friedman-Kien, A. E., Laubenstein, L. J., Rubinstein, P. *et al.* (1982). Disseminated Kaposi's sarcoma in homosexual men. *Ann. Intern. Med.*, **96**, 693–700
177. Mildvan, D., Mathur, U., Enlow, R. W. *et al.* (1982). Opportunistic infections and immune deficiency in homosexual men. *Ann. Intern. Med.*, **96**, 700–4
178. Taylor, J. M., Fahey, J. L., Detels, R. and Giorgi, J. V. (1989). CD4 percentage, CD8 number, and CD4:CD8 ratio in HIV infection: which to use and how to use. *J. AIDS*, **2**, 114–24
179. Goedert, J. J., Biggar, R. J., Melbye, M. *et al.* (1987). Effect of T4 count and cofactors on the incidence of AIDS in homosexual men infected with human immunodeficiency virus. *J. Am. Med. Assoc.*, **257**, 331–4
180. De Wolf, F., Lange, J. M. A., Houweling, J. T. M., Mulder, J. W., Beemster, J., Schellekens, P. T., Coutinho, R. A., van der Noorda, J. and Goudsmit, J. (1989). Appearance of predictors of disease progression in relation to the development of AIDS. *AIDS*, **3**, 563–9
181. Schwartz, K., Visscher, B., Detels, R., Taylor, J., Nishanian, P. and Fahey, J. L. (1985). Immunological changes in lymphadenopathy virus positive and negative symptomless male homosexuals. *Lancet*, **2**, 831–2
182. El-Sadr, W., Marmor, M., Zolla-Pazner, S. *et al.* (1987). Four prospective studies of homosexual men, correlation of immunologic abnormalities, clinical status, and serology to human immunodeficiency virus. *J. Infect. Dis.*, **155**, 789–93
183. Phillips, A., Lee, C. A., Elford, J., Janossy, G., Bofill, M., Timms, A. and Kernoff, P. B. A. (1989). Prediction of progression to AIDS by analysis of CD4 lymphocyte counts in a haemophiliac cohort. *AIDS*, **3**, 737–41
184. Reid, M. J., Goetz, D. W., Zajac, R. A., Houk, R. W. and Boswell, R. N. (1988). The natural history of human immunodeficiency virus infection in screened HIV positive US Air Force

personnel; a preliminary report. *J. AIDS*, **1**, 508–15
185. Fernandez-Cruz, E., Fernandez, A. M., Gutierez, C. *et al.* (1988). Progressive cellular immune impairment leading to development of AIDS; two year prospective study of HIV infection in drug-addicts. *Clin. Exp. Immunol.*, **72**, 190–5
186. Lang, W., Perkins, H., Anderson, R. E., Royce, R., Jewell, N. and Winkelstein, W. Jr (1989). Patterns of T-lymphocyte changes with human immunodeficiency virus infection from seroconversion to the development of AIDS. *J. AIDS*, **2**, 63–9
187. Munoz, A., Carey, V., Saah, A. J. *et al.* (1988). Predictors of decline in CD4 lymphocytes in a cohort of homosexual men infected with human immunodeficiency virus infection. *J. AIDS*, **1**, 396–404
188. Weber, J. N., Clapham, P. R., Weiss, R. A. *et al.* (1987). Human immunodeficiency virus infection in two cohorts of homosexual men neutralising sera and association of anti-gag antibody and prognosis. *Lancet*, **i**, 119–22
189. Lange, J., Coutinho, R., Krone, W. *et al.* (1986a). Distinct IgG recognition patterns during progression of clinical and subclinical infection with LAV/HTLV-III. *Br. Med. J.*, **292**, 228–30
190. Lange, J., Paul, D., Huisman, H. *et al.* (1986b). Persistent antigenaemia and decline of core antibodies associated with transition to AIDS. *Br. Med. J.*, **293**, 1459–62
191. Mayer, K. H., Falk, L. A., Paul, D. A. *et al.* (1987). Correlation of enzyme-linked immunosorbent assays for serum human immunodeficiency virus antigen and antibodies to recombinant viral proteins with subsequent clinical outcomes in a cohort of asymptomatic homosexual men. *Am. J. Med.*, **83**, 208–12
192. Forster, S. M., Osborne, L. M., Cheingsong-Popov, R. *et al.* (1987). Decline of anti-p24 antibody precedes antigenaemia as correlate of prognosis in HIV-1 infection. *AIDS*, **1**, 235–40
193. De Wolf, F., Lange, J. M. A., Houweling, J. T. M. *et al.* (1988). Numbers of CD4+ cells and levels of core antigens of, and antibodies to, the human immunodeficiency virus as predictors of AIDS among seropositive homosexual men. *J. Infect. Dis.*, **158**, 615–22
194. Allain, J.-P., Laurian, Y., Paul, D. *et al.* (1987). Long term evaluation of HIV antigen and antibodies to p24 and gp41 in patients with haemophilia. *N. Engl. J. Med.*, **317**, 1114–21
195. Pedersen, C., Moller, N. C., Nielsen, C., Vestergaard, B. F., Gerstoft, J., Krogsgaard, K. and Nielsen, J. O. (1987). Temporal relation of antigenaemia and loss of antibodies to core antigens to development of clinical disease in HIV infection. *Br. Med. J.*, **295**, 567–9
196. Montagnier, L., Clavel, F., Krust, B. *et al.* (1985). Identification and antigenicity of the major envelope glycoprotein of lymphadenopathy associated virus. *Virology*, **144**, 283–9
197. Lange, J. M. A., de Wolf, F., Krone, W. J. A., Danner, S. A., Coutinho, R. A. and Goudsmit, J. (1987). Decline of antibody reactivity to outer viral core protein p17 is an earlier serological marker of disease progression in human immunodeficiency virus infection than anti-p24 decline. *AIDS*, **1**, 155–9
198. Lefrere, J.-J., Courouce, A.-M., Lambin, P., Fine, J-M., Doinel, C. and Salmon, C. (1989). Clinical and biological features in the 12 months preceding onset of AIDS in HIV-infected subjects. *J. AIDS*, **2**, 100–1
199. Paul, D. A., Falk, L. A., Kessler, H. A., Chase, R. M. and Blaauw, B. (1987). Correlation of serum HIV antigen and antibody with clinical status in HIV-infected patients. *J. Med. Virol.*, **22**, 357–63
200. Goudsmit, J., Lange, J. M. A., Paul, D. A. and Dawson, G. J. (1987). Antigenaemia and antibody titres to core and envelope antigens in AIDS, AIDS related complex and subclinical human immunodeficiency virus infection, *J. Infect. Dis.* **155**, 558–60
201. Murray, H. W., Godbold, J. H., Jurica, K. B. and Roberts, R. B. (1989). Progression to AIDS in patients with lymphadenopathy or AIDS related complex: reappraisal of risk and predictive factors. *Am. J. Med.*, **86**, 533–8
203. Ho, D., Moudgil, T. and Alam, M. (1989). Quantification of HIV-1 in the blood of infected persons. *N. Engl. J. Med.*, **321**, 1621–5
203. Coombs, R., Collier, A., Allain, J.-P. *et al.* (1989). Plasma viraemia in HIV infection. *N. Engl. J. Med.*, **321**, 1626–31
204. Lelie, P. N., Reesink, H. W., Bakker, E., Huisman, J. G. and ten Veen, J. H. (1988). Clinical importance of HIV antigen and anti-HIV core markers in persons infected with HIV. *N. Engl. J. Med.*, **318**, 1204–5
205. Fahey, J. L., Taylor, J. M. G., Detels, R. *et al.* (1989). Enhanced prediction of AIDS in HIV seropositive asymptomatic men; relative value of 8 cellular and serologic markers

singly and in combination. V International Conference on AIDS, Montreal, June: Abstract WAP 62

206. Fahey, J. L., Taylor, J. M. G., Detels, R., Hofman, B., Melmed, R., Nishanian, P. and Giorgi, J. V. (1990). The prognostic value of cellular and serologic markers in infection with human immunodeficiency virus type 1. *N. Engl. J. Med.*, **322**, 166–72
207. Grey, H. M., Kubo, R. T., Colon, S. *et al.* (1973). The small subunit of HLA is β_2-microglobulin. *J. Exp. Med.*, **138**, 1608–12
208. Peterson, P. A., Rask, L. and Lindblom, J. B. (1974). Highly purified papain solubilised HLA antigens contain β_2-microglobulin. *Proc. Natl. Acad. Sci. USA*, **71**, 35–39
209. Cresswell, P., Springer, T., Stromiger, J. L., Turner, M. J., Grey, H. M. and Kubo, R. T. (1974). Immunological identity of the small subunit of the HLA-A antigens and β_2-microglobulin and its turnover on the cell membrane. *Proc. Natl. Acad. Sci. USA*, **71**, 2123–7
210. Lamelin, J-P., Vincent, C., Fontaine-Legrand, C. and Revillard, J-P. (1982). Elevation of serum β_2-microglobulin levels during infectious mononucleosis. *Clin. Immunol. Immunopathol.*, **24**, 55–62
211. Cooper, E. H., Forbes, M. A. and Hambling, M. H. (1984). Serum β_2-microglobulin and C-reactive protein concentrations in viral infections. *J. Clin. Pathol.*, **37**, 1140–3
212. Cooper, E. H., Forbes, M. A., Sutherland, S. and MacManus, T. J. (1989). Serum B2 M in intravenous drug abusers with HIV infection. V International Conference on AIDS, Montreal, June: Abstract WBP 81
213. Burkes, R. L., Sherrod, A. E., Stewart, M. L. *et al.* (1986). Serum β_2-microglobulin levels in homosexual men with AIDS and persistent generalised lymphadenopathy. *Cancer*, **57**, 2190–2
214. Lacey, C. J., Forbes, M. A., Waugh, M. A., Cooper, E. H. and Hambling, M. H. (1987). Serum β_2-microglobulin and human immunodeficiency virus infection. *AIDS*, **1**, 123–7
215. Sonnerborg, A. B., von Stedingk, L-V., Hansson, L-O. and Strannegard, O. O. (1989). Elevated neopterin and β_2-microglobulin levels in blood and cerebrospinal fluid occur early in HIV-1 infection. *AIDS*, **3**, 277–83
216. Jacobson, M. A., Adrams, D. I., Volberding, P. A. *et al.* (1989). Serum β_2-microglobulin decreases in patients with AIDS or ARC treated with azidothymidine. *J. Infect. Dis.*, **159**, 1029–36
217. Moss, A. R. (1988). Predicting who will progress to AIDS. *Br. Med. J.*, **297**, 1067–8
218. Grieco, M. H., Reddy, M. M., Fusillo, C. A., Sorrell, S. J., Buimovici-Klein, E., Gindi, E. J., Brown, D. K., Saxinger, W. C., Weiss, S. H. and Flaster, E. R. (1989). Cross-sectional study of immunologic abnormalities in intravenous drug abusers on methadone maintenance in New York City. *AIDS*, **3**, 235–7
219. Hofmann, B., Wang, Y., Cumberland, W. G., Detels, R., Bozorgmerhri, M. and Fahey, J. L. (1990). Serum β_2-microglobulin level increases in HIV infection: related to seroconversion, CD4 T-cell fall and prognosis. *AIDS*, **4**, 207–14
220 Anderson, R. E., Lang, W., Shiboski, S., Royce, R., Jewell, N. and Winkelstein, W. Jr (1990). Use of β_2-microglobulin level and CD3 lymphocyte count to predict development of acquired immune deficiency syndrome in persons with human immunodeficiency virus infection. *Arch. Intern. Med.*, **150**, 73–7
221. Huber, C. H., Batchelor, J. R., Fuchs, D. *et al.* (1984). Immune response associated production of neopterin release of macrophages primarily under the control of interferon-gamma. *J. Exp. Med.*, **160**, 310–16
222. Wachter, H., Fuchs, D., Hausen, A. *et al.* (1983). Elevated urinary neopterin levels in patients with the acquired immune deficiency syndrome. *Hoppe Seyler's Z. Physiol. Chem.*, **364**, 1345–6
223. Fuchs, D., Banekovich, M., Hausen, A. *et al.* (1988). Neopterin estimation compared with the ratio of T cell subpopulations in persons infected with the human immunodeficiency virus 1. *Clin. Chem.*, **24**, 2415–17
224. Fuchs, D., Hausen, A., Reibnegger, G. *et al.* (1988). Neopterin as a marker for activated cell-mediated immunity: application in HIV infection. *Immunol. Today*, **9**, 150–5
225. Bogner, J. R., Matuschke, A., Heinrich, B., Eberle, E. and Goebel, F. D. (1988). Serum neopterin levels as predictor of AIDS. *Klin. Wochenschr.*, **66**, 1015–18
226. Kramer, A., Wiktor, S. Z., Fuchs, D. *et al.* (1989). Neopterin, a predictive marker of AIDS in HIV infection. *J. AIDS*, **2**, 291–6
227. Melmed, R. N., Taylor, J. M., Detels, R. *et al.* (1989). Serum neopterin changes in

HIV-infected subjects: indicator of significant pathology, CD4 cell change, and the development of AIDS. *J. AIDS*, **2**, 70–6

228. Pui, C. H. (1989). Serum interleukin 2 receptor; clinical and biological implications. *Leukaemia*, **3**, 323–7
229. Pizzolo, G., Vinante, F., Sinicco, A., Chilosi, M., Agostini, C., Perini, A., Zuppini, B., Semenzato, G., Battistella, L. and Foa, R. (1987). Increased levels of soluble interleukin 2 receptor in the serum of patients with human immunodeficiency virus infection. *Diag. Clin. Immunol.*, **5**, 180–3
230. Lang, J. M., Levy, S., Coumaros, G., Lehr, L., Partisani, M., Dossou-Gbete, V., Steckmeyer, M. and Koehl, C. (1989). Follow-up, of soluble interleukin 2 receptor serum levels in non-progressing HIV infected people. *AIDS*, 673–4
231. Allen, J. B., McCartney-Francis, N., Smith, P. D., Simon, G., Gartner, S., Wahl, L. M., Popovic, M. and Wahl, S. M. (1990). Expression of interleukin 2 receptors by monocytes from patients with the acquired immunodeficiency syndrome and induction of monocyte interleukin 2 receptors by human immunodeficiency virus in vitro. *J. Clin. Invest.*, **85**, 192–9
232. Lang, J. M., Comaros, G., Falkenrodt, A., Steckmeyer, M., Partisani, M., Aleksijevic, A., Lehr, L. and Koehl, C. (1989). Elevated serum levels of soluble interleukin 2 receptors in HIV infection: correlation studies with markers of cell activation. *Immunol. Lett.*, **19**, 99–102
233. Schulte, C. and Meurer, M. (1989). Soluble IL2 receptor serum levels – a marker for disease progression in patients with HIV-1 infection. *Arch. Dermatol.*, **281**, 299–303
234. Honda, M., Kitamura, K., Matsuda, K., Yokota, Y., Yamamoto, N., Mitsuyasu, R., Chermann, J-C. and Tokunaga, T. (1989). Soluble IL-2 receptor in AIDS: correlation of its serum level with the classification of HIV-induced diseases and its characterization. *J. Immunol.*, **142**, 4248–55
235. Rothenberg, R., Woelfel, M., Stoneburner, R., Milberg, J., Parker and R., Truman, B. (1987). Survival with the acquired immunodeficiency syndrome. *N. Engl. J. Med.*, **317**, 1297–302
236. Verdegem, T. D., Sattler, F. R. and Boylen, C. T. (1988). Increased fatality from *Pneumocystis carinii* pneumonia (PCP) in women with AIDS. IV International Conference on AIDS, Stockholm, Sweden, 13–16 June: Abstract 7271
237. Kloser, P., Grigoriu, A. and Kapila, R. (1988). Women with AIDS: a continuing study 1987. IV International Conference on AIDS, Stockholm, Sweden, 13–16 June: Abstract 4065
238. Carpenter, C. C. J., Fisher, A., Desai, M., Durand, L., Indacochea, F. and Mayer, K. M. (1988). Clinical characteristics of AIDS in women in Southeastern New England. IV International Conference on AIDS, Stockholm, Sweden, 13–16 June: Abstract 7274
239. Young, M. A. and Pierce, P. (1990). Natural history of HIV disease in an urban cohort of women. VIth International Conference on AIDS, San Francisco: Abstract FB 432
240. Danila, R., Jones, D., Reier, D., Thomas, J., Osterholm, M. and MacDonald, K. (1990). A comparison of statewide Minnesota HIV/AIDS surveillance data with a population-based HIV seroprevalence study of childbearing women in Minnesota. VI International Conference on AIDS, San Francisco: Abstract FC 569
241. Willocks, L., Cowan, F. M., Brettle, R. P., MacCallum, L. R., McHardy, S. and Richardson, A. (1991). Early HIV infection in Scottish women. VII International Conference on AIDS, Florence, Italy: Abstract MB 2433
242. Schafer, A., Friedmann, W., Mielke, M., Schwartlander, B. and Koch, M. A. (1990). Increased frequency of cervical dysplasia/neoplasia in HIV infected women is related to the extent of immunosuppression. VI International Conference on AIDS, San Francisco: Abstract SB 519
243. Vermund, S. H., Kelley, K. F., Burk, R. D., Feingold, A. R., Schreiber, K., Munk, G., Schrager, L. K. and Klein, R. S. (1990). Risk of human papillomavirus (HPV) and cervical squamous intraepithelial lesions (SIL) highest among women with advanced HIV disease. VI International Conference on AIDS, San Francisco: Abstract SB 517
244. Batalla, J., Gatell, J., Cayla, J. A., Plasencia, A., Jansa, J. M. and Parellada, N. (1989). Predictors of the survival of AIDS in Barcelona, Spain. *AIDS*, **3**, 355–9
245. Lemp, G. F., Payne, S. F., Neal, D., Temelso, T. and Rutherford, G. W. (1990). Survival trends for patients with AIDS. *J. Am. Med. Assoc.*, **262**, 402
246. Harris, J. E. (1990). Improved short-term survival of AIDS patients initially diagnosed with *Pneumocystis carinii* pneumonia, 1984 through 1987. *J. Am. Med. Assoc.*, **263**, 397–401
247. Selik, R. M., Starcher, E. T. and Curran, J. W. (1987). Opportunistic diseases reported in AIDS patients; frequencies, associations and trends. *AIDS*, **1**, 175–82

248. Rutherford, G. W., Schwarcz, S. K., Lemp, G. F. *et al.* (1989). The epidemiology of AIDS-related Kaposi's sarcoma in San Francisco. *J. Infect. Dis.*, **159**, 567–71
249. Fischl, M. A., Richman, D. D., Grieco, M. H. *et al.* (1987). The efficacy of zidovudine (AZT) in the treatment of patients with AIDS and AIDS-related complex. *N. Engl. J. Med.*, **317**, 185–91
250. Fischl, M. A., Richman, D. D., Causey, D. M. *et al.* (1989). Prolonged zidovudine therapy in patients with AIDS and advanced AIDS related complex. *J. Am. Med. Assoc.*, **262**, 2405–10
251. Creagh-Kirk, T., Doi, P., Andrews, E. *et al.* (1988). Survival experience among patients with AIDS receiving zidovudine. *J. Am. Med. Assoc.*, **260**, 3009–15
252. Yarchoan, R., Berg, G., Brouwers, P. *et al.* (1987). Response of human-immunodeficiency virus associated neurological disease to 3-azido-3 deoxythymidine. *Lancet*, **1**, 132–5
253. Pizzo, P. A., Eddy, J., Falloon, J. *et al.* (1989). Effect of continuous intravenous zidovudine (AZT) in children with symptomatic HIV infection. *N. Engl. J. Med.*, **319**, 889–96
254. Schmitt, F. A., Bigley, J. W., McKinnis, R. *et al.* (1988). Neuropsychological outcome of zidovudine (AZT) treatment of patients with AIDS and AIDS related complex. *N. Engl. J. Med.*, **319**, 1573–8
255. Stambuk, D., Youle, M., Hawkins, D. *et al.* (1989). The efficacy of azidothymidine (AZT) in the treatment of patients with AIDS and AIDS related complex (ARC): an open uncontrolled treatment study. *Q.J. Med.*, **262**, 161–74
256. Montgomery, A. B., Leong, G. S., Wardlaw, L. A. *et al.* (1989). Effect of zidovudine on mortality rates and Pneumocystis cariniii pneumonia (PCP) incidence in AIDS and ARC patients on aerosolised pentamidine. *Am. Rev. Resp. Dis.*, **138**, A250 (abstract)
257. Peters, B. S., Beck, E. J., Coleman, D. G., Wadsworth, M. J. H., McGuinness, O., Harris, J. R. W. and Pinching, A. J. (1991). Changing disease patterns in patients with AIDS in a referral centre in the United Kingdom: the changing face of AIDS. *Br. Med. J.*, **302**, 203–7
258. Jacobson, M. A., Bachetti, P., Kolokathis, A. *et al.* (1991). Surrogate markers for survival in patients with AIDS and AIDS related complex treated with zidovudine. *Br. Med. J.*, **302**, 73–8
259. Peters, B. S., Matthews, J., Gompels, M., Hartley, R. C. and Pinching, A. J. (1990). Acute myeloblastic leukaemia in AIDS. *AIDS*, **4**, 367–8
260. Pluda, J. M., Yarchoan, R., Jaffe, E. S. *et al.* (1990). Development of non-Hodgkin lymphoma in a cohort of patients with severe human immunodeficiency virus (HIV) infection on long term antiretroviral therapy. *Ann. Intern. Med.*, **113**, 276–82
261. Ayers, K. M. (1988). Preclinical toxicity of zidovudine: an overview. *Am. J. Med.*, **85**, 186–8
262. Burroughs Wellcome Co. (1989). Lifetime bioassay studies. In *Comprehensive Information for Investigators*, RETROVIR (Research Triangle Park, NC: Burroughs Wellcome), p. 48
263. The Surveillance Program, Division of Cancer Prevention and Control. National Cancer Institute (1990). Table II-I. Summary of 15 year trends: age adjusted cancer incidence rates. In: Ries, L. A., Barrett, M. J. and Labbe, R. R. (eds), *Cancer Statistics Review* 1973–1987, (Bethesda, MD: National Cancer Institute), pp. 11–14
264. Larder, B. A., Darby, G. and Richmann, D. D. (1989). HIV with reduced sensitivity to zidovudine (AZT) isolated during prolonged therapy. *Science*, **243**, 1731–34
265. Boucher, C. A. B., Tersmette, M., Lange, J. M. A. *et al.* (1990). Zidovudine sensitivity of Human Immunodeficiency Viruses from high-risk, symptom-free individuals during therapy. *Lancet*, **336**, 585–90
266. Fischl, M. A., Richmann, D. D., Hansen, N. *et al.* (1990). The safety and efficacy of zidovudine (AZT) in the treatment of patients with mildly symptomatic human immunodeficiency virus type 1 (HIV) infection: a double-blind placebo controlled trial. *Ann. Intern. Med.*, **112**, 727–37
267. Volberding, P. A., Lagakos, S. W., Koch, M. A. *et al.* (1990). Zidovudine in asymptomatic human immunodeficiency virus infection. A controlled trial in persons with fewer than 500 CD4 positive cells per cubic millimetre. *N. Engl. J. Med.*, **322**, 941–9
268. Collier, A. C., Bozzette, S., Coombs, R. W. *et al.* (1990). A pilot study of low dose zidovudine in human immunodeficiency virus infection. *N. Engl. J. Med.*, **323**, 1015–21

2
The role of HIV variability in the pathogenesis of AIDS

M. TERSMETTE

INTRODUCTION

The human immunodeficiency virus (HIV) is the causative agent of the acquired immunodeficiency syndrome (AIDS). AIDS is the terminal phase of a prolonged infectious process, clinically characterized by a symptom-free period which may last for years. Recent investigations have demonstrated that during this phase the virus is not latent, as thought previously, but is chronically produced at a low, barely detectable level. In this chapter it will be described how the ability of HIV to assume different characteristics enables the virus to adapt itself to survive in the host, thus causing a persistent infection, and how HIV may finally induce the pathognomonic $CD4^+$ T-cell depletion resulting in the progression to AIDS.

BIOLOGY OF HIV

Taxonomy

The human immunodeficiency virus (HIV) is a member of the group of lentiviruses, one of the three subfamilies of the family of retroviruses, a group of single-stranded RNA viruses. The other two subfamilies are the group of neoplasma-inducing oncoviruses, to which belong the human T-cell leukaemia/lymphoma viruses I and II (HTLV I and II), and the group of spumaviruses which to date have not been associated with clinical disease. Other lentiviruses include the visna virus in sheep, equine infectious anaemia virus (EIAV), feline immunodeficiency virus (FIV), and simian immunodeficiency virus (SIV). Like HIV, these viruses cause chronic disease processes, which may eventually result in the death of the host. Two subtypes of HIV are known, HIV-1[1] and HIV-2[2]. The former is the major cause of the worldwide

AIDS epidemic. The latter virus is mainly found in West African countries and may also cause AIDS, although it is not certain whether it is equally pathogenic[3,4]. The studies discussed in this chapter are mainly concerned with HIV-1, but most of the conclusions probably also pertain to HIV-2.

Replication cycle

The replication cycle of HIV is shown in Figure 2.1. HIV enters the host cell via binding of its envelope glycoprotein gp120 to CD4, a membrane marker present on T-helper cells, but also on other cell types, e.g. monocytes. Following binding virus penetration occurs, probably mediated by yet unidentified accessory molecule(s) not present on all CD4 expressing cells (see below), and the viral nucleoprotein complex is released in the cytoplasm. Like all retroviruses HIV has the capacity to reverse transcribe its genomic RNA into double-stranded DNA by means of the viral enzyme reverse transcriptase. The proviral DNA subsequently may integrate in the host genome.

Unlike oncoviruses, which may immortalize the cell they have infected, lentiviruses do not transform their host cell but cause a persistent infection which may be silent or productive, depending on the combined effects of cellular and viral transcription factors on the long terminal repeat (LTR) of the virus, a non-coding viral sequence regulating viral expression. Viral offspring are produced by transcription of various mRNAs coding for early regulatory and late structural viral proteins, as well as transcription of genomic RNA. Free infectious virions are formed as the assembled viral capsid buds from the cell membrane, enveloping itself in a patch of viral glycoprotein-loaded cell membrane in the process. Depending upon the host cell type HIV expression may result in lysis of the cell (see below).

HIV VARIABILITY

HIV variability is the result of genomic mutations which may occur during the viral replication cycle. Unlike oncovirus infection, where disease results from the outgrowth of a limited number of cells immortalized by the virus, in lentivirus infection disease is caused by destruction of cells, a process demanding a much higher number of virus replication cycles. Most mutations are caused during reverse transcription of the viral genome because of the relatively high error frequency of the reverse transcriptase[5]. Two types of virus variability, antigenic variation and variation of biological phenotype, have been described for the group of lentiviruses. Present evidence indicates that both types may be pathogenically involved, and may in part share mechanisms at the molecular level.

Antigenic variation

The phenomenon of antigenic variation is well known in animal lentivirus infections, such as visna and equine infectious anaemia[6,7]. Sequential virus isolates from the same animal are differentially neutralized by the animal's sequential serum samples, suggesting antigenic drift caused by selective

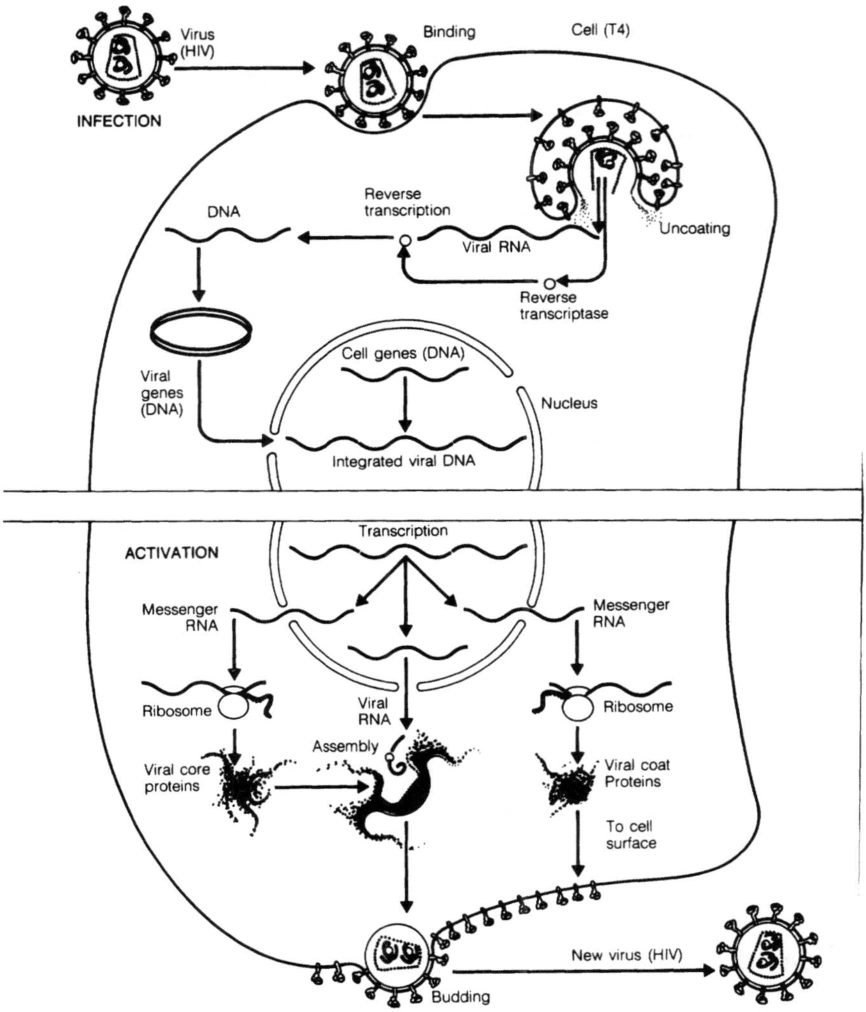

Figure 2.1 Replication cycle of HIV

pressure exerted by the immune system[7,8]. A number of neutralization epitopes on the HIV envelope have been described[9–11]. In the HIV envelope a major variable neutralization epitope has been identified within the third variable domain (V3 loop), which elicits a type-specific immune response[10,12–14]. *In vitro* neutralization with anti-V3 antibodies abolished infectivity of HIV in chimpanzees, indicating that antibodies to the V3 epitope may be protective *in vivo*[15]. Emergence of HIV variants resistant to neutralization by V3-specific antibodies that neutralized the inoculum virus, could be demonstrated in chimpanzees in 6–16 weeks after infection[16]. Also, differential neutralizing ability of sera of HIV-infected individuals against sequential HIV variants has been observed[17]. These results indicate that antigenic variation may be used by HIV to escape neutralization. Mutations resulting in neutralization-resistant variants did not necessarily have to occur within the V3 loop, indicating that the epitope is influenced by the overall conformation of gp120[16,18]. Similar findings have been reported for the foot-and-mouth disease virus[19]. Along with neutralization epitopes, T cell epitopes have been identified on HIV structural proteins, and variation in the peptide sequences critical for recognition by cytotoxic T cells (CTL) may allow HIV-infected cells to avoid lysis by these T cells. Indeed, peptide sequences corresponding to the V3 loop may be recognized by murine CTL[20].

Biological variation

Along with antigenic variation between HIV isolates, differences in biological properties such as replication rate, syncytium-inducing (SI) ability and cytotropism have been observed[21–23]. Similar biological variation exists between isolates from other lentiviruses[24] and feline leukaemia virus (FeLV)[25].

For the study of HIV biological variability we isolated HIV by cocultivation of patient peripheral blood mononuclear cells (PBMC) with phytohaemagglutinin (PHA)-stimulated PBMC (PBL) from healthy individuals. Virus replication in these cultures was detected with an enzyme immunoassay (EIA) for p24, the major HIV core protein. In this way virus could be recovered with over 90% efficiency. According to the first day of detection of virus replication in these cultures, the isolate could be classified as rapid or slow. Part of the high-replicating isolates induced cell fusion in PBL culture, resulting in the formation of typical multinucleated giant cells (syncytia). It appeared that only these syncytium-inducing (SI) isolates were able to replicate in the H9 cell line, a $CD4^+$ T cell line. This type of isolate was observed more often in PBMC from patients with AIDS-related complex (ARC) or AIDS than in asymptomatic individuals[22].

RELATION BETWEEN HIV BIOLOGICAL VARIABILITY AND CLINICAL COURSE

HIV biological phenotype and progression to AIDS

To investigate the prevalence of HIV phenotypes in a patient over time, longitudinal studies were performed among 34 participants in the Amsterdam cohort study over a 33-month period[26,27]. In general, properties of sequential isolates from the same individual were relatively stable with respect to replication rate. In 29 individuals only non-syncytium-inducing (NSI) isolates were observed, of these 22 had a low, and seven had a high replication rate. In five individuals SI isolates were detected. Among these three groups, mean levels of $CD4^+$ T cells differed significantly at the start of the study. Also the rate of $CD4^+$ T-cell decline was inversely related to the replication rate of the isolates of an individual[26]. The presence of SI isolates or high-replicating NSI isolates was associated with progression to AIDS (median lag times from first detection of the typical isolate to AIDS 15 and 22 months respectively). In contrast, persons with low-replicating isolates mostly remained asymptomatic (estimated lag time to AIDS >42 months). Also, survival of AIDS patients with SI isolates was reduced compared to the patients with NSI isolates[27]. Subsequent studies over longer time periods revealed that within an individual increases in viral virulence may occur over time. In particular, in persons followed from seroconversion generally SI isolates could not be detected initially, but emerged only during the course of infection[28].

HIV phenotype early in infection

In view of the considerable frequency of SI variant carriers in the population of asymptomatic seropositive individuals (see below) and the relatively high viral load of these individuals (own unpublished observations) a significant portion of newly infected individuals will be infected by SI variants. More detailed virological analysis, applying an adapted culture method in microtitre plates to obtain multiple HIV clones from a single PBMC sample[28], revealed that uncloned HIV isolates may comprise clones with heterogeneous biological phenotypes. The SI phenotype was found to be dominant *in vitro*, probably due to its high replication rate. Thus, whereas NSI isolates contain only NSI clones, SI isolates are made up of a mixture of clones with both NSI and SI phenotypes. Therefore individuals infected by an SI variant carrier will probably become infected with both types of clones.

In virus isolation studies in recently infected individuals, however, we detected only NSI isolates in the majority of persons. This seems to imply that newly infected, still immunocompetent individuals are able to selectively clear SI clones, mostly even before they can become detectable by virus isolation techniques. Confirmative evidence for this hypothesis comes from two mother–child transmission cases, in which SI-type viruses were detected in the mother[29,30]. An SI isolate was detected in one of the children at birth, but after 1 year only NSI isolates could be detected in these children. In three individuals with an exceptional clinical course ($CD4^+$ T cell decline to levels below $0.15–0.35 \times 10^9$ within 1 year after infection, one of them progressing to AIDS in 25 weeks), SI isolates were observed from the start of infection. Although temporary suppression of the SI phenotype was observed in one of the individuals, and a transient reduction in numbers of infected cells in another, apparently clearance of SI clones was inefficient in these individuals.

The inoculum with which these persons were infected probably was not exceptionally large. At the moment it is unclear whether this precipitous clinical course is caused by pre-existent host immune deficiency, concomitant exogeneous influences, or virulence of the particular HIV strain. Recently, two infectious molecular SIV clones were described able to cause AIDS-like disease in monkey species[31,32]. One of these clones, SIV_{SMM} – PBJ14, is cytopathic and tropic for human T cell lines[31]. The clinical course of monkeys infected with SIV_{SMM} – PBJ14 resembles the rapid progression to disease observed in three individuals described above, and further argues for a causative role of SI isolates in $CD4^+$ T cell depletion.

HIV monocytotropism

It has been suggested that in addition to the CD4$^+$ T cell, monocyte/macrophages may play an important role as host cells for HIV *in vivo*, in particular in the early phase of HIV infection[33,34] (see Chapter 3). In contrast to CD4$^+$ T cells, which are susceptible to lysis following HIV infection[35], monocytes may persistently produce HIV without being killed[33]. To investigate the relationship between monocytotropism of HIV isolates and the biological phenotypes described above, we tested a panel of SI and NSI isolates, established by PBL coculture, for their ability to infect monocytes[36]. Most of the NSI isolates were able to infect monocytes, compared to only a minority of the SI isolates. Moreover, NSI isolates infected a broader range of monocytes from different donors. Similar differences were observed with biological HIV clones. In longitudinal studies virus could be recovered from patient PBMC by coculture with monocytes in all phases of infection. The isolates, upon passage to PBL culture, were all NSI, even when they were obtained from a patient sample that yielded SI isolates in direct coculture with PBL[36]. These results indicate that monocytotropic isolates reside within the NSI population. Accumulation of HIV particles within intracellular vacuoles has been described for monocytes. This difference in monocytotropism between NSI and SI variants may be one of the reasons why following infection and the rise of an anti-HIV immune response SI clones are lost, whereas NSI clones persist.

Factors involved in the emergence of SI variants

Although we have shown that within an individual all kinds of HIV biological variants may evolve over time, SI isolates are observed in only half of the persons developing AIDS. At present it is unclear why this is the case. Possibly within the HIV population virulent strains with the intrinsic capacity to generate SI variants can be distinguished (strain here to be defined as 'a population of variants found within a cluster of patients with at least one stable common property'). Individuals infected with such strains would be at higher risk for progression to AIDS. Virulent SIV clones, as described above, could serve as representatives for such virulent strains. In epidemiological studies it has indeed been shown that infection by a person progressing to AIDS is associated with a higher risk for AIDS in the recipient[37,38]. Alternatively host factors may (co-)determine whether SI variants will develop in a given individual. The demonstration of an association between the HLA haplotype A1B8DR3 and rapid progression to AIDS[39,40] is compatible with this hypothesis.

Molecular analysis of HIV biological phenotype

The association between HIV biological variants and the clinical course of HIV infection has prompted a number of groups to generate infectious molecular HIV clones with distinct biological phenotypes to study in more detail which molecular determinants are responsible for the observed differences in biological phenotype[41–43]. In our own approach we took two points into consideration. First, we thought it necessary to obtain clones derived from the patient as directly as possible, avoiding prolonged culture and adaptation to cell lines. Second, in view of the considerable genetic variation of HIV, most of which probably is irrelevant for biological properties, the clones should be derived from a single patient, obtained at closely spaced time-points. Therefore we selected a frequently sampled individual with an NSI/SI conversion and obtained biological clones with distinct phenotypes from his sequential PBMC. Following minimal culture in PBL these biological clones were used as starting material for the molecular cloning. In this way eight infectious molecular clones were obtained. Four of these with distinct properties were selected for further analysis. Restriction mapping revealed a >96% homology among these clones[43]. Sequencing of the 3′ part of the viral genome, containing *env*, and the small regulatory and accessory genes, revealed that the latter were virtually 100% homologous in the domains known to be critical for their function, limiting the possibility that these genes were involved in the biological differences among the clones. On the other hand a sequence variation ranging from 0.2% to 8.0% was observed in the *env* gene. In biological assays we obtained evidence that cell tropism was restricted at the level of entry. In preliminary exchange experiments biological phenotype segregated with the *env* gene. Therefore the *env* gene seems to be the primary determinant for biological phenotype in these clones. Similar conclusions were drawn by other investigators. In particular a domain of gp120 located between the V3 loop and the CD4 binding site was shown to be involved by exchange studies[42]. So far there is little evidence for a major role of the HIV LTR in the determination of biological phenotype[44,45]. However, the acutely pathogenic SIV clone SIV_{SMM} – PBJ14 is characterized by the presence of an extra binding site in the LTR for NF kappa B, an inducible transcription enhancer[31]. At the moment it is not clear to what extent this extra binding site is critical for the pathogenic properties of this clone.

PATHOGENESIS OF HIV INFECTION

HIV infection, like other lentiviral infections, is characterized by its protracted clinical course. This has been thought to be the direct reflection of regulatory mechanisms that govern HIV expression, and determine latency or active replication at the cellular level. More recent evidence, however, indicates that the long-lasting asymptomatic phase is the result of a chronic interaction between HIV and the immune system, and not the consequence of true viral latency. First, HIV variation, genetic[46], antigenic[17] as well as biological[23,26,28], has been demonstrated during the asymptomatic phase. Second, the ability to culture HIV from plasma at all time-points of infection[47,48] provides direct proof that HIV replication occurs throughout infection. Extensive evidence, discussed in Chapter 5 of this volume, was obtained that immunological defects in HIV infection are not restricted to the pathognomonic $CD4^+$ T cell depletion. Instead, even early in infection qualitative defects are present in the B cell, T cell and monocyte compartments[49,50]. Of particular interest eis the early selective loss of antigen-primed T-memory cells, described by several groups[51–54].

A model for AIDS pathogenesis

Integration of virological and immunological data results in the following model of AIDS pathogenesis. Infection of an individual is achieved by a mixture of related HIV clones, possibly representing a more or less virulent HIV strain. In early rounds of replication in the initially unprotected host, further HIV variants may be generated. Following the development of an anti-HIV immune response, in the majority of individuals high-virulent clones are suppressed, either due to their high expression[55], or their lack of monocytotropism[36], and NSI/monocytotropic clones remain. These variants, because of their biological properties, are able to escape the immune system and maintain a low level of HIV replication, incessantly generating new antigenic variants which contribute to the persistence of HIV infection in the asymptomatic phase. In a manner still incompletely understood these HIV variants induce the early qualitative immune defects described in Chapter 5. Evidence from the SIV model indicates that SIV preferentially infects activated naive and memory $CD4^+$ T cells[56], which may in part explain the observed selective loss of memory T cells in early HIV infection. Similar results have been obtained for HIV[57]. Functional impairments of B cell and monocyte populations are best explained by indirect systemic effects of HIV infection, possibly caused by the early loss of critical $CD4^+$ T cell subpopulations. These qualitative immune defects, gradually increasing over time, will lead to an increasingly less efficient anti-HIV immune response. Also due to the continuous antigenic variation, eventually variants may be generated, against which in the specific host no efficient immune response can be mounted. The decreased capacity of the immune system to clear HIV is reflected by an increasing virus load with ongoing infection[47,48].

The gradual collapse of the immune system finally allows for overt replication of more virulent HIV variants. Severe $CD4^+$ T cell depletion may be achieved by several direct mechanisms including more rapid lysis of infected $CD4^+$ T cells, infection and lysis of precursor T cells and depletion of $CD4^+$ T cells by syncytium formation. Also indirect immunological mechanisms may be involved. For instance increased production of viral gp120 could lead to significant destruction of uninfected $CD4^+$ T cells, coated with gp120[58], or presenting processed gp120 fragments on their cell membrane[59]. Once virulent HIV variants can be detected, one or more of these mechanisms will result in $CD4^+$ T cell depletion and development of AIDS in $1\frac{1}{2}$–2 years.

CLINICAL IMPLICATIONS

The virological studies reviewed here indicate a role for slow NSI/monocytotropic HIV variants in the persistence of HIV infection, and for SI and rapid NSI variants in $CD4^+$ T cell depletion. These insights may have several implications for early diagnosis and treatment, as well as prevention, of HIV infection.

Early diagnosis

Since SI isolates are detectable well before AIDS diagnosis, at still low–normal $CD4^+$ T cell numbers, we investigated the possibility of using HIV biological phenotyping as a prognostic marker for progression to AIDS. Compared to coculture with PBL, rescue of HIV from patient PBMC by direct coculture with permanent T cell lines is less laborious but also less efficient. Comparative studies with a panel of T cell lines revealed that the MT2 cell line was most suitable for virus isolation. Rescue by direct coculture with MT2 was successful only in persons with SI isolates, in accordance with the previously observed correlation between SI ability and H9 cell line tropism. Using the MT2 coculture method we screened 213 individuals from the Amsterdam cohort study for the prevalence of the SI phenotype. MT2-tropic viruses were present in 31 (15%) asymptomatic seropositive individuals in 1988. Of these individuals 61% progressed to AIDS within 2 years, compared to 9% of the remaining individuals. In the subsequent 2 years a switch from NSI to SI phenotype occurred in 24 individuals, implying a conversion rate of 7% per year (Koot *et al.*, in preparation). This again demonstrates that as a rule SI isolates emerge in the course of HIV infection, heralding the progression to AIDS. This assay thus seems very promising for the early identification of about half of the individuals at risk for short-term progression to AIDS, and may be useful as a screening assay for seropositive individuals with low–normal $CD4^+$ T cell counts.

Treatment and prevention

In early intervention trials prevention of a switch to SI variants could be used as a measure of efficacy of treatment. In individuals with SI variants, zidovudine at best seems to delay progression to AIDS[27]. Moreover, treatment with zidovudine of asymptomatic individuals with NSI variants did not totally prevent a switch to SI variants. Remarkably, SI variants were found in over 80% of individuals who developed AIDS despite zidovudine treatment[27,60] (Koot *et al.*, in preparation). The relationship between the emergence of SI variants and the development of zidovudine resistance remains to be investigated.

In the model proposed above, the breakdown of the immune system by HIV is an active process from seroconversion onwards. This implies that early treatment is desirable, at least before irreversible damage has occurred. In cases of long-standing HIV infection, specific immune therapy, e.g. specific anti-HIV immunoglobulin, might assist the failing immune system to prevent or postpone the emergence of SI variants.

Finally, the probability that NSI/monocytotropic variants play an important role in the persistence of HIV infection implies that more detailed study of the antigenicity of these variants is required, and that candidate vaccines must also induce protective immunity to these HIV variants.

Acknowledgements

The studies described in this paper were funded in part by grant 28-1079 from The Netherlands Foundation for Preventive Medicine, grant 88005 from the Dutch Ministry of Public Health and grant 900-502-104 from the Netherlands Organization for Scientific Research.

References

1. Barre-Sinoussi, F., Chermann, J. C., Rey, R., Nugeyre, M. T., Chamaret, S., Gruest, J., Dauget, C., Rozenbaum, W. and Montagnier, L. (1983). Isolation of a T-lymphotropic retrovirus from a patient at risk for acquired immune deficiency syndrome. *Science*, **220**, 868–71
2. Clavel, F., Guetard, D., Brun-Vezinet, F., Chamaret, S., Rey, M. A., Santos-Ferreira, M. O., Laurent, A., Dauget, C., Katlama, C., Rouzioux, C., Klatzmann, D., Champalimaud, J. L. and Montagnier, L. (1986). Isolation of a new retrovirus from West African patients with AIDS. *Science*, **233**, 343–6
3. Clavel, F., Manshino, K., Chamaret, S., Favier, V., Nina, J., Santos-Ferreira, M. O., Champalimaud, J. L. and Montagnier, L. (1987). Human immunodeficiency virus type 2 infection associated with AIDS in West Africa. *N. Engl. J. Med.*, **316**, 1180–85
4. Schulz, T. F., Whitby, D., Hoad, J. G., Corrah, T., Whittle, H. and Weiss, R. A. (1990). Biological and molecular variability of human immunodeficiency virus type 2 isolates from The Gambia. *J. Virol.*, **64**, 5177–82
5. Roberts, J. D., Bebenek, K. and Kunkel, T. A. (1988). The accuracy of reverse transcriptase from HIV-1. *Science*, **242**, 1171–3
6. Clements, J. E., Pedersen, F. S., Narayan, O. and Haseltine, W. A. (1980). Genomic changes associated with antigenic variation of visna virus during persistent infection. *Proc. Natl. Acad. Sci. USA*, **77**, 4454–8
7. Clements, J. E., Gdovin, S. L., Montelaro, R. C. and Narayan, O. (1988). Antigenic variation in lentiviral diseases. *Ann. Rev. Immunol.*, **6**, 139–59
8. McGuire, T. C., Norton, L. K., O'Rourke, K. I. and Cheevers, W. P. (1988). Antigenic variation of neutralization-sensitive epitopes of caprine arthritis–encephalitis lentivirus during persistent arthritis. *J. Virol.*, **62**, 3488–92
9. Ho, D. D., Kaplan, J. C., Rackauskas, I. E. and Gurney, M. E. (1988). Second conserved domain of gp120 is important for HIV infectivity and antibody neutralisation. *Science*, **239**, 1021–3
10. Palker, T. J., Clark, M. E., Langlois, A. J., Matthews, T. J., Weinhold, K. J., Randall, R. R., Bolognesi, D. P. and Haynes, B. F. (1988). Type-specific neutralisation of the human immunodeficiency virus with antibodies to env-encoded synthetic peptides. *Proc. Natl. Acad. Sci. USA*, **85**, 1932–6
11. Ho, D. D., Sarngadharan, M. G., Hirsch, M. S., Schooley, R. T., Rota, T. R., Kennedy, R. C., Chanh, T. C. and Sato, V. L. (1987). Human immunodeficiency virus neutralizing antibodies recognize several conserved domains on the envelope glycoproteins. *J. Virol.*, **61**, 2024–8
12. Looney, D. J., Fischer, A., Putney, S. D., Rusche, J. R., Redfield, R. R., Burke, D. S., Gallo, R. C. and Wong-Staal, F. (1988). Type-restricted neutralization of molecular clones of human immunodeficiency virus. *Science*, **241**, 357–9
13. Goudsmit, J., Debouck, C., Meloen, R. H., Smit, L., Bakker, M., Asher, D. M., Wolff, A. X., Gibbs, C. J. and Gajdusek, D. C. (1988). Human immunodeficiency virus type 1 neutralization epitope with conserved architecture elicits early type-specific antibodies in experimentally infected chimpanzees. *Proc. Natl. Acad. Sci. USA*, **85**, 4478–82
14. LaRosa, G. J., Davide, J. P., Weinhold, K., Waterbury, J. A., Profy, A. T., Lewis, J. A., Langlois, A. J., Dreesman, G. R., Boswell, R. N., Shadduck, P., Holley, L. H., Karplus, M., Bolognesi, D. P., Matthews, T. J., Emini, E. A. and Putney, S. D. (1990). Conserved sequence and structural elements in the HIV-1 principal neutralizing determinant. *Science*, **249**, 932–5
15. Emini, E. A., Nara, P. L., Schleif, W. A., Lewis, J. A., Davide, J. P., Lee, D. R., Kessler, J., Conley, S., Matsushita, S., Putney, S. D., Gerety, R. J. and Eichberg, J. W. (1990). Antibody-mediated *in vitro* neutralization of human immunodeficiency virus type 1 abolishes infectivity for chimpanzees. *J. Virol.*, **64**, 3674–8
16. Nara, P. L., Smit, L., Dunlop, N., Hatch, W., Merges, M., Waters, D., Kelliher, J., Gallo, R. C., Fischinger, P. J. and Goudsmit, J. (1990). Emergence of virus resistant to neutralization

by V3-specific antibodies in experimental human immunodeficiency virus type 1 IIIB infection of chimpanzees. *J. Virol.*, **64**, 3779–91
17. Albert, J., Abrahamsson, B., Nagy, K., Aurelius, E., Gaines, H., Nystrom, G. and Fenyö, E. M. (1990). Rapid development of isolate-specific neutralizing antibodies after primary HIV-1 infection and consequent emergence of virus variants which resist neutralization by autologous sera. *AIDS*, **4**, 107–12
18. Willey, R. L., Ross, E. K., Buckler-White, A. J., Theodore, T. S. and Martin, M. A. (1989). Functional interaction of constant and variable domains of human immunodeficiency virus type 1 gp120. *J. Virol.*, **63**, 3595–600
19. Parry, N., Fox, G., Rowlands, D., Brown, F., Fry, E., Acharya, R., Logan, D. and Stuart, D. (1990). Structural and serological evidence for a novel mechanism of antigenic variation in foot-and-mouth disease virus. *Nature*, **347**, 569–72
20. Takahashi, H. J., Cohen, A., Hosmalin, A., Cease, K. B., Houghten, R., Cornette, J. L., DeLisi, C., Moss, B., Germain, R. N. and Berzofsky, J. A. (1988). An immunodominant epitope of the human immunodeficiency virus envelope glycoprotein gp160 recognized by class I major histocompatibility complex molecule-restricted murine cytotoxic T lymphocytes. *Proc. Natl. Acad. Sci. USA*, **85**, 3105–9
21. Asjo, B., Albert, J., Karlsson, A., Morfeld-Manson, L., Biberfeld, G., Lidman, K. and Fenyo, E. M. (1986). Replicative properties of human immunodeficiency virus from patients with varying severity of HIV infection. *Lancet*, **2**, 660–2
22. Tersmette, M., De Goede, R. E. Y., Al, B. J. M., Winkel, I. N., Gruters, R. A., Cuypers, H. T. M., Huisman, H. G. and Miedema, F. (1988). Differential syncytium-inducing capacity of human immunodeficiency virus isolates: frequent detection of syncytium-inducing isolates in patients with acquired immunodeficiency syndrome (AIDS) and AIDS-related complex. *J. Virol.*, **62**, 2026–32
23. Cheng-Mayer, C., Seto, D., Tateno, M. and Levy, J. A. (1988). Biologic features of HIV-1 that correlate with virulence in the host. *Science*, **240**, 80–2
24. Querat, G., Barban, V., Sauze, N., Filippi, P., Vigne, R., Russo, P. and Vitu, C. (1984). High lytic and persistent lentiviruses naturally present in sheep with progressive pneumonia are genetically distinct. *J. Virol.*, **52**, 672–9
25. Mullins, J. I., Chen, C. and Hoover, E. A. (1986). Disease-specific and tissue-specific production of unintegrated feline leukaemia virus variant DNA in feline AIDS. *Nature*, **319**, 333–6
26. Tersmette, M., Gruters, R. A., De Wolf, F., De Goede, R. E. Y., Lange, J. M. A., Schellekens, P. T. A., Goudsmit, J., Huisman, J. G. and Miedema, F. (1989). Evidence for a role of virulent HIV variants in the pathogenesis of AIDS obtained from studies on a panel of sequential HIV isolates. *J. Virol.*, **63**, 2118–25
27. Tersmette, M., Lange, J. M. A., De Goede, R. E. Y., De Wolf, F., Eeftink Schattenkerk, J. K. M., Schellekens, P. T. A., Coutinho, R. A., Huisman, J. G., Goudsmit, J. and Miedema, F. (1989). Differences in risk for AIDS and AIDS mortality associated with biological properties of HIV variants. *Lancet*, **1**, 983–5
28. Tersmette, M. and Miedema, F. (1990). Interactions between HIV and the host immune system in the pathogenesis of AIDS. *AIDS* **Suppl. 1**, 557–66
29. Baur, A., Schwarz, N., Ellinger, S., Korn, K., Harrer, T., Mang, K. and Jahn, G. (1989). Continuous clearance of HIV in a vertically infected child. *Lancet*, **2**, 1045
30. Rubsamen-Waigmann, H., Willems, W. R., Bertram, U. and Von Briessen, H. (1989). Reversal of HIV-phenotype to fulminant replication on macrophages in perinatal transmission. *Lancet*, **1**, 1155–56
31. Dewhurst, S., Embretson, J. E., Anderson, D. C., Mullins, J. I. and Fultz, P. N. (1990). Sequence analysis and acute pathogenicity of molecularly cloned $SIV_{SMM-PBj14}$. *Nature*, **345**, 636–40
32. Kestler, H., Kodama, T., Ringler, D., Marthas, M., Pedersen, N., Lackner, A., Regier, D., Sehgal, P., Daniel, M., King, N. and Desrosiers, R. (1990). Induction of AIDS in rhesus monkeys by molecularly cloned simian immunodeficiency virus. *Science*, **248**, 1109–12
33. Gartner, S., Markovits, P., Markovits, D. M., Kaplan, M. H., Gallo, R. C. and Popovic, M. (1986). The role of mononuclear phagocytes in HTLV-III/LAV infection. *Science*, **233**, 215–19
34. Popovic, M. and Gartner, S. (1987). Isolation of HIV-1 from monocytes but not T lymphocytes. *Lancet*, **2**, 916

35. Zagury, D., Bernard, J., Leonard, R., Cheynier, R., Feldman, M., Sarin, P. S. and Gallo, R. C. (1986). Long-term cultures of HTLV-III-infected T cells: a model of cytopathology of T-cell depletion in AIDS. *Science*, **231**, 850–3
36. Schuitemaker, H., Kootstra, N. A., De Goede, R. E. Y., De Wolf, F., Miedema, F. and Tersmette, M. (1991). Monocytotropic human immunodeficiency virus 1 (HIV-1) variants detectable in all stages of HIV infection predominantly lack T-cell line tropism and syncytium-inducing ability in primary T-cell culture. *J. Virol.*, **65**, 356–63
37. Polk, B. F., Fox, R., Brookmeyer, R. *et al.* (1987). Predictors of the acquired immunodeficiency syndrome developing in a cohort of seropositive homosexual men. *N. Engl. J. Med.*, **316**, 61–6
38. Ward, J. W., Bush, T. J., Perkins, H. A., Lieb, L. E., Allen, J. R., Goldfinger, D., Samson, S. M., Pepkowitz, S. H., Fernando, L. P., Holland, P. V., Kleinman, S. H., Grindon, A. J., Garner, J. L., Rutherford, G. W. and Holmberg, S. D. (1989). The natural history of transfusion-associated infection with human immunodeficiency virus: factors influencing the rate of progression to disease. *N. Engl. J. Med.*, **321**, 947–52
39. Kaslow, R. A., Duquesnoy, R., Van Raden, M., Kingsley, L., Marrari, M., Friedman, H., Su, S., Saah, A. J., Detels, R., Phair, J. and Rinaldo, C. (1990). A1, Cw7, B8, DR3 HLA antigen combination associated with rapid decline of T-helper lymphocytes in HIV-1 infection. *Lancet*, **335**, 927–30
40. Steel, C. M., Ludlam, C. A., Beatson, D., Peutherer, J. F., Cuthbert, R. J. G., Simmonds, P., Morrison, H. and Jones, M. (1990). HLA haplotype A1 B8 DR3 as a risk factor for HIV-related disease. *Lancet* **1**, 1185–88
41. Cheng-Mayer, C., Quiroga, M., Tung, J. W., Dina, D. and Levy, J. A. (1990). Viral determinants of human immunodeficiency virus type 1 T-cell or macrophage tropism, cytopathogenicity, and CD4 antigen modulation. *J. Virol.*, **64**, 4390–8
42. O'Brien, W. A., Koyanagi, Y., Namazie, A., Zhao, J. Q., Diagne, A., Idler, K., Zack, J. and Chen, I. S. Y. (1990). HIV-1 tropism for mononuclear phagocytes can be determined by regions of gp120 outside the CD4-binding domain. *Nature*, **348**, 69–73
43. Groenink, M., Fouchier, R. A. M., De Goede, R. E. Y., De Wolf, F., Cuypers, H. T. M., Gruters, R. A., Huisman, H. G. and Tersmette, M. (1991). Phenotypical heterogeneity in a panel of infectious molecular HIV-1 clones derived from a single individual. *J. Virol.*, **65**, 1968–75
44. Golub, E. I., Gongrong, L. and Volsky, D. J. (1990). Differences in the basal activity of the long terminal repeat determine different replicative capacities of two closely related human immunodeficiency virus type 1 isolates. *J. Virol.*, **64**, 3654–60
45. Pomerantz, R. J., Feinberg, M. B., Andino, R. and Baltimore, D. (1991). The long terminal repeat is not a major determinant of the cellular tropism of human immunodeficiency virus type 1. *J. Virol.*, **65**, 1041–5
46. Hahn, B. H., Shaw, G. M., Taylor, M. E., Redfield, R., Markham, P. D., Salahuddin, S. Z., Wong-Staal, F., Gallo, R. C., Parks, E. S. and Parks, W. P. (1986). Genetic variation in HTLV-III/LAV over time in patients with AIDS or at risk for AIDS. *Science*, **232**, 1548–53
47. Ho, D. D., Moudgil, T. and Alam, M. (1989). Quantitiation of human immunodeficiency virus type 1 in the blood of infected persons. *N. Engl. J. Med.*, **321**, 1621–25
48. Coombs, R. W., Collier, A. C., Allain, J. P., Nikora, B., Leuther, M., Gjerset, G. F. and Corey, L,. (1989). Plasma viremia in human immunodeficiency virus infection. *N. Engl. J. Med.*, **321**, 1626–31
49. Miedema, F., Petit, A. J. C., Terpstra, F. G., Schattenkerk, J. K. M. E., De Wolf, F., Al, B. J. M., Roos, M., Lange, J. M. A., Danner, S. A., Goudsmit, J. and Schellekens, P. T. A. (1988). Immunological abnormalities in human immunodeficiency virus (HIV)-infected asymptomatic homosexual men. HIV affects the immune system before $CD4^+$ T helper cell depletion occurs. *J. Clin. Invest.*, **82**, 1908–14
50. Terpstra, F. G., Al, B. J. M., Roos, M. Th. L., De Wolf, F., Goudsmit, J., Schellekens, P. T. and Miedema, F. (1989). Longitudinal study of leukocyte functions in homosexual men seroconverted for HIV: rapid and persistent loss of B-cell function after HIV infection. *Eur. J. Immunol.*, **19**, 667–73
51. Fletcher, M. A., Azen, S. P., Adelsberg, B., Gjerset, G., Hassett, J., Kaplan, J., Niland, J. C., Odom-Maryon, T., Parker, J. W., Stites, D. P., Mosley, J. W. and Transfusion Safety Study Group (1989). Immunophenotyping in a multicentre study: the transfusion safety study experience. *Clin. Immunol. Immunopathol.*, **52**, 38–47
52. Giorgi, J. V., Fahey, J. L., Smith, D. C., Hultin, L. E., Cheng, H. L., Mitsuyasu, R. T. and

Detels, R. (1987). Early effects of HIV on CD4 lymphocytes *in vivo*. *J. Immunol.*, **138**, 3725–30
53. Van Noesel, C. J. M., Gruters, R. A., Terpstra, F. G., Schellekens, P..T.A., Van Lier, R. A. W. and Miedema, F. (1990). Functional and phenotypic evidence for a selective loss of memory T cells in asymptomatic HIV-infected men. *J. Clin. Invest.*, **86**, 293–9
54. De Martini, R. M., Turner, R. R., Formenti, S. C., Boone, D. C., Bishop, P. C., Levine, A. M. and Parker, J. W. (1988). Peripheral blood mononuclear cell abnormalities and their relationship to clinical course in homosexual men with HIV infection. *Clin. Immunol. Immunopathol.*, **46**, 258–71
55. Asjo, B., Barkhem, T., Albert, J., Chiodi, F., Von Gegerfeldt, H., Biberfeld, P. and Fenyo, E. M. (1988). HIV-1 strains with differences in replicative capacities are distinguished by *in situ* hybridization of infected cells. IV International Congress on AIDS, abstract No. 1569
56. Willerford, D. M., Gale, M. J. Jr, Benveniste, R. E., Clark, E. A. and Gallatin, W. M. (1990). Simian immunodeficiency virus is restricted to a subset of blood $CD4^+$ lymphocytes that includes memory cells. *J. Immunol.*, **144**, 3779–83
57. Schnittman, S. M., Lane, H. C., Greenhouse, J., Justement, J. S., Baseler, M. and Fauci, A. S. (1990). Preferential infection of $CD4^+$ memory T cells by human immunodeficiency virus type 1: evidence for a role in the selective T-cell functional defects observed in infected individuals. *Proc. Natl. Acad. Sci. USA*, **87**, 6058–62
58. Weinhold, K. J., Lyerley, H. K., Stanley, S. D., Austin, A. A., Matthews, T. J. and Bolognesi, D. P. (1989). HIV-1 GP120-mediated immune suppression and lymphocyte destruction in the absence of viral infection. *J. Immunol.*, **142**, 3091–7
59. Siliciano, R. F., Lawton, T., Knall, C., Karr, R. W., Berman, P., Gregory, T. and Reinherz, E. L. (1988). Analysis of host–virus interactions in AIDS with anti-gp120 T cell clones: effect of HIV sequence variation and a mechanism for $CD4^+$ cell depletion. *Cell*, **54**, 561–75
60. Boucher, C. A. B., Tersmette, M., Lange, J. M. A., Kellam, P., De Goede, R. E. Y., Mulder, J. W., Darby, G., Goudsmit, J. and Larder, B. A. (1990). Emergence of human immunodeficiency virus with reduced sensitivity to zidovudine in asymptomatic 'high risk' individuals. *Lancet*, **2**, 585–90

3
Antigen presentation in HIV infection

S. C. KNIGHT, S. E. MACATONIA and S. PATTERSON

INTRODUCTION

Bone marrow-derived dendritic cells (DC), macrophages (Mϕ) and follicular dendritic cells (FDC) may be infected in individuals exposed to human immunodeficiency virus (HIV)[1-3]. These are all cell types that are involved in different ways in the presentation of antigen and the stimulation of immune responses. Consequently, if infection by HIV results in destruction or dysfunction of these cell types, this may affect the stimulation of immunity by inhibiting the entry of lymphocytes into immune responses. This chapter will, firstly, present evidence suggesting that the three cell types – DC, Mϕ and FDC – represent separate cell lineages. These different cells also fulfil different roles in the development and promotion of immune activity; the function of DC in stimulating immune responses in resting T cells and the effectiveness of all three cell types in promoting the proliferation of already activated T cell clones will be described. Finally, some of the evidence for infection, removal and dysfunction of these cells on exposure to HIV will be discussed.

In this chapter no attempt is made to repeat the thorough reviews of the literature on HIV-infection of these cells[1-3]. Instead the theory is presented that infection, depletion and dysfunction of DC is a fundamental defect in early HIV infection.

ONTOGENY OF DENDRITIC CELLS (DC) AND FOLLICULAR DENDRITIC CELLS (FDC)

Bone marrow-derived Mϕ were for many years considered to be the major antigen-presenting cell type[4]. However, recognition of the potency and importance of DC in presenting antigens to T cells has resulted, following the original descriptions of DC[5], in the recognition that Langerhans' cells

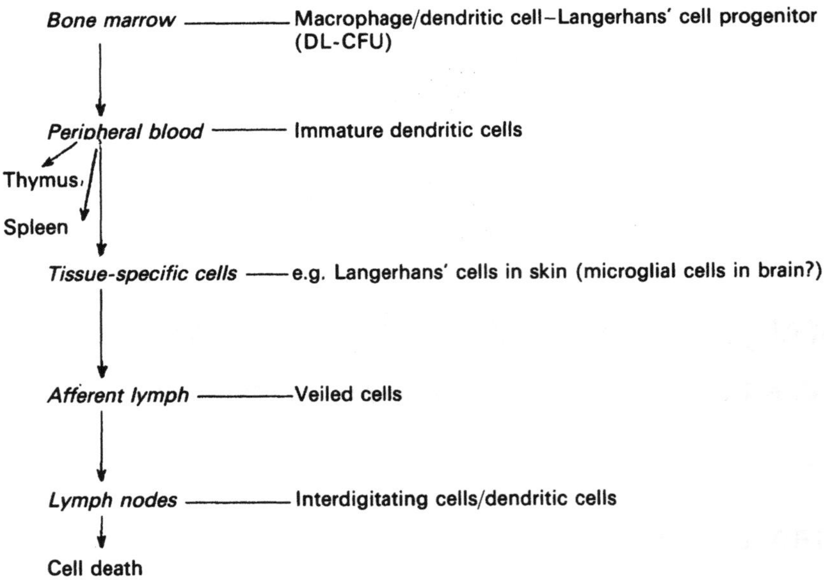

Figure 3.1 Life history of dendritic cells

of the skin may be involved in antigen presentation[6] and evidence for the relationship between Langerhans' cells and the DC/interdigitating cells within T cell areas of lymph nodes[7]. A second dendritic cell type, the FDC, found in the B cell areas of lymph nodes, has been implicated in antigen presentation during memory responses. These two cell types (DC and FDC) are often considered together with Mϕ and described as 'tissue macrophages'. There is now strong evidence that these cells, DC and FDC, are of separate lineages and perform different functions. The effects of HIV infection, therefore, are also different, and a new hypothesis on the mode of development of HIV-related immunosuppression can be developed on the basis of these differing effects.

Figure 3.1 describes the proposed life history of DC. DC, particularly those within tissues, share many markers with Mϕ (e.g. complement and Fc receptors FcR, HLA-DR expression)[8,9]. In addition, they are both derived from large mononuclear cells within the blood. There has therefore been a belief, and some supportive evidence[10], that the DC represent a stage in the life history of classical Mϕ. However, more recent evidence suggests that confusion about the lineage and relationships between these peripheral blood cells may come from the failure to recognize the separate cell types within a population of large mononuclear cells containing precursors of Mϕ and DC which have been loosely described as 'monocytes'. The major evidence for separate lineages of these cells comes from studies of bone marrow stem cells.

A bone marrow origin for DC has long been established (for references see ref. 11). Studies of rat bone marrow cells showed that DC were derived from an HLA-DR negative precursor after short-term culture (1–2 days).

These studies indicated that, if precursors of DC did belong to the granulocyte–macrophage lineage, they branched from the maturation pathway prior to the point of action of macrophage–colony-stimulating factor. There is now much evidence firstly that skin Langerhans' cells are the precursors of some interdigitating cells of the lymph nodes (see refs 12 and 13 for references) and secondly that the DC separated from lymph nodes are isolated interdigitating cells[14]. This supports the view that the Mϕ and DC lineages divide prior to the tissue-specific stage in their life history. The most convincing evidence of the separation of the Mϕ and DC early from bone marrow precursor cells comes from studies of human bone marrow[15]. DC/Langerhans' cell colony-forming units (DL-CFU) were identified in methylcellulose cultures. Small colonies of dividing cells with functional and phenotypic characteristics of DC – many including the Langerhans' cell marker CD1a – were identified. Some of these colonies were joint Mϕ/DC colonies, suggesting an early divergence of these cell types from a common stem cell. Small numbers of these colonies were also observed in human peripheral blood (1–3.7 per 10^5 mononuclear cells). The evidence is thus convincing that the separation of Mϕ and DC lineages occurs early from a bone marrow precursor cell, and that there are already distinct cell types within the population of large mononuclear cells in peripheral blood[16]. However, the changes in phenotype and function during maturation of these cells, and the properties they share with Mϕ, can make the clear separation and identification of these cells in humans problematical[8–12,17]. In mice there are specific anti-DC antibodies which make identification easier (see ref. 14 for references).

The bone marrow-derived cells are believed to be distributed to most tissues of the body[18,19] via peripheral blood. They have been reported to be present as 0.5–1% of the blood mononuclear cell population[20,21], although it is becoming apparent using improved separation and identification techniques that this may be an underestimate of their numbers, which may be 2–4%[22]. They were originally identified in small numbers in all tissues of the body except the brain[18,19]. Differences exist in the characteristics of DC within the interstitial tissues (e.g. Langerhans' cells) and those within lymphoid tissue. The former frequently express the CD1a marker in addition to many markers that are also expressed by Mϕ (e.g. CR3 complement receptor, FcRII receptors, F4/80 labelling in the mouse). By contrast, all these markers may be reduced during the maturation of tissue cells to become DC within the lymph nodes (for references see refs. 9–12). A feature seen at all stages of development is the expression of low levels of CD4[1,23,24]. The CD4 marker is up-regulated by treatment with γ-interferon in Langerhans' cells[23] or in DC from peripheral blood (Patterson, Gross, Bedford and Knight, in preparation).

The identification of any cells of the DC lineage within the brain has proved difficult. However, there is now evidence indicating that the microglial cells may be DC. The evidence for this comes mainly from phenotypic studies which show that microglia have a phenotype similar to that of other interstitial DC of the tissues. They show constitutive expression of MHC class II molecules (see ref. 25 for references). They also show low levels of CD1a expression and CD4[25]. They are also negative for non-specific esterase which is another feature distinguishing them from the non-specific esterase-positive Mϕ. Like other tissue-specific DC they express the CR1/C3b receptor[26] and in mice have Fc receptors and F4/80 labelling[27], which are features shared with Mϕ. If the preliminary evidence on the DC nature of the microglial cells in the brain is confirmed, the presence of a primary antigen-presenting cell in the brain may have implications for the pathogenesis of disease involving immunological activity within the brain. There is already evidence that small numbers of DC isolated from lymph nodes of rats with experimentally induced allergic encephalomyelitis can initiate symptoms of the disease in naive recipient rats[28].

DC in peripheral tissues, particularly after exposure to antigen, travel as veiled cells in the afferent lymphatics to the lymph nodes. Here they can cluster and activate T lymphocytes, so ensuring that major immunological developments occur in these specialized lymphoid tissues (for references see refs 12 and 13). There is no evidence that DC leave lymph nodes in any number and they may die at this site. Feedback mechanisms for this are not known, although DC can act as targets for natural killer cells[29], and we have evidence that DC can be killed by antigen-specific cytotoxic T lymphocytes (Macatonia, Askonas and Knight, in preparation).

In contrast to the bone-marrow derivation of DC and Mϕ the small amount of evidence available suggests that the FDC of the B cell areas are derived *in situ* within lymphoid organs from fibroblastic reticulum elements[30]. Thus, in pairs of parabiosed rats there was no evidence that the FDC were replaced from circulating cells. In addition, a precise histological study also suggests that the FDC develop locally within lymph nodes from reticulum cells[31]. The surface phenotype has been identified for these cells and shows distinctive features suggesting that they belong neither to Mϕ nor DC populations[32]. Thus, FDC express MHC class I and class II antigens, common leucocyte antigen, and have C3b and Fc receptors but lack many markers of Mϕ and lymphoctyes. From what is known of the ontogeny of the DC and FDC it is therefore apparent that they can be considered separately from each other and from classical Mϕ.

DC, Mϕ AND FDC MAY STIMULATE ALREADY-ACTIVATED T CELLS BUT ONLY DC STIMULATE RESTING T CELLS

DC are potent antigen-presenting cells, not only for promoting the growth of already-activated T cell clones but also for recruitment of resting T cells – both CD4 and CD8 – into immune responses. The efficient primary recruitment of resting T cells may be an exclusive property of DC, since only DC and not Mϕ or resting B cells were shown to function in this way either *in vitro*[33–35] or *in vivo*[36]. This is demonstrated in Figure 3.2, where human peripheral blood T cells have been stimulated with a variety of antigens. Stimulation of 'primary' responses to allogeneic DC in the mixed leucocyte reaction is shown to be a property of DC but not of Mϕ. Activated B cells may possibly have some activity in stimulating primary responses, but this

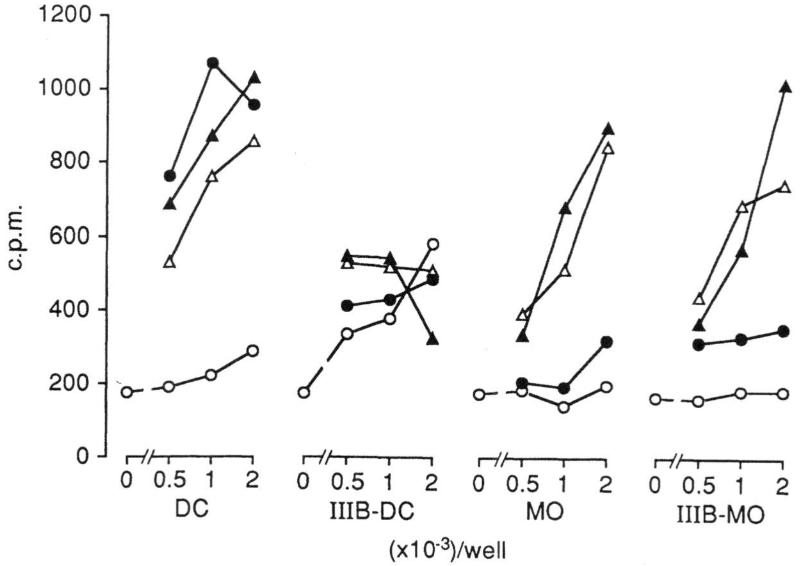

Figure 3.2 Stimulation of primary or secondary T cell responses by dendritic cells (DC) or monocytes (MO) infected with HIV-1 *in vitro*. Mononuclear cells isolated from peripheral blood of normal uninfected individuals were separated into T cells, low-density DC and adherent MO[62]; the antigen-presenting cells were either untreated or exposed to HIV-I (10^4 $TCID_{50}$ units of IIIB for 2 days). Primary responses were measured in mixed leucocyte reactions (MLR) using DC or MO to stimulate T cells from an unrelated donor. To stimulate responses to recall antigens autologous DC or MO were pulsed with either A/X47 influenza virus (100 HAU/10^6 cells at 37 °C for 1 h) or with tetanus toxoid (tetanus vaccine BP, in simple solution 10^4 dilution of stock 14Lf toxoid for 1 h at 37 °C). Proliferation of 5×10^4 T cells/well in 20 μl hanging drop cultures[81] was measured on day 4 by uptake of [^{3}H]thymidine: ○, untreated; △, tetanus toxoid; ▲, A/X47 influenza virus; ●, allogeneic MLR

is not clear since the presence of DC-contaminating cell populations has not been excluded in studies of activated B cells (see refs 37 and 38 for references). This is of particular importance since the potency of these cells means that DC at 0.1% of the lymphocyte number *in vitro* can cause stimulation[16] and *in vivo* as few as 100–10 000 allogeneic Langerhans' cells or DC can sensitize rodents to alloantigens[28,39]. It is not known what special properties of DC equip them to stimulate resting T cells so efficiently, but they appear to express constitutively all MHC class II antigens including DR, DP, DQ and the DQ-associated antigen identified by the antibody RFD1[40]. Mϕ express DR but may require stimulation for high-level expression of other MHC class II products. The life history of DC with their migrating properties and capacity to cluster T cells non-specifically also distinguishes the DC from Mϕ, and may be instrumental in allowing them to recruit resting T cells.

Once T cells are activated both DC and Mϕ are then able to cause promotion of the growth of the recently activated T cell clone[5,33,35], although once the cells return to the 'resting' stage DC are again required for activation[33]. However, there is little information on the important question of the precise characteristics of primed cells which make them susceptible to restimulation by different antigen-presenting cells. It is clear that using human cells both Mϕ and DC will stimulate secondary responses to many common recall antigens. This is demonstrated in Figure 3.2, where stimulation of secondary responses to the recall antigens influenza virus and tetanus toxoid can be stimulated not only by DC but also by Mϕ. Indeed, the promotion of growth of T cells already stimulated by antigen may be a property of any cell type bearing MHC class II molecules, and many routes of expanding ongoing immune responses are then available.

In contrast to the central role of DC in initiating primary immune responses, the FDC play a unique part in memory responses. On secondary exposure to an antigen, immune complexes of antigen/antibody form. Much of this material may be cleared by internalization and removed by classical Mϕ. However, some immune complexes are carried on the surface of non-phagocytic cells into lymph nodes where they are acquired by FDC (see ref. 32 for references). The formation of immune complexes in coated bodies which form 'beads' or icosomes occurs, and these appear to bud from the dendritic processes of FDC. There is evidence that these icosomes may be internalized by B lymphocytes which are then stimulated. The further stimulation of helper T lymphocytes via the B cells activated through FDC has been reported (see ref. 32 for references). This mechanism for B cell stimulation and restimulation of T cells is believed to be an integral part of long-term memory responses, since FDC may retain antigen over long periods of time. The FDC may thus provide an efficient method not only of promoting, but also of maintaining, secondary immune responses.

HIV INFECTION OF ANTIGEN-PRESENTING CELLS

A reduction in MHC class II molecules and in ATPase activity in the skin in patients with HIV infection was the first clue that Langerhans' cells of the skin might be affected by HIV[41]. The report did not distinguish whether these changes resulted from loss of Langerhans' cells from the skin or whether the phenotypes of the individual cells were changed. However, other work showed that early in HIV infection the Langerhans' cells show morphological abnormalities, with many having condensation of nuclear and cytoplasmic material and vacuolation and even cytolysis of cells[42]. This study also gave direct evidence of viral infection from staining of some biopsies with antibodies to HIV protein, and electron microscopical evidence of viral particles associated with the Langerhans' cells. A further study also reported viral particles in or around a proportion of Langerhans' cells[43]. A reduction of the number of Langerhans' cells in the skin has also been observed which may correlate with disease state[44,45]. Although some studies have failed to find evidence that the Langerhans' cells are major targets of HIV[46,47] there is nevertheless considerable evidence that infection of this cell type occurs *in vivo. In vitro* susceptibility of Langerhans' cells to infection has also been described[48].

Following evidence that DC from peripheral blood were susceptible to infection with HIV *in vitro*[49,50], it was shown that a population of low-density cells usually enriched for DC, when taken from peripheral blood of HIV-infected patients, showed lower expression of MHC class II[51]. Evidence now indicates that this reflected a loss of DC from this low-density population, since the numbers of DC is significantly reduced in HIV infection[22]. HIV seropositive individuals who are asymptomatic show this loss of DC, and all individuals with AIDS had numbers below the normal range. By contrast, in persistent generalized lymphadenopathy the number of circulating DC were in the normal range. Infected DC, as assessed by *in situ* hybridization to identify viral RNA and DNA[22,52] were detected in approximately half the asymptomatic and PGL patients and in all patients in the AIDS category of the disease. The proportion of infected DC was between 3% and 25%. Less than 0.2% infection of lymphocytes or macrophages was found.

In vitro infection resulted in the productive infection of some DC within 3 days[49,50], and occurred mainly via the CD4 receptors in these cells (Patterson, in preparation). The productively infected cells appeared to be those of a more mature phenotype, e.g. those with a 'veiled' morphology similar to that of afferent lymph DC[1,53]. *In situ* hybridization studies for viral RNA and DNA showed that a much greater proportion of cells (as many as 65% in some experiments)[53] were infected. The number of positive cells was also higher when DNA was identified in addition to RNA, which was suggestive of a latent infection in many cells. It may be that cells are latently infected and that, as they are stimulated to mature, productive infection may result.

Further support for the idea of Langerhans' cells as targets for HIV infection comes from studies of transgenic mice. In mice transgenic either for the HIV-LTR[54] or for HIV-tat[55] there is preferential expression of the gene in skin Langerhans' cells.

Much available evidence therefore points to the DC lineage being a major target for HIV infection. Perhaps the most surprising aspect in the light of this information of infection by DC in the blood and in the skin is that infection of the interdigitating cells within the lymph nodes has not been reported.

In contrast to the lack of evidence for infection by DC within the lymph nodes, the FDC are a major site of infection in late AIDS patients[56,57]. The presence of viral particles is seen in FDC, particularly in late disease, and there is also a loss of FDC and destruction of the organization of the follicles themselves. Destruction of follicles can also be seen in other severe virus infections and is not, therefore, a property exclusive to HIV infection, so that the relevance of this observation to the peculiar immunosuppressive properties of HIV is not clear.

Mϕ infection *in vitro*, usually seen most clearly when cells are exposed to HIV in the presence of granulocyte–macrophage colony-stimulating factor or with macrophage colony-stimulating factor, has shown that virus assembly and release does not occur by budding through the plasma membrane as seen in DC and FDC. Instead, the virus buds internally into vesicles, apparently via the Golgi complex[2]. This has been suggested as a mechanism for viral replication in a privileged site where immune reactivity is prevented.

However, these cells should still be recognized by MHC class I restricted CTLs. Some 'lymphotropic' strains have been reported not to grow in Mϕ, although those strains derived from Mϕ grow in both Mϕ and lymphocytes (see refs 2 and 3 for references).

Descriptions of Mϕ infection *in vivo* have included descriptions of infection in different cell populations. Thus, 0.001–0.2% of peripheral blood Mϕ are infected (see ref. 2 for references). Brain isolates of HIV have properties consistent with those of macrophage trophic strains of HIV[2], but in contrast to the low infection rate in blood monocyte/Mϕ there is a much higher infection rate in 'brain macrophages'. In the brain the main infected cell is the microglial cell[58,59], and the infection is reported to occur via CD4 expression in these cells[60]. Other types of glial cells within the central nervous system – astrocytes or oligodendrocytes – have not shown consistent HIV infection, although sporadic reports of infection of these cells exist. The suggestive evidence from the phenotype of microglial cells that these cells are of the DC lineage has already been described in the previous section, and such tentative data relying on cell phenotype require further confirmation. Thus, it is not clear at present whether the explanation of the enormous variation in infection levels between Mϕ from other areas (e.g. peripheral blood) might be related to differences in cell lineage or to differences in the stage of macrophage differentiation in the tissues. In the peripheral blood itself there is a disparity of two orders of magnitude between the low infection rate in Mϕ and the higher rate in the DC. A high rate of HIV infection is also reported in 'lung macrophages'[61], but precise analysis of the phenotype and function of the cell type within the airways[19] that are involved is not clear.

ANTIGEN PRESENTATION IN HIV INFECTION

The differential effects of HIV infection on DC, Mϕ and FDC can explain the immunological effects of the virus. Exposure of DC + Mϕ either *in vivo*[22,52] or *in vitro* to a lymphotropic strain of HIV[49,50,53,62] results in infection of a high proportion of DC but of few Mϕ, as judged from studies using peripheral blood cells. The infection of cells is accompanied by a block in the functional capacity of DC to present antigen in primary or secondary stimulation of T cell responses[22,50,52,62,63]. The block in stimulation is still apparent when DC are infected and infection of lymphoctyes is blocked[50]. In addition, the block in antigen presentation is not reversed by the presence of soluble CD4[1]. Thus, the effect does not appear to function through infection of T cells via DC, and does not work through blocking T cell receptors. The block may thus operate directly through an effect on DC. The blocked responses are demonstrated in Figure 3.2, where DC exposed *in vitro* to HIV fail to stimulate responses to alloantigens or to the recall antigens, influenza or tetanus toxoid. By contrast, Mϕ which function only in the secondary responses are effective in stimulating responses to influenza and tetanus toxoid[62] (Figure 3.2). A similar pattern of responsiveness is seen using cells from HIV-infected individuals who are asymptomatic or who have persistent generalized lymphadenopathy (Macatonia, Patterson, Pinching and Knight, in preparation). In contrast to the non-responsiveness to HIV itself, DC infected with HIV stimulate responses to HIV antigens[1,64] (Macatonia, Patterson and Knight, submitted). This presentation of antigen by DC presumably forms the basis for the development of immune responses to the virus *in vivo*[3], and it may also underlie the reported primary stimulation *in vitro* of normal cells by virus-infected cells[61,65].

The block in the capacity of DC in HIV infection to present antigens other than HIV itself, and the continuing capacity of Mϕ to function as antigen-presenting cells, can be used to describe the spectrum of immunological abnormalities and their slow evolution. Thus, there have been reports that T cell function is deficient before there are many indications of loss of T cell numbers[66,67]. A block in the capacity of DC to stimulate primary responses, as well as the loss in their contribution to secondary responses (e.g. as in Figure 3.2) could account for this loss in responsiveness. However, many reports show that antigen presentation still occurs in HIV-infected monocytes[65–70], although defects in responses have been reported, particularly when 'limiting' culture conditions have been used[69,70] or when using a 'monocyte' cell line[71]. The relative importance of DC and Mϕ in contributing to 'accessory' defects is not clear from these papers. As demonstrated in Figure 3.2, a defect in DC and not Mϕ combined with variations in the number of memory T cells would provide an explanation for the varying effects on antigen presentation.

Another feature of the early defects in T cell function during HIV infection has been the loss of responsiveness to recall antigens without defects in responses to alloantigen or to mitogen[72–74]. In response to alloantigens the stimulus to T cells is provided by allogeneic DC, and it has been shown that T cells still function if normal allogeneic DC are used as a stimulus[22,50]. The responses to mitogens are also partially independent of accessory cell function. It is only the responses to recall antigens, therefore, that rely on accessory cells that are likely to show some loss of responsiveness via DC. Maintenance of secondary responsiveness via Mϕ would explain the responses that still occur.

A further feature of the loss of immunological activity in HIV infection is that the 'T cell defects' seem to be related to loss of memory T cells[75] (see also Chapter 5). This at first sight seems paradoxical, because the early effect of HIV on DC will be most critical for the stimulation of naive cells and recruitment of T cells into immune responses. However, it is likely that most ongoing responses in asymptomatic individuals will be occurring via the Mϕ, which will stimulate secondary responses to recall antigens (e.g. Figure 3.2). It may only be as the memory cell pool is depleted that the complete loss of responses will occur. Without activated T cell clones the Mϕ will become ineffective. Loss of memory T cells will therefore be associated with the loss of T cell activation. This loss may proceed through many mechanisms previously discussed[3]. For example, memory, rather than naive T cells, are infected when the low-level T cell infection is analysed[76]. This is consistent with the many observations that viruses may infect and inactivate stimulated lymphocytes but not resting cells. Another mechanism effective in reducing the number of memory cells may be the loss of the FDC and the destruction of germinal centres late in infection. Loss of FDC may remove the major stimulus for long-term persistence of activated 'memory cells'. Without adequate numbers of recently activated memory cells the Mϕ will become impotent. It appears that loss of T cell activity may not be a primary defect but a consequence of the loss of antigen-presenting function of DC and of FDC in HIV infection.

A final speculation on the role of antigen-presenting cells in the spectrum of HIV-associated disease can be made. It seems likely that persistent B cell stimulation and the proliferation of T cells – particularly CD8 cells in persistent generalized lymphadenopathy – could be stimulated by persistent presentation of HIV by DC. The concept that the major infected cell type within the brain, the microglial cells, may be of the DC type leads to the speculation that these cells, when infected, may represent a primary lymphocyte stimulation system for recruitment of T cells within the brain. There is evidence that DC exposed *in vitro* or *in vivo* to autoantigens can initiate autoimmune disease; a role for DC has been seen not only in the development of experimental allergic thyroiditis[77] but also in arthritis[78] and in experimental allergic encephalomyelitis[28]. In the latter disease the involvement of cells of dendritic morphology presenting antigen within the brain has been suggested, and these cells have the features of microglial cells[79]. In multiple sclerosis itself, where the involvement of a retrovirus remains possible, the suggestion has been made that presentation of antigen occurs within the brain, in part by microglial cells within the plaques[80]. Thus, in addition to strong evidence that antigen presentation defects may be involved in the development of the immunosuppressive aspects of HIV infection, there is also some circumstantial evidence that presentation of HIV antigens themselves by DC may occur, and could underlie the unusual immunological activity of the immune system systemically and in the localized lesions within the brain.

Acknowledgements

We are grateful to Norma Saunders for her help in preparing the manuscript.

References

1. Knight, S. C., Macatonia, S. E. and Patterson, S. (1990). HIV-I infection of dendritic cells. *Int. Rev. Immunol.*, **6**, 163–75
2. Meltzer, M. S., Skillman, D. R., Gomatos, P. J., Kalter, D. C. and Gendelman, H. E. (1990). Role of mononuclear phagocytes in the pathogenesis of human immunodeficiency virus infection. *Ann. Rev. Immunol.*, **8**, 169–94
3. Rosenberg, Z. F. and Fauci, A. S. (1989). The immunopathogenesis of HIV infection. *Adv. Immunol.*, **47**, 377–31
4. Unanue, E. R. (1983). Regulatory functions of mononuclear phagocytes. *Prog. Immunol.*, **V**, 973–83
5. Steinman, P. M. and Cohn, Z. A. (1973). Identification of a novel cell type in peripheral organs of mice. I. Morphology, qualitative tissue distribution. *J. Exp. Med.*, **137**, 1142–62
6. Silberberg, I. (1971). Studies of electron microscopy of epidermis after topical application of mercuric chloride. Morphological and histochemical findings in epidermal cells of human subjects who do not show allergic sensitivity or primary irritant reaction to mercuric chloride. *J. Invest. Dermatol.*, **64**, 37–51
7. Silberberg-Sinakin, I., Gigli, I., Baer, R. L. and Thorbecke, G. J. (1980). Langerhans' cells: role in contact hypersensitivity and relationship to lymphoid dendritic cells and macrophages. *Immunol. Rev.*, **53**, 203–37

8. Macpherson, G. G. (1989). Lymphoid dendritic cells: their life history and roles in immune responses. *Res. Immunol.*, **140**,. 877–926
9. Freudenthal, P. S. and Steinman, R. M. (1991). The distinct surface of human blood dendritic cells as observed after an improved isolation method. *Proc. Natl. Acad. Sci.*, **87**, 7698–702
10. Kabel, P. J., Haan-Meulman, M. de, Voorby, H. A. M., Kleingold, M., Knol, E. F. and Drexhage, H. A. (1989). Accessory cells with a morphology and marker pattern of dendritic cells can be obtained from elutriator purified blood monocyte fractions. An enhancing effect of metrizamide in this differentiation. *Immunobiology*, **179**, 335–41
11. Bowers, W. E. and Goodell, E. M. (1989). Dendritic cell ontogeny. *Res. Immunol.*, **140**, 880–3
12. Romani, N. and Schuler, G. (1989). Structural and functional relationships between epidermal Langerhans' cells and dendritic cells. *Res. Immunol.*, **140**, 895–8
13. Knight, S. C. (1989). Dendritic cells in contact sensitivity. *Res. Immunol.*, **140**, 907–10
14. Kraal, G. (1989). Immunocytochemistry of dendritic cells. A clue to their function? *Res. Immunol.*, **140**, 891–5
15. Reid, C. D. L., Fryer, P. R., Clifford, C., Kirk, A., Tikerpae, J. and Knight, S. C. (1990). Identification of hematopoietic progenitors of macrophages and dendritic Langerhans cells (DL-CFU) in human bone marrow and peripheral blood. *Blood*, **76**, 1139–49
16. Knight, S. C., Farrant, J., Bryant, A., Edwards, A. J., Burman, S., Lever, A., Clarke, J. and Webster, D. B. (1986). Non-adherent, low density cells from human peripheral blood contain dendritic cells and monocytes both with veiled morphology. *Immunology*, **57**, 595–603
17. Wood, G. S., Turner, R. R., Shiurba, R. A., Eng, L. and Warnke, R. A. (1985). Human dendritic cells and macrophages: in situ immunophenotypic definition of subsets that exhibit morphologic and microenvironmental characteristics. *Am. J. Pathol.*, **119**, 73–92
18. Hart, D. N. J. and Fabre, J. W. (1981). Demonstration and characterisation of la-positive dendritic cells in the interstitial connective tissues of rat heart and other tissues, but not brain. *J. Exp. Med.*, **154**, 347–61
19. Sertl, K., Takemura, T., Tschachler, E., Ferrans, V. J., Kaliner, M. A. and Shevach, E. M. (1986). Dendritic cells with antigen presenting capability reside in airway epithelium, lung parenchyma, and visceral pleura. *J. Exp. Med.*, **163**, 436–51
20. Kuntz-Crow, M. and Kunkel, H. C. (1982). Human dendritic cells: major stimulators of the autologous and allogeneic mixed leukocyte reactions. *Clin. Exp. Immunol.*, **49**, 338–46
21. Van Voorhis, W. C., Hair, L. S., Steinman, R. M. and Kaplan, G. (1982). Human dendritic cells: Enrichment and characterisation from peripheral blood. *J. Exp. Med.*, **155**, 1172–87
22. Macatonia, S. E., Lau, R., Patterson, S., Pinching, A. J. and Knight, S. C. (1990). Dendritic cell infection, depletion and dysfunction in HIV-infected individuals. *Immunology*, **71**, 38–45
23. Walsh, L. J., Parry, A., Scholes, A. and Seymour, G. J. (1987). Modulation of CD4 antigen expression on human gingival Langerhans' cells by gamma interferon. *Clin. Exp. Immunol.*, **70**, 379–85
24. Knight, S. and Patterson, S. (1989). Effect of human immunodeficiency virus on dendritic cells isolated from human peripheral blood. In Dupont, B. (ed.), *Immunobiology of HLA, Tenth International Histocompatibility Workshop*, vol. II, (Springer Verlag), p. 378
25. Lowe, J., Maclennan, K. A., Powe, D. G., Pound, J. D. and Palmer, J. B. (1989). Microglial cells in human brain have phenotypic characteristics related to possible function as dendritic antigen presenting cells. *J. Pathol.*, **159**, 143–9
26. Hayes, G. M., Woodroofe, M. N. and Cuzner, M. L. (1987). Microglia are the major cell type expressing MHC class II in human white matter. *J. Neurol. Sci.*, **80**, 25–37
27. Perry, V. H., Hume, D. A. and Gordon, S. (1985). Immunohistochemical localisation of macrophages and microglia in the adult and developing mouse brain. *Neuroscience*, **15**, 313–26
28. Knight, S. C., Mertin, J., Stackpoole, A. and Clarke, J. (1983). Induction of immune responses *in vivo* with small numbers of veiled (dendritic) cells. *Proc. Natl. Acad. Sci.*, **80**, 6032–5
29. Shah, P. D., Gilbertson, S. M. and Rowley, D. A. (1985). Dendritic cells that have interacted with antigen are targets for natural killer cells. *J. Exp. Med.*, **162**, 625–36
30. Klaus, G. G. B., Humphrey, J. H., Kunkl, A. and Dongworth, D. W. (1980). The follicular dendritic cell: Its role in antigen presentation and the generation of immunological memory. *Immunol. Rev.*, **53**, 2–28
31. Villena, A., Zapata, A., Rivera-Pomov, J. M., Barrutia, M. G. and Fonfria, J. J. (1983). Structure of the non-lymphoid cells during the postnatal development of the rat lymph nodes. *Cell Tissue Res.*, **229**, 219–32

32. Szakal, A. K., Kosco, M. H. and Tew, J. G. (1989). Microanatomy of lymphoid tissues during humoral immune responses: structure–function relationships. *Am. Rev. Immunol.*, **7**, 91–109
33. Inaba, K. and Steinman, R. M. (1984). Resting and sensitised T lymphocytes exhibit distinct stimulatory (antigen-presenting cell) requirements for growth and lymphokine release. *J. Exp. Med.*, **160**, 1717–1735
34. Young, J. W. and Steinman, R. M. (1990). Dendritic cells stimulate primary human cytolytic lymphocyte responses in the absence of $CD4^+$ helper cells. *J. Exp. Med.*, **171**, 1315–32
35. Macatonia, S. E., Taylor, P. M., Knight, S. C. and Askonas, B. A. (1989). Primary stimulation by dendritic cells induces antiviral proliferative and cytotoxic T cell responses *in vitro*. *J. Exp. Med.*, **169**, 1255–64
36. Macatonia, S. E., Edwards, A. J. and Knight, S. C. (1986). Dendritic cells and the initiation of contact sensitivity to fluorescein isothiocyanate. *Immunology*, **59**, 509–14
37. Metlay, J. R., Pure, E. and Steinman, R. M. (1990). Control of immune responses at the level of antigen-presenting cells: a comparison of the function of dendritic cells and B lymphocytes. *Adv. Immunol.*, **45**, 45–116
38. Sprent, J. and Schaefer, M. (1989). Antigen-presenting cells for unprimed T cells. *Immunology Today*, **10**, 17–22
39. Rico, M. J. and Streilein, J. W. (1987). Comparison of alloimmunogenicity of Langerhans' cells and keratinocytes from mouse epidermis. *J. Invest. Dermatol.*, **89**, 607–10
40. Knight, S. C., Fryer, P., Griffiths, S. and Harding, B. (1987). Class II histocompatibility antigens on human dendritic cells. *Immunology*, **61**, 21–7
41. Belsito, D. V., Sanchez, R., Baer, M. D., Valentine, F. and Thorbecke, G. J. (1984). Reduced Langerhans' cell 1a antigen and ATPase activity in patients with the acquired immunodeficiency syndrome. *N. Engl. J. Med.*, **310**, 1279–81
42. Tschachler, E., Groh, V., Popovic, M., Mann, D. L., Konrad, K., Sofai, B., Eron, L., Veronese, F., Wolff, K. and Stingl, G. (1987). Epidermal Langerhans' cells – a target for HTLV-III/LAV infection. *J. Invest. Dermatol.*, **88**, 233–7
43. Rappersberger, K. S., Gartner, S., Schenk, P., Stingl, G., Groh, V., Tschachler, E., Mann, D. P., Wolff, K., Konrad, K. and Popovic, M. (1988). Langerhans' cells are an actual site of HIV replication. *Intervirology*, **29**, 185–90
44. Oxholm, P., Helweg-Larsen, S. and Permin, H. (1986). Immunohistological skin investigations in patients with the acquired immune deficiency syndrome. *Acta Pathol. Microbiol. Immunol. Scand.* (*Sect. A*), **94**, 113–16
45. Dreno, B., Milpied, B., Bignon, J., Stadler, J. F. and Litoux, P. (1988). Prognostic value of Langerhans' cells in the epidermis of HIV patients. *Br. J. Dermatol.*, **118**, 481–6
46. Kanitakis, J. and Thivolet, J. (1990). Infection of human epidermal Langerhans' cells by HIV. *AIDS*, **4**, 266
47. Kalter, D. C., Gendelman, H. E. and Meltzer, M. S. (1990). Infection of human epidermal Langerhans' cells by HIV. *AIDS*, **4**, 266
48. Braathen, L. R., Ramirez, G., Kunze, R. O. and Gelderblom, H. (1987). Langerhans' cells as primary target cells for HIV infection. *Lancet*, **2**, 1094
49. Patterson, S. and Knight, S. C. (1987). Susceptibility of human peripheral blood dendritic cells to infection by human immunodeficiency virus. *J. Gen. Virol.*, **68**, 1177–81
50. Macatonia, S. C., Patterson, S. and Knight, S. C. (1989). Suppression of immune responses by dendritic cells infected with HIV. *Immunology*, **67**, 285–9
51. Eales, L. J., Farrant, J., Herbert, M. and Pinching, A. J. (1988). Peripheral blood dendritic cells in persons with AIDS and AIDS related complex: loss of high intensity class II antigen expression and function. *Clin. Exp. Immunol.*, **71**, 423–7
52. Hughes, R., Macatonia, S. E., Keat, A. S. and Knight, S. C. (1990). The detection of human immunodeficiency virus in dendritic cells from the joints of patients with aseptic arthritis. *Br. J. Rheumatol.*, **29**, 166–70
53. Patterson, S., Gross, J., Bedford, P. A. and Knight, S. C. (1991). Morphology and phenotype of dendritic cells from peripheral blood and productive and non-productive infection with human immunodeficiency virus type 1. *Immunology*, **72**, 361–7
54. Leonard, J., Khillan, J. S., Gendelman, H. E., Adachi, A., Lorenzo, S., Westphal, H., Martin, M. A. and Meltzer, M. S. (1989). The human immunodeficiency virus long terminal repeat is preferentially expressed in Langerhans cells in transgenic mice. *AIDS Res. Hum. Retrov.*,

5, 421–30

55. Vogel, J., Hinrichs, S. H., Reynolds, R. K., Luciw, P. A. and Jay, G. (1988). The HIV tat gene induces dermal lesions resembling Kaposi's sarcoma in transgenic mice. *Nature*, **335**, 606–11
56. Armstrong, J. A. and Horne, R. (1984). Follicular dendritic cells and virus-like particles in AIDS-related lymphadenopathy. *Lancet*, **2**, 370–2
57. Tenner-Racz, K., Racz, P., Gartner, S., Ramsauer, J., Dietrich, M., Gluckman, J. C. and Popovic, M. (1989). Ultrastructural analysis of germinal centers in lymph nodes of patients with HIV-induced persistent generalised lymphadenopathy: evidence for persistence of infection. *Progr. AIDS Pathol.*, **1**, 29–40
58. Koenig, S., Gendelman, H. E., Orenstein, J. M., Dal Canto, M. C., Pezeshkpour, G. H., Yungbluth, M., Janotta, F., Aksamit, A., Martin, M. A. and Fauci, A. S. (1986). Detection of AIDS virus in macrophages in brain tissue from AIDS patients with encephalopathy. *Science*, **233**, 1089–93
59. Vazeux, R., Brousse, N., Jarry, A., Henin, D., Marche, C., Vedrenne, C., Mikol, J., Wolff, M., Michon, C., Rozenbaum, W., Bureau, J.-F., Montagnier, L. and Brahic, M. (1987). AIDS subacute encephalitis. *Am. J. Pathol.*, **126**, 403–10
60. Jordan, C. A., Watkins, B. A., Kufta, C. and Dubois-Dalcq, M. (1991). Infection of brain microglial cells by human immunodeficiency virus type 1 is CD4 dependent. *J. Virol.*, **65**, 736–42
61. Plata, F., Autran, B., Martins, L. P., Wain Hobson, S., Raphael, M., Mayaud, C., Denis, M., Guillon, J. M. and Debre, P. (1987). AIDS virus specific cytotoxic T lymphocytes in lung disorders. *Nature*, **328**, 348–53
62. Knight, S. C. and Macatonia, S. E. (1991). Effect of HIV on antigen presentation by dendritic cells and macrophages. *Res. Virol.*, **142**, 123–8
63. Knight, S. C., Patterson, S. and Macatonia, S. E. (1988). Dendritic cells and viruses. *Immunol. Lett.*, **19**, 177–81
64. Knight, S. C., Macatonia, S. E., Bedford, P. A. and Patterson, S. (1991). Peripheral blood dendritic cells in HIV infection. In Racz, P. (ed.), *Morphological and Functional Aspects of Accessory Cells in Retroviral Infections* (Basel: Karger) (in press)
65. Mann, D. C., Gartner, S., Le Sane, F., Buchow, H. and Popovic, M. (1990). HIV-I transmission and function of virus-infected monocytes/macrophages. *J. Immunol.*, **144**, 2152–8
66. Miedema, F., Petit, A. J. C., Terpestra, F. G., Schuttenkerk, J. K. M. E., Wolf, F. De, Roos, B. J. M. Al. M., Lange, J. M. A., Panner, S. A., Goudsmit, J. and Schellekens, P. T. A. (1988). Immunological abnormalities in human immunodeficiency virus (HIV)-infected asymptomatic homosexual men. HIV affects the immune system before CD4$^+$ T helper function depletion occurs. *J. Clin. Invest.*, **82**, 1908–14
67. Lane, H. C., Depper, J. L., Greene, W. C., Whalen, G., Waldmann, T. A. and Fauci, A. S. (1985). Qualitative analysis of immune function in patients with acquired immunodeficiency syndrome. *N. Engl. J. Med.*, **313**, 79–84
68. Manca, F., Habeshaw, J. A. and Dalgleish, A. G. (1990). HIV-envelope glycoprotein, antigen-specific T cell responses and soluble CD4. *Lancet*, **335**, 811–15
69. Ennen, J., Seipp, I., Norley, S. G. and Kurth, R. (1990). Decreased accessory cell function of macrophages after infection with human immunodeficiency virus type 1 *in vitro*. *Eur. J. Immunol.*, **20**, 2451–6
70. Prince, H., Moody, D., Shubin, B. and Fahey, J. L. (1985). Defective monocyte function in acquired immune deficiency syndrome (AIDS): evidence from a monocyte-dependent T cell proliferative system. *J. Clin. Immunol.*, **5**, 215
71. Petit, A. J. C., Tersmette, M., Terpestra, F. G., Goode, R. E. Y., Lier, R. A. W. van L. and Miedema, F. (1988). Decreased accessory cell function by human monocytic cells after infection with HIV. *J. Immunol.*, **140**, 1485–9
72. Shearer, G. M., Payne, S. M., Joseph, L. J. and Biddison, W. E. (1984). Functional T lymphocyte immune deficiency in a population of homosexual men who do not exhibit symptoms of acquired immune deficiency syndrome. *J. Clin. Invest.*, **74**, 496–506
73. Shearer, G. M., Salahuddin, S. Z., Markham, P. D., Joseph, L. J., Payne, S. M., Kriebel, P., Bernstein, D. C., Biddison, W. E., Sarngadharan, M. G. and Gallo, R. C. (1985). Prospective study of cytotoxic T lymphocyte responses to influenza and antibodies to human T lymphotropic virus III in homosexual men. *J. Clin. Invest.*, **76**, 1699–1704
74. Shearer, G. M., Bernstein, D. C., Tung, K. D. K., Via, C. S., Redfield, R., Salahuddin, S. Z. and Gallo, R. C. (1986). A model for the selective loss of major histocompatibility complex

self-restricted T cell immune responses during the development of acquired immune deficiency syndrome (AIDS). *J. Immunol.*, **137**, 2514–21

75. Van Noesel, C. J. M., Gruters, R. A., Terpstra, F. G., Shellekens, P. A., van Lier, R. A. W. and Miedema, F. (1990). Functional and phenotypic evidence for a selective loss of memory T cells in asymptomatic HIV-infected men. *J. Clin. Invest.*, **86**, 293–9
76. Schnittman, S. M., Lane, H. C., Greenhouse, J., Justement, J. S., Baseler, M. and Fauci, A. S. (1990). Preferential infection of $CD4^+$ memory T cells by human immunodeficiency virus type 1: evidence for a role in the selective T-cell functional defects observed in infected individuals. *Proc. Natl. Acad. Sci.*, **87**, 6058–62
77. Knight, S. C., Farrant, S. C., Chan, J., Bryant, A., Bedford, P. A. and Bateman, C. (1988). Induction of autoimmunity with dendritic cells: Studies on thyroiditis in mice. *Clin. Immunol. Immunopathol.*, **48**, 277–89
78. Verschure, P. J., Van Noorden, C. J. F. and Dijkstra, C. D. (1989). Macrophages and dendritic cells during the early stages of antigen-induced arthritis in rats: immunohistochemical analysis of cryostat sections of the whole knee joint. *Scand. J. Immunol.*, **29**, 371–81
79. Matsumoto, Y., Hara, N., Tanaka, R. and Fujiwara, M. (1986). Immunohistochemical analysis of the rat central nervous system during experimental allergic encephalomyelitis with special reference to Ia-positive cells with dendritic morphology. *J. Immunol.*, **136**, 3668–76
80. Woodroofe, M. N., Bellamy, A. S., Feldmann, M., Davison, A. N. and Cuzner, M. L. (1986). Immunocytochemical characterisation of the immune reaction in the central nervous system in multiple sclerosis. Possible role for microglia in lesion growth. *J. Neurol. Sci.*, **74**, 135–52
81. Knight, S. C. (1988). Lymphocyte proliferation assays. In Klaus, G. G. B. (ed.), *Lymphocytes: A Practical Approach* (Oxford–Washington DC: IRL Press), pp. 189–207

4
The cytotoxic T cell response to HIV

D. F. NIXON

INTRODUCTION

The normal immune response to an infectious organism involves both non-specific and antigen-specific immunity. Virus infections stimulate specific antibodies, T-helper cells and cytotoxic T cells (CTL). The importance of virus-specific CTL in the clearance of viral infections has been increasingly recognized over the past decade, and it is likely that CTL form the major specific defence against primary virus infections. Evidence for the *in vivo* role of virus-specific CTL comes from experimental animal models and, in addition, a few studies in humans. Following influenza A virus infection, CTL specific for influenza are generated, detectable before the primary IgM response[1], and help in the clearance of the infection. In experimental mouse models of influenza infection, cloned influenza-specific CTL have been adoptively transferred to infected mice with resulting clearance of the virus from the lungs[2], and in a comparison of humoral and cell-mediated immunity, antibody failed to clear the virus infection whereas CTL cultures eliminated the virus[3]. $CD4^+$ T cell-depleted mice generate viral-specific CTL which clear influenza virus from the lungs[4] and assist in recovery from ectromelia virus infection[5]. $CD8^+$ T cells have also been shown to be actively involved in the elimination of retrovirus-induced tumours[6]. In humans the rapid clearance of nasal virus after deliberate infection with influenza A virus has been correlated with specific CTL activity[7], and control of primary and latent Epstein–Barr virus (EBV) and cytomegalovirus (CMV) infections has also been associated with circulating CTL activity[8–10]. This accumulating evidence points to a major role of CTL in the elimination of virally infected cells. As retrovirus-specific CTL have been shown to be of great importance in the immune attack against retrovirus-induced mouse tumours[6,11], and human HTLV-I-specific CTL have been detected from HTVL-I-infected patients[12–14], several groups of scientific investigators looked for HIV-specific CTL in HIV-infected individuals.

Cytotoxic T cells (CTL) are thymus-derived lymphocytes which usually have the CD8 antigen on their cell surface. The major histocompatibility complex (MHC) antigens are crucial in the targeting of infected cells by CTL, and this phenomenon has been called MHC restriction. CTL will recognize virally infected targets only if the targets share HLA molecules with the CTL. For $CD8^+$ CTL, targets have to share class I antigens and for $CD4^+$ helper and cytotoxic T cells, targets have to share class II antigens. These fundamental observations[15] can now be considered at a molecular level because of the exciting experiments in cellular immunology over the past 10 years which have increased the understanding of the molecular basis for CTL recognition, both through knowledge of the structure of the HLA molecule, and the processing and presentation of virus antigens. A brief summary of current knowledge allows better understanding of the CTL recognition process.

CTL RECOGNITION OF VIRAL ANTIGENS

CTL recognize processed viral peptides

In the early 1980s it was thought that CTL recognized virus glycoproteins expressed on the surface of infected cells. However, when cloned influenza-specific CTL were assayed on genetically reassorted viruses, their specificity was mapped to polymerase PB1,2[16] and nucleoprotein[17], both internal influenza proteins. In influenza infection the majority of CTL in a bulk culture preparation have been found to recognize internal proteins[18]. The recognition of such internal proteins implied that CTL were recognizing processed antigen, and this was demonstrated by Townsend and colleagues who found that influenza nucleoprotein (NP)-specific CTL recognized fragments of NP cDNA expressed in target cells[19]; they then used synthetic peptides to identify sites of CTL recognition[20]. This was done by adding short synthetic peptides of about 15 amino acids long, taken from the virus amino acid sequence, into the CTL assay. CTL could recognize certain peptides and these became known as the CTL 'peptide' epitopes; these were the exact sequences of the virus that the CTL receptor was recognizing. In a virally infected cell the virus is processed into peptide-sized fragments which associate with an HLA molecule, and this complex of peptide plus MHC is presented on the cell surface. Confirmation of these processes has come from the X-ray crystallographic analysis of HLA molecules[21–23] and recent experiments on antigen processing[24–27].

The HLA molecule contains a 'peptide-binding' groove

The X-ray crystallographic structures of two HLA class I molecules, HLA-A2 and Aw68, have been defined to a fine resolution[21–23]. Class I MHC molecules are composed of heavy and light polypeptide chains which are non-covalently attached. The heavy chain, molecular weight 44 KDa, spans the membrane bilayer, and the extracellular part is divided into three domains, α_1, α_2 and α_3, which are encoded on separate exons. The light chain is a 12 KDa polypeptide called β_2-microglobulin, β_2m. The structure of HLA-A2, as shown by X-ray crystallography, consists of two pairs of structurally similar domains – α_3 with β_2-microglobulin and α_1 with α_2. The α_3 and β_2m domains are β-sandwich structures connected by a disulphide bond. The α_1 and α_2 domains each consisted of an antiparallel β-pleated sheet spanned by a long α-helical region. A deep groove, approximately 2.5 nm long and 1.0 nm wide, runs between the two long α-helices of the α_1 and α_2 domains. In this molecule the groove contains a region of electron density which is thought to be a 'self-peptide'[21]. This groove has become known as the peptide binding groove and its size suggests that antigenic peptides of between 8 and 20 amino acids could fit into it, depending on the folding of the peptide. The location, size and shape of this region were consistent with the idea that the groove binds a processed antigen in the form of a peptide. The HLA-Aw68 structure[23] was extremely similar to HLA-A2. However analysis of the X-ray structures showed that the polymorphic amino acids in the class I molecule pointed into the peptide binding groove, and this gave a rational basis for understanding how the amino acid polymorphism of HLA class I molecules would affect peptide binding by implying that each allelic product would bind a different peptide.

Peptides stabilize HLA molecules

The self peptide identified in the HLA structures led to the idea that peptide is an integral part of the class I molecule and endogenous peptides are constantly being presented at the cell surface by class I molecules. Recent experiments have shown that peptides are important for the stability, conformation and cell surface expression of the class I molecules themselves. Townsend and colleagues[20] have found that adding exogenous specific peptides allowed cell surface expression of class I on a mutant cell line that lacked class I surface expression. Although class I molecules are stabilized by peptide, they can be expressed at the cell surface without peptide in an unstable form. Peptide added exogenously stabilizes these empty MHC molecules[25]. The exact subcellular compartment of the peptide–class I association is unclear, but is likely to be in a pre-Golgi compartment[24]. Proof for the processing of viral proteins into short peptides which bind to MHC molecules has recently been obtained[26–28]. Peptides isolated in these experiments have shown peptides of 9 amino acids in length.

THE CYTOTOXIC T CELL ASSAY

An assay to detect virus-specific cytotoxic T cells requires a primed virus-specific CTL population (effector or killer cells), target cells and a detection system to measure lysis of target cells. The most commonly used assay is the chromium release assay which involves the radioactive labelling of target cells with ^{51}Cr[29].

Effector (killer) cell population

The CTL has usually been detected from the peripheral blood mononuclear cell population, but CTL from other sources such as spleen, lymph node, CSF or bronchoalveolar lavage have also been used as a source of killer cells. In most virus infections the frequency of specific CTL is low enough that restimulation and expansion with virus is necessary to increase the numbers of specific CTL to a level that can be detected in the assay. In the detection of influenza-specific CTL, PBMC from a patient who has previously had influenza are set up in culture and incubated with influenza virus[30]. The virus stimulates memory CTL which divide and expand. After about a week, sufficient cells are present in the culture to use in the CTL assay.

Target cells

Because CTL recognize peptide fragments of a virus in assocition with an MHC class I molecule, the target cell must have the correct MHC type for cytotoxicity to be detected. If the HLA type of the patient is known, target cells can also be used that match or mismatch at HLA antigens, and this can help in showing that a CTL response is MHC-restricted. A number of target cells have been used; perhaps the commonest target cell used is the EBV transformed B lymphoblastoid cell line (BCL), usually from the patients themselves – an autologous BCL target. These cells are easy to grow in culture and have been found to be good target cells. Fibroblasts, macrophages, PHA lymphoblasts and mouse cells transfected with MHC genes have also been used for targets. A second essential component for the target cell is expression of the viral antigen. In some cases the virus has been used to infect the target cells, i.e. with influenza or CMV. However, it is often of interest to narrow the response down to specific proteins so methods of expressing single proteins have been used. These include using protein fragments or expression of the virus gene in a recombinant molecule. One of the commonest systems used is to insert the virus gene of interest in vaccinia virus. This recombinant vaccinia virus (rVV) is used to infect target cells which then express the foreign protein.

DETECTION OF HIV-SPECIFIC CTL FROM SEROPOSITIVE PEOPLE

The first descriptions of HIV-specific CTL were in 1987 from two groups. Bruce Walker and colleagues used a CTL assay based on rVV expressing HIV gene products[31]. They found that eight out of eight seropositive donors had CTL specific for HIV envelope, and three out of eight also had *gag*-specific CTL. Five HIV seronegative donors tested did not recognize either rVV-*env* or rVV-*gag*-infected targets. Freshly isolated peripheral blood mononuclear cells had been used as the source of CTL, without any restimulation *in vitro*. The other group, led by Fernando Plata, used CTL found in bronchoalveolar lavage washings obtained from seropositive patients with lymphocytic alveolitis, again without any *in vitro* restimulation[32]. They tested bronchoalveolar lavage CTL on autologous (HIV-infected) macrophage targets or on P815 targets transfected with HLA-A2 and HIV-*env*. These HIV-specific CTL were $CD8^+$ T cells restricted by class I HLA antigens, the same phenotype as CTL found in most other viral systems.

Many other groups of investigators have confirmed these original findings. Several HIV proteins have now been shown to contain CTL epitopes, and some peptide epitopes have been mapped within these proteins.

HIV-SPECIFIC CTL ARE DIRECTED TO ANTIGENS FOUND IN SEVERAL HIV PROTEINS

HIV-specific CTL have been isolated from peripheral blood, lymph node, cerebrospinal fluid and bronchoalveolar lavage washings of seropositive patients. One striking feature of the HIV-specific CTL response has been the ability to detect CTL directly isolated from freshly separated PBM[31] or alveolar lymphocytes[33], without the need to restimulate memory CTL *in vitro*, which is required for most other virus systems studied. There is discrepancy between various groups as to what proportion of patients have freshly detectable responses, and this probably depends on the clinical status of the patient, time since infection, the target antigen and the assay system. The range appears to be between 15% and 85% of healthy seropositive patients. Nixon and colleagues devised a restimulation strategy to boost the number of HIV-specific CTL in the patients who did not have fresh responses[34]. This has allowed the identification of HIV-specific CTL in the majority of healthy seropositive donors. CTL have been found to *env*, *gag*, *pol*, *nef* and *vif*. It is likely that other proteins such as tat or vpr also contain CTL epitopes. This is in contrast to what had been expected from study of the influenza system where few CTL epitopes had been identified, which had led to the concept of a restricted repertoire of CTL epitopes[35]. HIV-1 contains multiple CTL-reactive sites, in all the structural genes and also some of the regulatory genes.

HIV-SPECIFIC CTL RESPONSES ARE DIRECTED TO PEPTIDE EPITOPES AND ARE HLA RESTRICTED

Identification of peptide epitopes within the proteins was an immediate target for investigation as the knowledge of these peptide epitopes would allow easier growth of CTL clones and their analysis, simplify the CTL assay by shortening it, and give a rational basis for stimulation of HIV-specific CTL based on knowledge of these peptide epitopes.

Peptide epitopes have been defined using restimulated or cloned CTL[36,37], or from fresh PBM[38], tested on target cells incubated with short synthetic peptides covering the protein of interest. A potential problem using cloned CTL is that rare CTL clones may have been expanded in culture, and epitopes defined by this method may not be found in all individuals. Several CTL epitopes have been identified from HIV proteins (see Table 4.1). As most epitopes have been discovered in the past 2 years, confirmation of published epitopes defined by different groups is limited. The identification of these epitopes has led to changes in thinking about CTL epitopes. Firstly, there appear to be many potential CTL sites within HIV proteins, in contrast to predictions from mouse experiments where single epitope sites were identified in *env* or *pol* from immunized mice[39,40]. Secondly, one peptide may be restricted by more than one HLA antigen[41], particularly between distant HLA molecules. Thirdly, several peptide epitopes within one epitope can be restricted by one HLA molecule, i.e. HLA-A11[36], or HLA-B8[37]. CTL epitopes are found in a wide range of sites within the protein, and the existing algorithms devised to predict epitope sites have a low predictive value for the actual epitopes identified. Newer methods for identifying CTL epitopes – such as analysis of naturally produced peptides[26,27], direct binding assays between purified HLA molecules and peptides[42,43] or peptide-induced assembly of class I molecules in mutant cell lines[24,25,44] – when related to the results from *in vitro* assays should rapidly generate information on HIV CTL epitopes.

HIV-2-specific CTL have not been described, but it is likely that the epitope sites are similar in that virus. HIV-1 *gag*-specific CTL recognize the HIV-2 sequence for the HLA-B27 restricted 265-279 *gag* epitope[45].

Table 4.1 CTL peptide epitodes from HIV

Restriction	*A.A. no.*	*Sequence*	*Reference*
GAG			
HLA-B27	265–279	KRWIILGLNKIVRMY	34
HLA-A2	193–203	GHQAAMEMLKE	89
HLA-A2	219–233	HAGPIAPGQMREPRG	89
HLA-A2	446–460	GNFLQSRPEPTAPPA	89
HLA-A2	418–433	KEGHQMKDCTERQANF	89
HLA-B8	255–269	NPPIPVGEIYKRWII	72
POL			
HLA-B8	172–196	IETVPVKLKPGMDGPKVKQPLTEE	36
HLA-Bw60	359–383	DLEIGQHRTKIEELRQHLLRWGLTT	36
HLA-A2	461–485	PLTEEAELELAENREILKEPVHGVY	36
HLA-A11	495–519	EIQKQGQGQWTYQIYQEPFKNLKTG	36
HLA-A11	342–349	NPDIVIYQ	36
HLA-A3.1	203–219	EICTEMEKEGKISKIGP	40
NEF			
HLA-B17/37	113–128	WIYHTQGYFPDWQNYT	41
ENV			
HLA-A2	381–392	RGEFFYCNTTQL	90

CD4$^+$ CLASS II RESTRICTED CTL

The majority of CTL isolated from virally infected animals and humans are CD8$^+$ and MHC class I restricted. CD4$^+$ class II restricted T cells with cytolytic potential have been isolated after *in vitro* culture following some viral infections – measles[46], influenza[47,48], herpes simplex[49], VSV[50], and HIV[51]. Primary $CD4^+$ class II restricted CTL have also been generated *in vitro* to HIV envelope protein[52,53]. The *in vivo* significance of such cytotoxic cells, which are usually detected after *in vitro* culture, is uncertain, although there are important theoretical consequences of such cells, both in a possible immunoregulatory role and as a way that viruses might exploit to generate a systemic immunosuppression[54]. The compartmentalization of processing requirements for presentation to class I- or class II-restricted T cells[55], with class I recognition of endogenously synthesized antigens and class II recognition of exogenous antigens, is not likely to be absolute – Rock and colleagues have shown that certain splenic antigen-presenting cells incubated with exogenous native ovalbumin can take up, process and present this protein in association with MHC class I molecules[56].

Certain vaccination protocols have stimulated $CD4^+$ CTL, and these include vaccination of chimpanzees[57] and humans[58] with a recombinant vaccinia virus containing the HIV-1 envelope gene. $CD4^+$ CTL specific for HIV appear to be very rare following HIV infection, and the role of these cells in the natural infection is unclear. If they were infected by HIV they might themselves become targets for CTL lysis.

SOME SERONEGATIVE PATIENTS APPEAR TO HAVE HIV-SPECIFIC CTL

An unusual and unexpected finding was that some HIV seronegative patients could have HIV-specific CTL induced in *in vitro* culture by stimulation with irradiated HIV superinfected lymphoblasts[32,33,59] and tested on P815-A2-*env*, *gag* or *nef* transfectants in an 18-h ^{51}Cr release assay. These CTL, apparently class I restricted, are in contrast to the *env*-specific class II restricted $CD4^+$ T cells that have been generated in seronegative donors with repeated *in vitro* stimulation with gp120[52,53] or to the T-helper cells from seronegative donors which proliferated specifically to HIV peptides (P. Beverley, personal communication). CTL specific for *env* and *nef*, but not *gag*, can be detected by the specific restimulation method used by this group from seronegative donors[59]. No other group has directly compared stimulation strategies with this group for seronegatives, but without stimulation CTL cannot be detected in seronegative low-risk individuals (Nixon *et al.*, unpublished observations; Y. Riviere, B. Walker and S. Koenig, personal communication).

THE ROLE OF HIV-SPECIFIC CTL IN HIV DISEASE

CTL have anti-HIV activity

Preliminary evidence suggests that HIV-specific CTL are mainly beneficial in HIV disease. The majority of long-term survivors in a cohort of

HIV-infected homosexuals had *gag*-specific CTL[60], as did a group of long-term HIV-infected patients in Africa (F. Gotch, personal communication). Healthy seropositive patients have a very high frequency of *gag*-specific CTL over a period of 2 years. Such an active level of CTL declines with disease progression (Nixon *et al.*, unpublished observations[33,61]), as does the CTL precursor frequency[33,61]. Possible reasons for the decline in CTL response are discussed below. $CD8^+$ T cells have been shown to have anti-HIV or anti-SIV activity *in vitro* – Kannagi and colleagues[62] initially showed that Con-A activated PBM of SIV_{mac}-infected monkeys did not generate reverse transcriptase activity, unless $CD8^+$ T cells were deleted from those cultures. Addition of autologous $CD8^+$ cells to the $CD8^+$-depleted cultures inhibited the viral replication. These investigators then extended their observations using cultures from SIV-infected monkeys or HIV-infected humans, and demonstrated that the $CD8^+$-dependent virus inhibition was MHC restricted and could be inhibited by anti-CD8 and anti-LFA mAbs, suggesting that the cell responsible was a CTL and that cell-to-cell contact was necessary[63]. In another experimental system Kannagi and colleagues[64] showed that PBM from healthy seropositive humans showed no virus replication following addition of exogenous HIV in contrast to PBM from seronegatives or patients with AIDS. When $CD8^+$ T cells were removed prior to adding exogenous HIV, PBM from healthy seropositives lost their ability to suppress virus replication. These studies implicated the class I restricted CTL in the control of virus replication but did not formally prove this. Johnson and colleagues[65] demonstrated anti-HIV activity of cloned CTL by showing *in vitro* reduction of p24 antigen production when cloned *pol*-specific CTL were mixed with HLA-matched, but not mismatched, activated T lymphoblasts infected with HIV. Reduction of viral titre occurred in those cultures with added CTL in an MHC-restricted manner. It is not known if virus was eliminated from these cultures as detection of viral genome by polymerase chain reaction was not performed. Collectively these studies suggest that HIV-specific CTL can suppress virus replication *in vitro*, and thus may be the major control of virus replication *in vivo*. The mechanisms of CTL control of virus replication is not known. Two groups have investigated possible soluble factors released by T cells with anti-HIV 'suppressive' activity[66,67]. Not all HIV-infected healthy seropositives appear to have this factor[68]. Brinchmann and colleagues[67] have used positive magnetic bead selection of $CD8^+$ T cells from healthy seropositives to isolate a factor from them responsible for reducing virus replication. The suppressive factor did not function in an MHC-restricted manner, suggesting a non-antigen-specific factor. Confirmation of such a factor, and analysis of the mechanism for reduction in virus replication, are important to establish, for such anti-HIV activity may be of great benefit for the infected individual.

The evidence for a beneficial role for HIV-specific CTL is strong, but will require careful analysis of CTL specificity. Evidence of an *in vivo* role for lentivirus-specific CTL in virus reduction may come from adoptive transfer experiments in the HIV-infected reconstituted immunodeficient SCID-hu mouse and SIV-infected primates, or a direct demonstration of reduction in virus titre after selective CTL stimulation *in vivo*.

CTL ACTIVITY DECLINES WITH DISEASE PROGRESSION

Several investigators have shown a decline in CTL activity with disease progression in the small number of patients studied (Nixon *et al.*, unpublished observations[33,61,69]), or a failure in the ability of AIDS patients' $CD8^+$ PBM to control virus replication[64]. If the $CD8^+$ T cell population is predominantly responsible for maintaining a low virus load, what factors lead to the loss of this control? One possibility is that $CD8^+$ HIV-specific CTL can be infected with HIV[63] and therefore become potential targets for CTL attack themselves. A possible mechanism for HIV entry into these cells has been demonstrated by Lusso *et al*: infection of $CD8^+$ cells with the herpes virus HHV-6 induces CD4 expression on these $CD8^+$ cells[70]. Another possibility is suppression of CTL by suppressor cells[61]. Joly *et al.* identified a population of 'suppressive' $CD8^+HNK1^+CD4^-CD16^-$ T cells from AIDS patients which inhibited anti-HIV CTL, as well as anti-HLA CTL, in an MHC-unrestricted manner. In contrast to this broad suppression of CTL reactivity Pantaleo and colleagues[69] found a selective decline in HIV-specific CTL but not broad cytolytic activity in AIDS patients. They also looked for $CD8^+HNK1^+$ cells in their patients, and found no difference in numbers of these cells between AIDS patients and healthy seropositives. They suggest $CD8^+$ T cells in AIDS patients have a defective clonogenic potential[71]. Gotch and colleagues[72] have also suggested the high level of circulating HIV-specific CTL in healthy HIV seropositive patients represents a terminally differentiated population of effector cells, perhaps through constant antigenic stimulation.

Possible immunopathological role for HIV-specific CTL

It has been shown that gp120 can also selectively bind to activated $CD4^+$ T cells in a way that results in its capture, processing and selective class II restricted presentation[52,53]. These gp120-specific T cells could then be recognized and killed by gp120-specific class II restricted cytotoxic T cells, as has been suggested by Lanzavecchia[54]. This mechanism has now been shown to occur post-vaccination with vac-*env*. Orentas and colleagues[58] detected $CD4^+$ class II restricted *env*-specific CTL clones in vac-*env* immunized individuals which could lyse non-infected autologous $CD4^+$ lymphoblasts pulsed with supernatants from infected cultures. $CD4^+$ CTL following natural infection have been detected only from cloned PBM from the CSF of an infected patient[51]. It is possible that these cells are contributing to neuropathology. The rarity of $CD4^+$ CTL detected from peripheral blood mononuclear cell preparations may only reflect the *in vitro* culture conditions or pool of effector cells in the blood. If this mechanism was found to operate in HIV infection selective suppression of *env*-specific CTL could be advantageous. CTL lysis of uninfected $CD4^+$ cells by envelope-specific CTL have been observed in HIV seropositive humans but not HIV-infected chimpanzees[73]. Such lysis could contribute to the decline in CD4 cell numbers. Cells expressing antigen in a form that can be recognized by CTL, but not producing virus, could also become targets for lysis and reduce the CD4 cell pool.

Possible target cells could be quiescent T cells[74] or T cells containing HIV mutants[75]. If defective HIV particles are produced, then taken up and processed by antigen-presenting cells, these cells could also be targets for CTL lysis.

Selective stimulation of CTL

$CD8^+$ CTL usually recognize viral antigen presented by class I molecules. Live virus infection primes a strong class I restricted response by endogenous expression of protein. Secondary CTL responses *in vitro* have been attempted with proteins with variable results. Influenza haemagglutinin could stimulate CTL response *in vitro*[76,77]. Protein could be presented to CTL when it was inserted in the cytoplasm by pinosome fusion[78]. Proteins could also sensitize target cells at high concentrations[79]. The uptake and compartmentalization of proteins is not absolute, and the antigen-presenting cells in the culture could be crucial in determining the fate of such proteins[56]. For vaccine development it is important to understand the delivery conditions necessary to induce CTL by non-infectious pathogens or components of protein fragment or peptides. Most proteins are able to induce $CD4^+$ T-helper cells. Chemically inactivated viruses with strong membrane fusion activity can induce specific CTL *in vivo*[80]. A primary CTL response to simian virus 5 was elicited by a peptide presented on killed and fixed *Staphylococcus aureus* coated with anti-SV5 MAb, which then trapped components of SV5[81].

Definition of peptide epitopes has led to many attempts to prime class I restricted CTL in animal models by inoculation of known peptide epitopes into responder animals. The responses have been variable[82]. Carbone and Bevan used a long ovalbumin peptide in high concentration to induce CTL[83].

Other successful approaches have used peptide coupled to palmitic acid and inserted into a liposome structure[84], emulsified in incomplete Freund's adjuvant[85], with an added lipid tail[86] or immunizing with peptides complexed in an ISCOM[87]. Other delivery systems able to replicate *in vivo*, such as recombinant *Salmonella typhimurium*[88], may be of use. Selective stimulation of class I restricted CTL is an area of current active research interest.

Immunoprophylaxis based on stimulation of HIV-specific CTL

Stimulation of selective parts of the immune system, based on the knowledge of epitopes, may help patients in prolonging effective anti-HIV activity and slow up the progression to AIDS. Experimental therapy along these lines has been tried for antibody responses. Such a therapy based on adoptive transfer of autologous CTL would be feasible, but presents formidable problems. A simpler approach could use peptide vaccines to specifically stimulate HIV CTL.

FUTURE TRENDS

The understanding of the HIV-specific CTL response is crucial in the development of therapeutic strategies for boosting immune responses in infected individuals, and in developing effective vaccines to prevent infection with all types of HIV. Longitudinal study of CTL responses to all known target antigens would provide information on responses to each antigen in individual patients, and correlation with disease progression might relate to presence or absence of CTL to a particular antigen. The knowledge of HIV CTL epitopes will allow formulation of subunit vaccines based on these sites, which can be tried both prophylactically and therapeutically.

Stages of the disease where little information is available on the HIV-specific CTL response include the CTL response to HIV in infants born to seropositive mothers, and the CTL response immediately after infection. Acute HIV infection is associated with an HIV viraemia which is reduced prior to the rise in specific HIV antibodies, suggesting cell-mediated immunity is important in the initial suppression of virus load. HIV-specific CTL may also be important in preventing transmission of HIV from mother to child. The role of HIV-specific CTL in the pathogenesis of HIV disease, and their influence on vaccines, should become apparent in the near future.

References

1. Yap, K. L. and Ada, G. L. (1978). Cytotoxic T cells in the lungs of mice infected with influenza A virus. *Scand. J. Immunol.*, **7**, 73–80
2. Lin, Y. and Askonas, B. A. (1981). Biological properties of an influenza A virus specific killer T cell clone. *J. Exp. Med.*, **154**, 225–34
3. Wells, M. A., Albrecht, P. and Ennis, F. A. (1981). Recovery from a viral respiratory infection. I. Influenza pneumonia in normal and T-deficient mice. *J. Immunol.*, **126**, 1036–41
4. Lightman, S., Cobbold, S., Waldmann, H. and Askonas, B. A. (1987). Do $L3T4^+$ T cells act as effector cells in protection against influenza virus infection? *Immunology*, **62**, 139–44
5. Buller, R. M. L., Holmes, K. L., Hugin, A., Frederickson, T. N. and Morse, H. C. (1987). Induction of cytotoxic T-cell responses *in vivo* in the absence of CD4 helper cells. *Nature*, **328**, 77–9
6. Engers, H. D., La Haye, T., Sorensen, G. D., Glasebrook, A. L., Horvath, C. and Brunner, K. T. (1984). Functional activity in vivo of effector T cell populations. II. Anti-tumor activity exhibited by syngeneic anti-MoMuLV-specific cytolytic T cell clones. *J. Immunol.*, **154**, 951–63
7. McMichael, A. J., Gotch, F. M., Noble, G. R. and Beare, P. A. S. (1983). Cytoxic T-cell immunity to influenza. *N. Engl. J. Med.*, **309**, 13–17
8. Moss, D. J., Rickinson, A. B. and Pope, J. H. (1978). Long-term T cell mediated immunity to Epstein–Barr virus in man. 1. Complete regression of virus-induced transformation in cultures of seropositive donor leukocytes. *Int. J. Cancer*, **22**, 662–8
9. Rickinson, A. B., Moss, D. J., Allen, D. J., Wallace, L. E., Rowe, M. and Epstein, M. A. (1981). Reactivation of Epstein–Barr virus-specific cytotoxic T cells by in vitro stimulation with autologous lymphoblastoid cell line. *Int. J. Cancer*, **27**, 593–601
10. Borysiewicz, L. K., Morris, S. M., Page, J. and Sissons, J. G. (1983). Human cytomegalovirus-specific cytotoxic T-lymphocytes: requirements for in vitro generation and specificity. *Eur. J. Immunol.*, **13**, 804–9
11. Schultz, K. R., Klarnet, J. P., Gieni, R. S., Hay Glass, K. T. and Greenberg, P. D. (1990). The role of B cells for *in vivo* T cell responses to a Friend virus-induced leukaemia. *Science*, **249**, 921–2
12. Mitsuya, H., Matis, L. A., Megson, M., Bunn, P. A., Murray, C., Mann, D. L., Gallo, R. C. and Broder, S. (1983). Generation of an HLA-restricted cytotoxic T cell line reactive against cultured tumor cells from a patient infected with human T cell leukaemia/lymphoma virus. *J. Exp. Med.*, **158**, 994–9

13. Kannagi, M., Sugamura, K., Sato, H., Okochi, K., Uchino, H. and Hinuma, Y. (1983). Establishment of human cytotoxic T cell lines specific for human adult T cell leukaemia virus-bearing cells. *J. Immunol.*, **130**, 2942–6
14. Jacobson, S., Shida, H., McFarlin, D. E., Fauci, A. S. and Koenig, S. (1990). Circulating $CD8^+$ cytotoxic T lymphocytes specific for HTLV-1 pX in patients with HTLV-1 associated neurological disease. *Nature*, **348**, 245–8
15. Zinkernagel, R. M. and Doherty, P. C. (1974). Restriction of in vitro cell-mediated cytotoxicity in lymphocytic choriomeningitis within a syngeneic or semiallogeneic system. *Nature*, **248**, 701–2
16. Bennink, J. R., Yewdell, J. W. and Gerhard, W. (1982). A viral polymerase involved in recognition of influenza-infected cells by a cytotoxic T cell clone. *Nature*, **296**, 75–6
17. Townsend, A. R. M., McMichael, A. J., Carter, N. P., Huddleston, J. A. and Brownlee, G. G. (1984). Cytotoxic T cell recognition of the influenza nucleoprotein and haemagglutinin expressed in transfected mouse L cells. *Cell*, **39**, 13–25
18. Kees, U. and Krammer, P. H. (1984). Most influenza A-virus specific memory cytotoxic T lymphocytes react with antigenic epitopes associated with internal virus determinants. *J. Exp. Med.*, **159**, 365–77
19. Townsend, A. R. M., Gotch, F. M. and Davey, J. (1985). Cytotoxic T cells recognize fragments of influenza nucleoprotein. *Cell*, **42**, 457–67
20. Townsend, A. R. M., Rothbard, J., Gotch, F. M., Bahadur, G., Wraith, D. and McMichael, A. J. (1986). The epitopes of influenza nucleoprotein recognised by cytotoxic T lymphocytes can be defined with short synthetic peptides. *Cell*, **44**, 959–68
21. Bjorkman, P. J., Saper, M. A., Samraoui, B., Bennet, W. S., Strominger, J. L. and Wiley, D. C. (1987). Structure of the human class 1 histocompatibility antigen, HLA-A2. *Nature*, **329**, 506–12
22. Bjorkman, P. J., Saper, M. A., Samraoui, B., Bennett, W. S., Strominger, J. L. and Wiley, D. C. (1987). The foreign antigen binding site and T cell recognition regions of class 1 histocompatibility antigens. *Nature*, **329**, 512–18
23. Garrett, T. P. J., Saper, M. A., Bjorkman, P. J., Strominger, J. L. and Wiley, D. C. (1989). Specificity pockets for the side chains of peptide antigens in HLA-Aw68. *Nature*, **342**, 692–6
24. Townsend, A., Ohlen, C., Bastin, J., Ljunggren, H. G., Foster, L. and Karre, K. (1989). Association of class 1 major histocompatibility heavy and light chains induced by viral peptides. *Nature*, **340**, 443–8
25. Ljunggren, H.-G., Stan, N. J., Ohlen, C., Neefjes, J. J., Hoglund, P., Heemels, M.-T., Bastin, J., Schumacher, T. N. M., Townsend, A., Karre, K. and Pleogh, H. L. (1990). Empty MHC class 1 molecules come out in the cold. *Nature*, **346**, 476–80
26. Van Bleek, G. M. and Nathenson, S. G. (1990). Isolation of an endogenously processed immunodominant viral peptide from the class 1 H-$2K^b$ molecule. *Nature*, **348**, 213–16
27. Rotzschke, O., Falk, K., Deres, K., Schild, H., Norda, M., Metzger, J., Jung, G. and Rammensee, H.-G. (1990). Isolation and analysis of naturally processed viral peptides as recognized by cytotoxic T cells. *Nature*, **348**, 252–4
28. Falk, K., Rotzschke, O. and Rammensee, H.-G. (1990). Cellular peptide composition governed by major histocompatibility complex class 1 molecules. *Nature*, **348**, 248–51
29. Brunner, K. T., Mauel, J., Cerottini, J. C. and Chapuis, B. (1968). Quantitative assay of the lytic action of immune lymphoid cells on ^{51}Cr-labelled allogeneic target cells *in vitro*: inhibition by isoantibody and by drugs. *Immunology*, **14**, 181–96
30. McMichael, A. J., Ting, A., Zweerink, H. J. and Askonas, B. A. (1977). HLA restriction of cell mediated lysis of influenza virus infected human cells. *Nature*, **270**, 524
31. Walker, B. D., Chakrabarti, S., Moss, B., Paradis, T. J., Flynn, T., Durno, A. G., Blumberg, R., Kaplan, J. C., Hirsch, M. S. and Schooley, R. T. (1987). HIV-specific cytotoxic T lymphocytes in seropositive individuals. *Nature*, **328**, 345–8
32. Plata, F., Autran, B., Martins, L. P., Wain-Hobson, S., Raphael, M., Mayaud, C., Denis, M., Guillon, J.-M. and Debre, P. (1987). AIDS virus-specific T lymphocytes in lung disorders. *Nature*, **328**, 348–51
33. Hoffenbach, A., Langlade-Demoyen, P., Dadaglio, G., Vilmer, E., Michel, F., Mayaud, C., Autran, B. and Plata, F. (1989). Unusually high frequencies of HIV-specific cytotoxic T lymphocytes in humans. *J. Immunol.*, **142**, 452–62
34. Nixon, D. F., Townsend, A. R. M., Elvin, J. G., Rizza, C. R., Gallwey, J. and McMichael, A. J. (1988). HIV-1 gag-specific cytotoxic T lymphocytes defined with recombinant vaccinia

virus and synthetic peptides. *Nature*, **336**, 484–7
35. Bennink, J. R. and Yewdell, J. W. (1988). Murine cytotoxic T lymphocyte recognition of individual influenza virus proteins. High frequency of nonresponder MHC class 1 alleles. *J. Exp. Med.*, **168**, 1935–9
36. Walker, B. D., Flexner, C., Birch-Limberger, K., Fisher, L., Paradis, T. J., Aldovini, A., Young, R., Moss, B. and Schooley, R. T. (1989). Long-term culture and fine specificity of human cytotoxic T-lymphocyte clones reactive with human immunodeficiency virus type 1. *Proc. Natl. Acad. Sci.*, **86**, 9514–18
37. Nixon, D. F. and McMichael, A. J. (1991). Cytotoxic T cell recognition of HIV proteins and peptides. *AIDS* (in press)
38. Koenig, S., Fuerst, T. R., Wood, L. V., Woods, R. M., Suzich, J. A., Jones, G. M., de la Cruz, V. F., Davey, R. T., Venkatesan, S., Moss, B., Biddison, W. E. and Fauci, A. S. (1990). Mapping the fine specificity of a cytolytic T cell response to HIV-1 nef protein. *J. Immunol.*, **145**, 127–35
39. Takahashi, H., Chen, J., Hosmalin, A., Cease, K. B., Houghton, R., Cornette, J. L., DeLisi, C., Moss, B., Germain, R. N. and Berzofsky, J. A. (1988) An immunodominant epitope of the human immunodeficiency virus envelope glycoprotein gp160 recognized by class 1 major histocompatibility complex molecule-restricted murine cytotoxic T lymphoctyes. *Proc. Natl. Acad. Sci.*, **85**, 3105–9
40. Hosmalin, A., Clerici, M., Houghten, R., Pendleton, C. D., Flexner, C., Lucey, D. R., Moss, B., Germain, R. N., Shearer, G. M. and Berzofsky, J. A. (1990). An epitope in human immunodeficiency virus 1 reverse transcriptase recognized by both mouse and human cytotoxic T lymphocytes. *Proc. Natl. Acad. Sci.*, **87**, 2344–8
41. Culmann, B., Gomard, E., Kieny, M.-P., Guy, B., Dreyfus, F., Saimot, A.-G., Sereni, D. and Levy, J.-P. (1989). An antigenic peptide of the HIV-1 NEF protein recognized by cytotoxic T lymphocytes of seropositive individuals in association with different HLA-B molecules. *Eur. J. Immunol.*, **19**, 2383–6
42. Frelinger, J. A., Gotch, F. M., Zweerink, H., Wain, E. and McMichael, A. J. (1990). Evidence of widespread binding of HLA class 1 molecules to peptides. *J. Exp. Med.*, **172**, 827–34
43. Choppin, J., Martinon, F., Gomard, E., Bahraoui, E., Connan, F., Bouillot, M. and Levy, J.-P. (1990). Analysis of physical interactions between peptides and HLA molecules and application to the detection of human immunodeficiency virus 1 antigenic peptides. *J. Exp. Med.*, **172**, 889–99
44. Cerundolo, V., Alexander, J., Lamb, C., Cresswell, P., McMichael, A., Gotch, F. M. and Townsend, A. (1990). Presentation of viral antigen controlled by a gene in the MHC. *Nature*, **345**, 449–52
45. Nixon, D. F., Huet, S., Rothbard, J., Kieny, M.-P., Delchambre, M., Thiriart, C., Rizza, C. R., Gotch, F. M. and McMichael, A. J. (1990). An HIV-1 and HIV-2 cross-reactive cytotoxic T-cell epitope. *AIDS*, **4**, 841–5
46. Jacobson, S., Richert, J. R., Biddison, W. E., Satinsky, A., Hartzman, R. J. and McFarland, H. F. (1984). Measles virus-specific $T4^+$ human cytotoxic T cell clones are restricted by class II HLA antigens. *J. Immunol.*, **133**, 754–7
47. Kaplan, D. R., Griffith, R., Braciale, V. L. and Braciale, T. J. (1984). Influenza virus-specific human cytotoxic T cell clones: heterogeneity in antigenic specificity and restriction by class II MHC products. *Cell. Immunol.*, **88**, 193–206
48. Hioe, C. E. and Hinshaw, V. S. (1989). Induction and activity of class II-restricted, $LyT\text{-}2^+$ ctytolytic T lymphocytes specific for the influenza H5 hemagglutinin. *J. Immunol.*, **142**, 2482–8
49. Yasukawa, M. and Zarling, J. M. (1984). Human cytotoxic T cell clones directed against herpes simplex virus-infected cells. 1. Lysis restricted by HLA class II MB and DR antigens. *J. Immunol.*, **133**, 422–27
50. Browning, M. J., Huang, A. S. and Reiss, C. S. (1990). Cytolytic T lymphocytes from the $BALB/C\text{-}H\text{-}2^{dm^2}$ mouse recognize the vesicular stomatitis virus glycoprotein and are restricted by class II MHC antigens. *J. Immunol.*, **145**, 985–94
51. Sethi, K. K., Naher, H. and Stroehmann, I. (1988). Phenotypic heterogeneity of cerebrospinal fluid-derived HIV-specific and HLA-restricted cytotoxic T-cell clones. *Nature*, **335**, 178–81
52. Lanzavecchia, A., Roosnek, E., Gregory, T., Berman, P. and Abrignani, S. (1988). T cells can present antigens such as HIV gp120 targeted to their own surface molecules. *Nature*, **334**, 530–2

53. Siliciano, R. F., Lawton, T., Knall, C., Karr, R. W., Berman, P., Gregory, T. and Reinherz, E. L. (1988). Analysis of host-virus interactions in AIDS with anti-gp120 T cell clones: effect of HIV sequence variation and a mechanism for CD4$^+$ cell depletion. *Cell*, **54**, 561–75
54. Lanzavecchia, A. (1989). Is suppression a function of class II-restricted cytotoxic T cells? *Immunol. Today*, **10**, 157–9
55. Germain, R. N. (1986). The ins and outs of antigen processing and presentation. *Nature*, **322**, 687–9
56. Rock, K. L., Gamble, S. and Rothstein, L. (1990). Presentation of exogenous antigen with class 1 major histocompatibility complex molecules. *Science*, **249**, 918–21
57. Zarling, J. M., Eichberg, J. W., Moran, P. A., McClure, J., Sridhar, P. and Hu, S.-L. (1987). Proliferative and cytotoxic T cells to AIDS virus glycoproteins in chimpanzees immunized with a recombinant vaccinia virus expressing AIDS virus envelope glycoproteins. *J. Immunol.*, **139**, 988–90
58. Orentas, R. J., Hildreth, J. E. K., Obah, E., Polydefkis, M., Smith, G. E., Clements, M. L. and Siliciano, R. F. (1990). Induction of CD4$^+$ human cytolytic T cells specific for HIV-infected cells by a gp160 subunit vaccine. *Science*, **248**, 1234–7
59. Chenciner, N., Michel, F., Dadaglio, G., Langlade-Demoyen, P., Hoffenbach, A., Leroux, A., Garcia-Pons, F., Rautmann, G., Guy, B., Guillon, J.-M., Mayaud, C., Girard, M., Autran, B., Kieny, M.-P., and Plata, F. (1989). Multiple subsets of HIV-specific cytotoxic T lymphocytes in humans and in mice. *Eur. J. Immunol.*, **19**, 1537–44
60. Mawle, A. C., Ridgeway, M. R., Kieny, M.-P. and Lifson, A. R. (1990). CTL response to p24 (gag) in long-term asymptomatic seropositive individuals infected with HIV-1. 6th International Conference on AIDS, San Francisco, USA: Abstract SA 254
61. Joly, P., Guillon, J.-M., Mayaud, C., Plata, F., Theodorou, I., Denis, M., Debre, P. and Autran, B. (1989). Cell-mediated suppression of HIV-specific cytotoxic T lymphocytes. *J. Immunol.*, **143**, 2193–201
62. Kannagi, M., Chalifoux, L. V., Lord, C. I. and Letvin, N. L. (1988). Suppression of simian immunodeficiency virus replication *in vitro* by CD8$^+$ lymphocytes. *J. Immunol.*, **140**, 2237–42
63. Tsubota, H., Lord, C. I., Watkins, D. I., Morimoto, C. and Letvin, N. L. (1989). A cytotoxic T lymphocyte inhibits acquired immunodeficiency syndrome virus replication in peripheral blood lymphocytes. *J. Exp. Med.*, **169**, 1421–34
64. Kannagi, M., Masuda, T., Hattori, T., Kanoh, T., Nasu, K., Yamamoto, N. and Harada, S. (1990). Interference with human immunodeficiency virus (HIV) replication by CD8$^+$ T cells in peripheral blood leukocytes of asymptomatic HIV carriers in vitro. *J. Virol.*, **64**, 3399–406
65. Johnson, R. P., Trocha, A., Mazzara, G., Panicali, D. and Walker, B. D. (1990). Propagation and analysis of HIV-1 gag-specific cytotoxic T cell clones. 6th International Conference on AIDS, San Francisco, USA: Abstract SA 261
66. Walker, C. M., Moody, D. J., Stites, D. P. and Levy, J. A. (1986). CD8$^+$ lymphocytes can control HIV infection *in vitro* by suppressing virus replication. *Science*, **234**, 1563–6
67. Brinchmann, J. E., Gaudernack, G. and Vartdal, F. (1990). CD8$^+$ T cells inhibit HIV replication in naturally infected CD4$^+$ T cells. Evidence for a soluble inhibitor. *J. Immunol.*, **144**, 2961–6
68. Walker, C. M., Moody, D. P., Stites, D. P. and Levy, J. A. (1989). CD8$^+$ lymphocyte control of HIV replication in cultured CD4$^+$ cells varies among infected individuals. *Cell. Immunol.*, **119**, 470–5
69. Pantaleo, G., De Maria, A., Koenig, S., Butini, L., Moss, B., Baseler, M., Lane, H. C. and Fauci, A. S. (1990). CD8$^+$ T lymphocytes of patients with AIDS maintain normal broad cytolytic function despite the loss of human immunodeficiency virus-specific cytotoxicity. *Proc. Natl. Acad. Sci.*, **87**, 4818–22
70. Lusso, P., De Maria, A., Malnati, M., Lori, F., DeRocco, S. E., Baseler, M. and Gallo, R. C. (1991). Induction of CD4 and susceptibility to HIV-1 infection in human CD8$^+$ T lymphocytes by human herpesvirus 6. *Nature*, **349**, 533–5
71. Pantaleo, G., Koenig, S., Baseler, M., Lane, H. C. and Fauci, A. S. (1990). Defective clonogenic potential of CD8$^+$ T lymphocytes in patients with AIDS. *J. Immunol.*, **144**, 1696–704
72. Gotch, F. M., Nixon, D. F., Alp, N., McMichael, A. and Borysiewicz, L. K. (1990). High frequency of memory and effector gag specific cytotoxic T lymphocytes in HIV seropositive individuals. *Int. Immunol.*, **2**, 707–12
73. Zarling, J. M., Ledbetter, J. A., Sias, J., Fultz, P., Eichberg, J., Gjerset, G. and Moran, P.

A. (1990). HIV-infected humans, but not chimpanzees, have circulating cytotoxic T lymphocytes that lyse uninfected CD4$^+$ cells. *J. Immunol.*, **144**, 2992–8

74. Zack, J. A., Arrigo, S. J., Weitsman, S. R., Go, A. S., Haislip, A. and Chen, I. S. Y. (1990). HIV-1 entry into quiescent primary lymphocytes: molecular analysis reveals a labile, latent viral structure. *Cell*, **61**, 213–22
75. Stevenson, M., Haggerty, S., Lamonica, C. A., Meier, C. M., Welch, S.-K., and Wasiak, A. J. (1990). Integration is not necessary for expression of human immunodeficiency virus type 1 protein products. *J. Virol.*, **64**, 2421–5
76. Braciale, T. J. (1979). Specificity of cytotoxicity T cells directed to influenza virus hemagglutinin. *J. Exp. Med.*, **149**, 856–69
77. Zweerink, H. J., Askonas, B. A., Millican, D., Courtneidge, S. A. and Skehel, J. J. (1977). Cytotoxic T cells to type A influenza virus; viral hemagglutinin induces A-strain specificity while infected cells confer cross-reactive cytotoxicity. *Eur. J. Immunol.*, **7**, 630–5
78. Moore, M. W., Carbone, F. R. and Bevan, M. J. (1988). Introduction of soluble protein into the class I pathway of antigen processing and presentation. *Cell*, **54**, 777–85
79. Bastin, J.,, Rothbard, J., Davey, J., Jones, I. and Townsend, A. (1987). Use of synthetic peptides of influenza nucleoprotein to define epitopes recognized by class 1 restricted cytotoxic T lymphocytes. *J. Exp. Med.*, **165**, 1508–23
80. Bangham, C. R., Cannon, M. J., Karzan, D. T. and Askonas, B. A. (1985). Cytotoxic T cell response to respiratory syncytial virus in mice. *J. Virol.*, **56**, 55–9
81. Randall, R. E. and Young, D. F. (1988). Humoral and cytotoxic T cell immune responses to internal and external structural proteins of simian virus 5 induced by immunization with solid matrix–antibody–antigen complexes. *J. Gen Virol.*, **69**, 2505–16
82. McMichael, A. J. (1991). The role of class 1 molecules of the major histocompatibility complex in cytotoxic T cell function in health and disease. *Springer Sem. Immunopathol.* (in press)
83. Carbone, F. R. and Bevan, M. J. (1989). Induction of ovalbumin-specific cytotoxic T cells by *in vivo* peptide immunization. *J. Exp. Med.*, **169**, 603–12
84. Watanari, E., Dietzchold, B., Szokan, G. and Heber-Katz, E. (1987). A synthetic peptide induces long-term protection from lethal infection with herpes simplex virus 2. *J. Exp. Med.*, **165**, 459–70
85. Aichele, P., Hengartner, H., Zinkernagel, R. M. and Schulz, M. (1990). Antiviral cytotoxic T cell response induced by in vivo priming with a free synthetic peptide. *J. Exp. Med.*, **171**, 1815–20
86. Deres, K., Schild, H., Weismuller, K. H., Jung, G. and Rammensee, H. G. (1989). In vivo priming of virus-specific cytotoxic T lymphocytes with synthetic lipopeptide vaccine. *Nature*, **342**, 561–4
87. Takahashi, H. H., Takeshita, T., Morein, B., Putney, S., Germain, R. N. and Berzofsky, J. A. (1990). Induction of CD8$^+$ cytotoxic T cells by immunization with purified HIV-1 envelope protein in ISCOMs. *Nature*, **344**, 873–5
88. Aggarwal, A., Kumar, S., Jaffe, R., Hone, D., Gross, M. and Sadoff, J. (1990). Oral salmonella: malaria circumsporozoite recombinants induce specific CD8$^+$ cytotoxic T cells. *J. Exp. Med.*, **172**, 1083–90
89. Claverie, J.-M., Kourilsky, P., Langlade-Demoyen, P., Chalufour-Prochnicka, A., Dadaglio, G., Tekaia, F., Plata, F. and Bougueleret, L. (1988). T-immunogenic peptides are constituted of rare sequence patterns. Use in the identification of T epitopes in the human immunodeficiency virus gag protein. *Eur. J. Immunol.*, **18**, 1547–53
90. Plata, F., Dadaglio, G., Chenciner, N., Hoffenbach, A., Wain-Hobson, S., Michel, F. and Langlade-Demoyen, P. (1989). T lymphocytes in HIV-induced disease: implications for therapy and vaccination. *Immunodef. Rev.*, **1**, 227–46

5
Lymphocyte functional analysis in HIV infection: mechanisms and clinical relevance

R. A. GRUTERS and F. MIEDEMA

INTRODUCTION

Acquired immunodeficiency syndrome (AIDS) is the collective name for many disease manifestations in the final stages of an infection with the human immunodeficiency virus (HIV)[1]. Development of disease is associated with a severe depletion of $CD4^+$ T cells[2,3], which have been shown to be the main target for HIV[4–6]. The central role of T-helper cells with this $CD4^+$ phenotype in regulation of several immune responses may explain the severe immune dysfunction in AIDS. However, it is unlikely that the mere depletion of $CD4^+$ T cells can explain the wide range of humoral and cellular abnormalities, including T-helper function[2,3,7,8], specific and non-specific cytotoxic activities[9–11], B-cell[2,3,8] and monocyte function[8,9,12,13]. Furthermore, immunological abnormalities have been observed in asymptomatic HIV-infected people with normal $CD4^+$ T cell numbers, indicating that HIV affects the immune system before T cell depletion ensues.

IMMUNE DYSFUNCTION IN EARLY HIV INFECTION

B cell function

Immunological abnormalities can be demonstrated not only in patients showing clinical signs of HIV infection, but also in asymptomatic HIV-infected individuals. Indeed, evidence has been obtained that HIV infection affects the immune system before $CD4^+$ T cell depletion occurs.

The number of circulating B cells in HIV-infected individuals is within the normal range, but phenotypical changes are observed. An increase in the

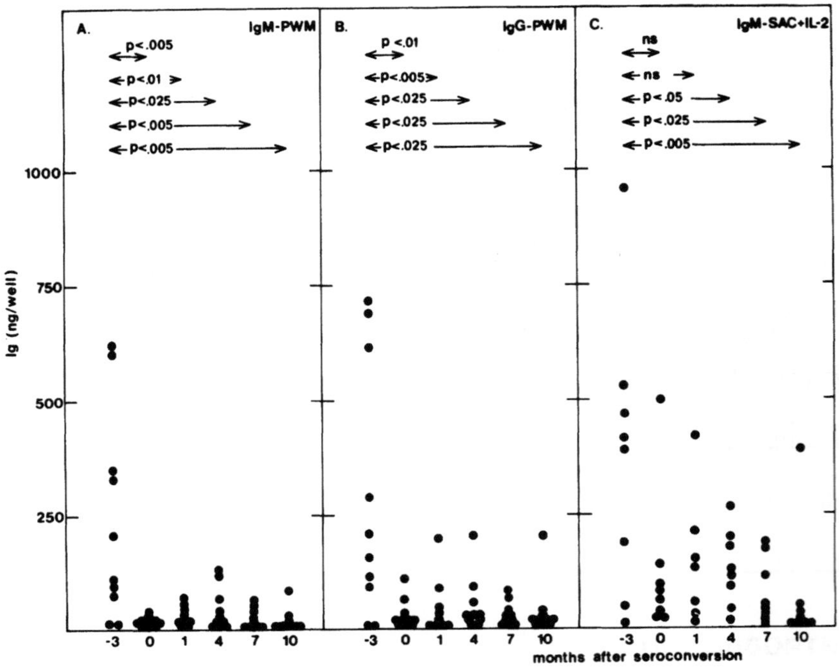

Figure 5.1 Ig production by peripheral blood mononuclear cells from 10 homosexuals prior to and after seroconversion. Cultures (80 000 cells/well) were stimulated with PWM, or formaldehyde-fixed Cowan strain I (SAC) as indicated. Secreted IgG and IgM was measured after 7 days of culture. Zero denotes the first immunoblot-positive anti-HIV antibody reaction

percentage of B cells expressing transferrin receptors and a decrease in the percentage of Leu-8 expressing cells indicates that B cells are activated[14]. However, elevated levels of serum IgD and *in vitro* spontaneous IgD production in early and late HIV infection are indicative of circulating immature B cells[14,15]. AIDS patients have increased numbers of CD10-expressing B cells, and this is also a marker of immature cells[14].

Elevated levels of serum immunoglobulin (Ig) indicate a chronic B cell activation in HIV infection[16,17]. However, upon immunization HIV-infected individuals show a decreased T-helper-dependent and T-helper-independent antibody response[18–20]. Activated B cells are also observed *in vitro* by spontaneous IgG and IgM synthesis[20–22]. This constitutive Ig production is at least in part induced by HIV, since 20–50% of the antibodies is directed against HIV[22,23]. Already early after infection, PWM-induced Ig synthesis is defective and cannot be restored by addition of normal $CD4^+$ T cells (Figure 5.1)[8,24]. Similar findings with other mitogens inducing activation or proliferation of B cells have been reported[18,20,24]. B cell abnormalities may be due to failing immune regulation, may be induced by activating effects of HIV proteins[22,25] or by up-regulation of expression of cytokines (e.g. interleukin-6 (IL-6) in monocytes[26]. It is, however, unlikely that B cells are a direct target for HIV *in vivo* as has been reported for EBV-transformed B cells *in vitro*[27,28], since PCR analysis of patient B cells never indicates the presence of proviral sequences[29].

Antigen-presenting cell function

Monocytes/macrophages and dendritic cells can be infected with HIV *in vitro*[30–33] and *in vivo*[34,35] (see also Chapter 3). The role of these antigen-presenting cells (APC) in the immunopathogenesis of HIV infection may be dual. First monocytes/macrophages may be persistently infected *in vivo* and function as a reservoir in virus dissemination to lungs and brains[34]. Second, HIV infection may induce severe defects in APC functions mediated by these cells. Indeed, studies from our and other laboratories demonstrate functional defects in these cells in symptomatic and asymptomatic HIV-infected persons[8,12,24,36]. In early infection, however, APC and monocyte function do not seem to be affected[24,37].

T cell function

$CD4^+$ T cells are progressively lost in HIV infection and the $CD4^+$ T cell count varies from normal levels in early asymptomatics to severely decreased levels in AIDS patients[2,38–40]. Functional analysis of T cells from early asymptomatic HIV-infected men shows that HIV also disturbs T cell function before depletion of $CD4^+$ T cells has occurred. T cell proliferation can be induced using monoclonal antibodies (MAb) directed against the monomorphic CD3 part of the CD3/T cell receptor (TCR) complex[41,42]. This stimulation signal bypasses the polymorphic TCR that recognizes its specific antigen in the context of self MHC[43]. Anti-CD3-induced proliferation thus reflects the total capacity of the T cell compartment irrespective of specific antigen.

Using soluble anti-CD3 Mab we and others have shown that T cell proliferation is affected before any $CD4^+$ T cell depletion can be observed[8,24,44]. The decreased response has been shown to be due to intrinsic T cell defects since the addition of monocytes from healthy donors does not restore T cell function[8]. This is further confirmed in an assay using immobilized anti-CD3 MAb, inducing monocyte-independent T cell proliferation, which is also decreased[45,46]. Furthermore, stimulation with a mitogenic combination of anti-CD2 MAb also results in decreased T cell proliferation in asymptomatic HIV-infected men[45]. In contrast to T cell proliferation, T cell differentiation to cytotoxic T lymphocytes (CTL), induced by immobilized anti-CD3 MAb, is not affected in early HIV infection[46].

Hofmann *et al.* observed that T cell proliferation induced by the lectin pokeweed mitogen (PWM) is also decreased in early infection[21]. In contrast, the response to the mitogen phytohaemagglutinin (PHA) is not affected in asymptomatic individuals with stable $CD4^+$ cell numbers[47]. Loss of T cell responsiveness is also observed for T-helper activity in *in-vitro* PWM-driven B cell differentiation assays[8,24].

Shearer and co-workers demonstrated a selective loss of T cell reactivity with respect to both proliferation and generation of CTL in response to nominal antigen (Ag) presented by self MHC molecules[48–50] in asymptomatic HIV-infected men, in contrast to normal responsiveness to alloantigens (ALLO). This non-responsiveness to nominal Ag can be restored by recombinant interleukin-2 (rIL-2) or by co-stimulation by nominal Ag plus ALLO[49]. This indicates that antigen-specific T cells are present that cannot be properly activated by nominal Ag alone. Shearer *et al.* have interpreted these data as a selective $CD4^+$ T cell defect, based on findings in the mouse that responses to nominal Ag are strictly dependent on functional $CD4^+$ T-helper cells, whereas responses to ALLO class I antigens can also be initiated by $CD8^+$ cells via an alternative helper pathway[49].

In contrast to stimulation assays described above, T cell activation via other receptors is not affected in early HIV infection. Stimulation via CD28, an activation molecule that utilizes a signal transduction pathway independent of the CD3/TCR route[51–53], results in normal enhancement of T cell proliferation[45,46].

The mechanism underlying this unresponsiveness has been investigated but no evidence for biochemical defects in signal transduction pathways, such as Ca^{2+} flux or pH increase, has been found[45]. Expression of CD25, the IL-2 receptor, is normal, but IL-2 production is decreased in T cells from asymptomatic HIV-infected men[46,54]. Proliferation can be restored to near-normal levels by the addition of exogenous IL-2[46].

Selective loss of memory T cells in early HIV infection

T cells from HIV-infected men in early infection largely resemble naive T cells with respect to their functional properties. This subset within the peripheral blood T cells is characterized by the expression of CD45RA, whereas the memory subset expresses CD45RO and CD29[55–60]. Antigen-reactive T cells and T cells that provide helper activity for polyclonal and antigen-specific antibody synthesis are mainly in the memory subset[55,56,58,59,61]. These mutually exclusive subsets do not exist independently, but rather a transition of naive to memory is observed after T cells first encounter their specific antigen[61,62]. The increased expression of various adhesion molecules by memory cells may facilitate recognition and enhance proliferation upon secondary activation by specific antigen[58,62].

Memory cells readily respond to anti-CD3 and anti-CD2 MAb, whereas naive cells respond poorly. Both groups, however, respond well to anti-CD28 MAb, PHA, and IL-2 as observed in early HIV infection[45,59]. Phenotypic analysis of T cells from early asymptomatics, indeed, shows a significant decrease in CD29 expressing memory cells in peripheral blood[45,46,63–65]. The complementary subset of $CD45RA^+$ T cells, however, is not dramatically increased in early infection[45,46,63,64,,66–68]. Results for subset changes from seroconversion to time of diagnosis of AIDS are shown for a typical patient in Figure 5.2. Similar changes in subsets have been observed in SIV-infected monkeys[69].

The loss of memory cells in early infection can be explained by the preferential infection of proliferating cells by retroviruses[70]. This implies that upon antigenic stimulation *in vivo*, memory cells are the main target for

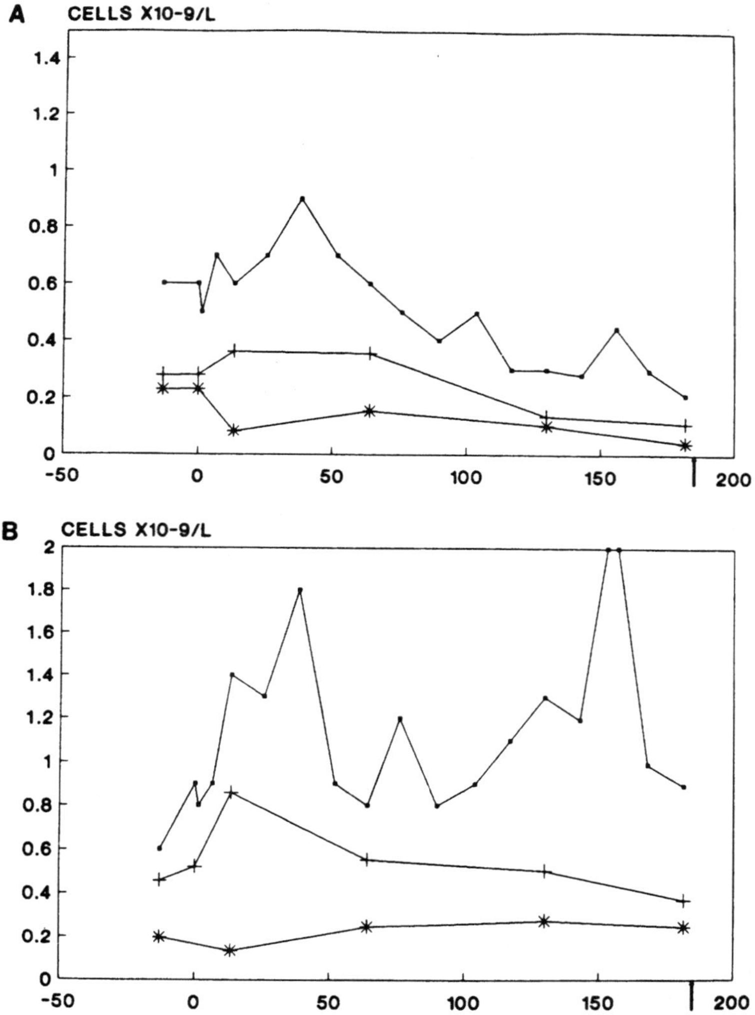

Figure 5.2 Naive CD45 RA⁺ (+) and memory CD29⁺ (*) subpopulations within the CD4 (panel A) or CD8 (panel B) (·) subsets in a typical patient from seroconversion to AIDS. Zero denotes the first Western blot positive sample. The arrow indicates the time AIDS was diagnosed. Time on the *x*-axis is in weeks

infection. Indeed, both in SIV and HIV infection evidence for a specific infection of memory cells has been obtained[69,71,72]. In addition, naive cells that are activated by primary antigen may be infected and cleared, thus abrogating the renewal of the memory pool. Cells may subsequently die via direct cytopathic effects of the virus, or virus-specific cytotoxic activities[35,73,74].

On the other hand, HIV may interfere indirectly with T cell education and

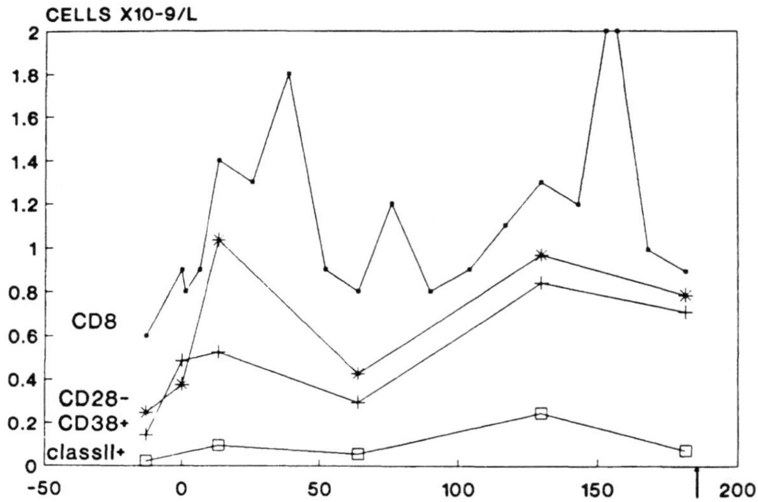

Figure 5.3 Changes in CD8 subpopulations in a patient from seroconversion to AIDS. Zero denotes the first Western blot positive sample; the arrow indicates the time of AIDS diagnosis. Time on the *x*-axis is in weeks

maturation by infection of antigen-presenting cells, resulting in decreased MHC class II expression[36,75,76], and diminished accessory cell function[8,36,77]. Interference with T cell outgrowth as a result of infection of precursor cells in the bone marrow has also been proposed[78–81].

T CELL FUNCTION IN LATER STAGES OF HIV INFECTION

As HIV infection progresses towards clinical symptoms $CD4^+$ T cell numbers decrease, $CD8^+$ T cell numbers increase and immune functions further deteriorate (schematically depicted in Figure 5.4). The causes of the further deterioration of the immune system in advanced HIV infection are less clear. The loss of both memory and naive T cells in late infection results in a normal naive to memory ratio[46]. However, in contrast to the remaining memory cells in early HIV-infected men[45], memory cells from men in later stages have become unresponsive. Severely decreased $CD4^+$ helper numbers may explain disturbance of immune function in other compartments including $CD8^+$ cells and APC[2,21].

In *in-vitro* assays this is reflected in further decrease of proliferative responses to anti-CD3 MAb, PWM and nominal antigen[21,46,48,49,82]. Remarkably, during asymptomatic infection anti-CD3-induced proliferation remains stable, but declines to very low levels in progression to AIDS[68,83]. This deterioration is further characterized by a rapid decrease in $CD4^+$ T cell numbers and decreased proliferative response to PHA and ALLO MHC[21,47–49,82]. Phenotypic changes in the T cell compartment include a further loss of memory cells, loss of naive cells and increase of absolute numbers of relatively unresponsive $CD8^+$ T cells[46,48]. Phenotypic analysis of these $CD8^+$ cells shows that a large percentage expresses CD57 and CD38 and lacks expression of CD11b, CD28 and 5′-nucleotidase activity[65,68,84–87]. The increase of this CD8 population during infection is shown in Figure 5.3 for a patient followed from seroconversion to diagnosis of AIDS[68]. It should be noted that at the time AIDS was diagnosed the CD8 population was composed almost solely of $CD28^-$ and $CD38^+$ T cells.

The $CD57^+$ subset has been shown to suppress T cell proliferation, T-helper function, CTL function and B cell differentiation by release of a soluble factor[84] (Sadat-Sowti and Autran, unpublished observation). T cells with a similar phenotype have been observed after bone marrow transplantation, possibly linked to immune dysregulation[88]. Pantaleo *et al.* describe a large percentage of $CD8^+$ T cells that express HLA-DR and lack expression of CD25[86]. These cells are refractory to stimulation via CD3, CD2 and CD28, which cannot be overcome by IL-2 or IL-4[86]. HIV-specific cytotoxicity by $HLA\text{-}DR^+CD8^+$ T cells is lost in AIDS patients, but non-specific cytotoxicity can still be measured[46,87].

Several groups have reported immune suppressive effects of HIV proteins in lymphocyte functions. Frankel and co-workers demonstrated that *tat* can inhibit proliferation to specific antigens[89,90]. The viral envelope protein gp120, however, is a more likely candidate, since this is produced and may be shed in large amounts in late stage infection. In initial experiments, investigating the effects of gp120 on lymphocyte function, large quantities of gp120 were required[91,92], but recently small amounts of gp120 have been shown to suppress $CD4^+$ T cell function[93]. A possible mechanism for immune dysfunction after CD4 crosslinking has recently been described in thymocytes and mature T cells in a murine model[94,95]. It can be envisaged that analogous

$CD4^+$ no's	0.8	0.8	0.6	0.3	0.2	0.1
T-cell response:						
nominal Ag	+	+	−	−	−	−
PWM	+	+	−	−	−	−
anti-CD3	+	+	+	−	−	−
ALLO	+	+	+	+	+	−
PHA	+	+	+	+	+	−
B-cell function Ig production:						
spontaneous	−	+	+	+	+	+
PWM-induced	+	−	−	−	−	−
APC function	+	+	+	−	−	−

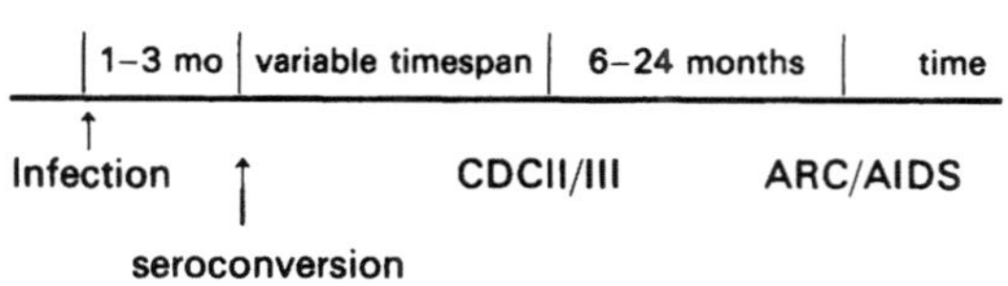

Figure 5.4 Gradual loss of immune functions in HIV infection

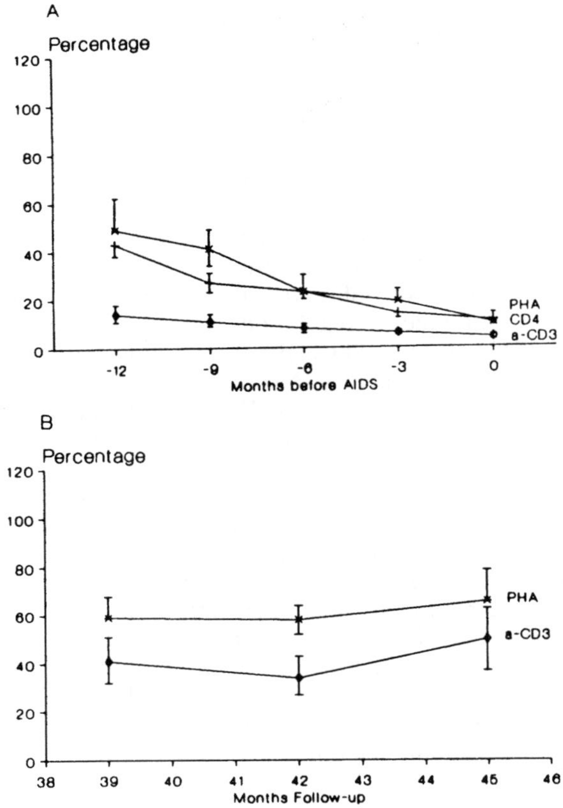

Figure 5.5 Proliferative T cell responses in whole blood cultures induced by PHA (×) and anti-CD3 antibodies (●) in individuals that progressed to AIDS (**A**) and in stable asymptomatics (**B**). The results are presented as the mean reactivity per T cell (±SE) related to the response of normal controls cultured in parallel

to crosslinking by anti-CD4 Mab, gp120 plus anti-gp120 Mab may efficiently crosslink CD4 molecules, after which T cell activation results in cell death via apoptosis. Obviously this mechanism involves only $CD4^+$ cells, but it may account for $CD4^+$ T cell depletion *in vivo* and unresponsiveness because of cell death *in vitro*.

PROGNOSTIC RELEVANCE OF IMMUNOLOGICAL MARKERS

Prognostic markers that are currently used to evaluate the risk of developing AIDS include $CD4^+$ T cell counts and p24 antigenaemia[96–98]. The results recently obtained with anti-CD3 and PWM-induced proliferation assays indicate that these may be used as an additional marker for progression of disease. Retrospective evaluation of T-cell proliferation in large cohort studies shows a highly significant difference between stable asymptomatics and people that progress to AIDS[46,99]. Analysis of T cell function using specific antigen or PWM has the disadvantage of APC dependency and the fact that antigen stimulates only a minor fraction of T cells. Anti-CD3 Mab induce polyclonal T cell proliferation irrespective of TCR specificity and accessory cells. Thus the total T cell proliferative capacity is assessed, regardless of previously encountered antigen and independent of other cellular functions that may also be affected in their function. For a larger-scale diagnostic purpose a T cell proliferation culture system has been developed using only 50 μl of whole blood per culture well[100]. An additional advantage of using the whole blood anti-CD3-driven culture system is the circumvention of laborious cell separation procedures[83,100]. In a prospective study in a large cohort of HIV-infected men, T cell responsiveness to anti-CD3 Mab has been shown to be a marker of progression independent of $CD4^+$ T cell numbers and antigenaemia[83] (Schellekens *et al.* in preparation). In the group that developed AIDS the anti-CD3 reactivity per T cell was already extremely low (< 10% of the normal response) at least 1 year before diagnosis (Figure 5.5A). At that time CD4 T cell numbers and the response to PHA was still comparable with the values observed in stable non-progressors (Figure 5.5B). These results suggest that anti-CD3-induced proliferation may be of use for evaluation and monitoring of therapeutic intervention. Currently $CD4^+$ T cell numbers and p24 antigenaemia are used as intake criteria to select individuals to receive early therapy. However, low or rapidly decreasing $CD4^+$ T cell counts occur relatively shortly before the diagnosis of AIDS, leaving a relatively short window for early treatment[83]. Intervention with therapeutic agents, such as zidovudine, based on severely decreased $CD4^+$ T cell numbers, therefore, may be rather late[46]. Furthermore, p24 antigenaemia, although an independent prognostic marker, occurs in a limited number of HIV-infected people progressing to AIDS and therefore has restricted applicability[46,101] (see also Chapter 6). Since anti-CD3-induced proliferation is low, for a relatively long period before the onset of disease[83,99], it may prove valuable, in combination with $CD4^+$ T cell numbers, to identify groups at high risk for disease progression when therapy may be most beneficial. Indeed, we have recently analysed T cell function in a group of asymptomatic HIV-infected men that were treated with zidovudine. In this group, selected for p24 antigenaemia, no significant differences in $CD4^+$ T cell numbers were observed at intake. Retrospective analysis shows that the clinical outcome after a 2-year follow up correlated significantly with T cell function at intake[99]. Similar studies are now being performed in a large double-blind zidovudine trial in asymptomatic HIV-infected men.

Acknowledgement

This work was supported by a grant from the Netherland Foundation for Preventive Medicine. Frank Miedema is a senior fellow of the Royal Netherlands Academy of Arts and Sciences.

References

1. CDC (1987). Revision of the CDC surveillance case definition for acquired immunodeficiency syndrome. *Morbid. Mortal. Weekly Rep.*, **36** (Suppl.), 1S–15S
2. Fahey, J. L., Prince, H. E., Weaver, M., Groopman, J., Visscher, B., Schwartz, K. and Detels, R. (1984). Quantitative changes in T helper or suppressor/cytotoxic lymphocyte subsets that distinguish acquired immune deficiency syndrome from other immune subsets disorders. *J. Am. Med. Assoc.*, **76**, 95–100
3. Melbye, M., Biggar, R. J., Ebbesen, P., Goedert, J. J., Faber, V., Lorenzen, I., Skinhoj, P., Gallo, R. C. and Blattner, W. A. (1986). Long-term seropositivity for Human T-lymphotropic Virus type III in homosexual men without the acquired immunodeficiency syndrome: development of immunologic and clinical abnormalities. *Ann. Intern. Med.*, **104**, 496–500
4. Klatzmann, D., Champagne, E., Chamaret, S., Gruest, J., Guetard, D., Hercend, T., Gluckman, J. C. and Montagnier, L. (1984). T-lymphocyte T4 molecule behaves as the receptor for human retrovirus LAV. *Nature*, **312**, 767–8
5. Dalgleish, A. G., Beverly, P. C. L., Clapham, P. R., Crawford, D. H., Greaves, M. F. and Weiss, R. A. (1984). The CD4 (T4) antigen is an essential component of the receptor for the AIDS retrovirus. *Nature*, **312**, 763
6. McDougal, J. S., Mawle, A., Cort, S. P., Nicholson, J. K. A., Cross, D., Schleppler-Campbell, J. A., Hicks, D. and Sligh, J. (1985). Cellular tropism of the human retrovirus HTLV-III/LAV. I. Role of T cell activation and expression of the T4 antigen. *J. Immunol.*, **135**, 3151–62
7. Clerici, M., Stocks, N., Zajac, R. A., Boswell, R. N., Lucey, D. R., Via, C. S. and Shearer, G. M. (1989). Detection of three different patterns of T helper cell dysfunction in asymptomatic, human immunodeficiency virus-seropositive patients. *J. Clin. Invest.*, **84**, 1892–9
8. Miedema, F., Petit, A. J. C., Terpstra, F. G., Schattenkerk, J. K. M. E., De Wolf, F., Al, B. J. M., Roos, M., Lange, J. M. A., Danner, S. A., Goudsmit, J. and Schellekens, P. T. A. (1988). Immunological abnormalities in human immunodeficiency virus (HIV)-infected asymptomatic homosexual men. HIV affects the immune system before $CD4^+$ T helper cell depletion occurs. *J. Clin. Invest.*, **82**, 1908–14
9. Rook, A. H., Masur, H., Lane, H. C. *et al.* (1983). Interleukin-2 enhances depressed natural killer and cytomegalovirus-specific cytotoxic activity of lymphocytes from patients with the acquired immunodeficiency syndrome. *J. Clin. Invest.*, **72**, 398–403
10. Murphey-Corb, M., Martin, L. N., Davison-Fairburn, B., Montelaro, R. C., Miller, M., West, M., Ohkawa, S., Baskin, G. B., Zhang, J. Y., Putney, S. D., Allison, A. C. and Eppstein, D. A. (1989). A formalin-inactivated whole SIV vaccine confers protection in macaques. *Science*, **246**, 1293–7
11. Bonavida, B., Katz, J. and Gottlieb, M. (1986). Mechanism of defective NK cells activity in patients with acquired immunodeficiency syndrome (AIDS) and AIDS-related complex. *J. Immunol.*, **137**, 1157–63
12. Prince, H. E., Moody, D. J., Shubin, B. I., Fahey, J. L. (1985). Defective monocyte function in acquired immune deficiency syndrome (AIDS): evidence from a monocyte dependent T-cell proliferative system. *J. Clin. Immunol.*, **5**, 21–5
13. Smith, P. D., Ohura, K., Masur, H., Lane, H. C., Fauci, A. S. and Wahl, S. M. (1984). Monocyte function in the acquired immune deficiency syndrome defective chemotaxis. *J. Clin. Invest.*, **74**, 2121–8
14. Martinez-Maza, O., Crabb, E., Mitsuyasu, R. T., Fahey, J. L. and Girogi, J. V. (1987). Infection with the human immunodeficiency virus (HIV) is associated with *in vivo* increase in B lymphocyte activation and immaturity. *J. Immunol.*, **138**, 3720–4
15 .Rogers, L. A., Forster, S. M. and Pinching, A. J. (1989). IgD production and other lymphocyte functions in HIV infection: Imunity and activation of B cells at different clinical stages. *Clin. Exp. Immunol.*, **75**, 7–11
16. Pahwa, S., Pahwa, R., Saxinger C., Gallo, R. C. and Good, R. A. (1985). Influence of the human T-lymphotropic virus/lymphadenopathy-associated virus on functions of human lymphocytes: evidence for immunosuppressive effects and polyclonal B-cell activation by banded viral preparations. *Proc. Natl. Acad. Sci. USA*, **82**, 198–202
17. Pahwa, S., Pahwa, R., Good, R. A. *et al.* (1986). Stimulatory and inhibitory influences of human immunodeficiency virus on normal B lymphocytes. *Proc. Natl. Acad. Sci. USA*, **83**, 9124–8

18. Lane, H. C., Masur, H., Edgar, L. C., Whalen, G., Rook, A. H. and Fauci, A. S. (1983). Abnormalities of B-cell activation and immunoregulation in patients with acquired immunodeficiency syndrome. *N. Engl. J. Med.*, **309**, 453–8
19. Ammann, A. J., Schiffman, G., Abrams, D., Volberding, P., Ziegler, J. and Conant, M. (1984). B-cell immunodeficiency in acquired immunodeficiency syndrome. *J. Am. Med. Assoc.*, **251**, 1447–9
20. Teeuwsen, V. J. P., Logtenberg, T., Siebelink, K. H. J., Lange, J. M. A., Goudsmit, J., Uytdehaag, F. G. C. M. and Osterhaus, A. D. M. E. (1987). Analysis of the antigen- and mitogen-induced differentiation of B lymphocytes from asymptomatic human immunodeficiency virus-seropositive male homosexuals. *J. Immunol.*, **139**, 2929–35.
21. Lane, H. C., Depper, J. L., Greene, W. C., Whalen, C., Waldmann, T. A. and Fauci, A. S. (1985). Qualitative analysis of immune function in patients with the acquired immunodeficiency syndrome. *N. Engl. J. Med.*, **313**, 79–84
22. Yarchoan, R., Redfield, R. and Broder, S. (1986). Mechanism of B-cell activation in patients with the acquired immunodeficiency syndrome and related disorders. *J. Clin. Invest.*, **78**, 439–447
23. Amadori, A., Zamarchi, R., Ciminale, V., Del Mistro, A., Siervo, S., Alberti, A., Colombatti, M. and Chieco-Bianchi, L. (1989). HIV-1-specific B cell activation: A major constituent of spontaneous B cell activation during HIV-1 infection. *J. Immunol.*, **143**, 2146–52
24. Terpstra, F. G., Al, B. J. M., Roos, M. Th. L., De Wolf, F., Goudsmit, J., Schellekens, P. T. and Miedema, F. (1989). Longitudinal study of leukocyte functions in homosexsual men seroconverted for HIV: rapid and persistent loss of B-cell function after HIV infection. *Eur. J. Immunol.*, **19**, 667–73
25. Schnittman, S. M., Lane, H. C., Higgins, S. E., Folks, T. and Fauci, A. S. (1986). Direct polyclonal activation of human B lymphocytes by the acquired immunodeficiency syndrome virus. *Science*, **233**, 1084–6
26. Nakajima, K., Martínez-Maza, O., Hrano, T., Breen, E. C., Nishanian, P. G., Salazar-Gonzalez, J. F., Fahey, J. L. and Kishimoto, T. (1989). Induction of IL-6 (B cell stimulatory factor-2/IFN-β_2) production by HIV. *J. Immunol.*, **142**, 531–6
27. Montagnier, L., Gruest, J., Chamaret, S., Dauget, C., Axler, C., Guetard, D., Nugeyre, T., Barre-Sinoussi, F., Chermann, J. C., Brunet, J. B., Klatzmann, D. and Gluckman, J. C. (1984). Adaption of lymphadenopathy-associated virus (LAV) to replication on EBV-transformed B-lymphoblastoid cell lines. *Science*, **225**, 63
28. Tersmette,. M., Miedema, F., Huisman, J. G., Goudemit, J. and Melief, C. J. M. (1985). Productive HTVL-III infection of human cell lines. *Lancet*, **1**, 815–16
29. Schnittman, S. M., Psallidopoulos, M. C., Lane, H. C., Thompson, L., Baseler, M., Massari, F., Fox, C. H., Salzman, N. P. and Fauci, A. S. (1989). The reservoir for HIV-1 in human peripheral blood is a T cell that maintains expression of CD4. *Science*, **245**, 305–8
30. Ho, D. D., Rota, T. R. and Hirsch, M. S. (1986). Infection of monocyte/macrophages by human T lymphotropic virus type III. *J. Clin. Invest.*, **77**, 1712–15
31. Gartner, S., Markovits, P., Markovits, D. M., Kaplan, M. H., Gallo, R. C. and Popovic, M. (1986). The role of mononuclear phagocytes in HTVL-III/LAV infection. *Science*, **233**, 215–19
32. Armstrong, J. A. and Horne, R. (1984). Follicular dendritic cells and virus-like particles in AIDS-related lymphadenopathy. *Lancet*, **1**, 370–2
33. Knight, S. C. and Macatonia, S. E. (1988). Dendritic cells and viruses. *Immunol. Lett.*, **19**, 177–82
34. Koenig, S., Orenstein, H. E., Gendelman, J. M., Dal Canto, M. C., Pezeshkpour, G. H., Yungbluth, M., Janotta, F., Aksamit, A., Martin, M. A. and Fauci, A. S. (1986). Detection of AIDS virus in macrophages in brain tissue from AIDS patients with encephalopathy. *Science*, **233**, 1089–93
35. Plata, F., Autran, B., Martins, L. P., Wain-Hobson, S., Raphael, M., Mayaud, C., Denis, M., Guillon, J. M. and Debre, P. (1987). AIDS virus-specific cytotoxic T lymphocytes in lung disorders. *Nature*, **328**, 348–51
36. Eales, L. J., Farrant, J., Helbert, M. and Pinching, A. J. (1988). Peripheral blood dendritic cells in persons with AIDS and AIDS related complex: loss of high intensity class II antigen expression and function. *Clin. Exp. Immunol.*, **71**, 423–7
37. Clerici, M., Stocks, N. I., Zajac, R. A., Boswell, R. N. and Shearer, G. M. (1990). Accessory cell function in asymptomatic human immunodeficiency virus-infected patients. *Clin.*

Immunol. Immunopathol., **54**, 168–73

38. Gottlieb, M. S., Schroff, R., Schanker, H. M., Weisman, J. D., Thim Fan, P., Wolf, R. A. and Saxon, A. (1981). *Pneumocystis carinii* pneumonia and mucosal candidiasis in previously healthy homosexual men: evidence of a new acquired cellular immunodeficiency. *N. Engl. J. Med.*, **305**, 1425–31
39. Masur, H., Michelis, M. A., Greene, J. B., Onorato, I., Vande Stouwe, R. A., Holzman, R. S., Wormser, G. P., Brettman, L., Lange, M., Murray, H. W. and Cunningham-Rundles, S. (1981). An outbreak of community-acquired pneumocystis carinii pneumonia: initial manifestation of cellular immune differentiation. *N. Engl. J. Med.*, **305**, 1431–8
40. Siegal, F. P., Lopez, C. and Hammer, G. S. (1981). Severe acquired immunodeficiency in male homosexuals, manifested by chronic perianal ulcerative herpes simplex lesions. *N. Engl. J. Med.*, **305**, 1439–44
41. Van Lier, R. A. W., Brouwer, M., Rebel, V. I., Van Noesel, C. J. M. and Aarden, L. A. (1989). Immobilized anti-CD3 monoclonal antibodies induce accessory cell-independent lymphokine production, proliferation and helper activity in human T lymphocytes. *Immunology*, **68**, 45–50
42. Imboden, J. B. and Stobo, J. D. (1985). Transmembrane signalling by T-cell antigen receptor. *J. Exp. Med.*, **161**, 446–56
43. Clevers, H., Alarcon, B., Wileman, T. and Terhorst, C. (1988). The T cell receptor/CD3 complex: a dynamic protein ensemble. *Ann. Rev. Immunol.*, **6**, 629–62
44. Bentin, J., Tsoukas, C., McCutchan, J. A., Spector, S. E., Richman, D. D. and Vaughan, J. H. (1989). Impairment in T-lymphocyte responses during early infection with the human immunodeficiency virus. *J. Clin. Immunol.*, **9**, 159–68
45. Van Noesel, C. J. M., Gruters, R. A., Terpstra, F. G., Schellekens, P. T. A., Van Lier, R. A. W. and Miedema, F. (1990). Functional and phenotypic evidence for a selective loss of memory T cells in asymptomatic HIV-infected men. *J. Clin. Invest.*, **86**, 293–9
46. Gruters, R. A., Terpstra, F. G., De Jong, R., Van Noesel, C. J. M., Van Lier, R. A. W. and Miedema, F. (1990). Selective loss of T-cell functions in different stages of HIV infection. *Eur. J. Immunol.*, **20**, 1039–44
47. Roos, M. Th. L., Miedema, F., Eeftink Schattenkerk, J. K. M., De Wolf, F., Goudsmit, J., Lange, J. M. A., Danner, S. A., Out, T. A. and Schellekens, P. T. A. (1989). Cellular and humoral immunity in various cohorts of male homosexuals in relation to infection with human immunodeficiency virus. *Neth. J. Med.*, **34**, 132–41
48. Shearer, G. M., Payne, S. M., Joseph, L. J. and Biddison, W. E. (1984). Functional T lymphocyte immune deficiency in a population of homosexual men who do not exhibit symptoms of acquired immune deficiency syndrome. *J. Clin. Invest.*, **74**, 496–506
49. Shearer, G. M., Bernstein, D. C., Tung, K. S. K., Via, C. S., Redfield, R., Salahuddin, S. Z. and Gallo, R. C. (1986). A model for the selective loss of major histocompatibility complex self-restricted T cell immune responses during the development of acquired immune deficiency syndrome (AIDS). *J. Immunol.*, **137**, 2514–21
50. Shearer, G. M., Salahuddin, S. Z., Markham, P. D., Joseph, L. J., Payne, S. M., Kriebel, P., Bernmstein, D. C., Biddison, W. E., Sarngadharan, M. G. and Gallo, R. C. (1985). Prospective study of cytotoxic T lymphocyte responses to influenza and antibodies to human T lymphotropic virus-III in homosexual men. *J. Clin. Invest.*, **76**, 1699–704
51. Weiss, A., Manger, B. and Imboden, J. B. (1986). Synergy between the T3/antigen receptor complex and TP44 in activation of human T cells. *J. Immunol.*, **137**, 819–25
52. Pantaleo, G., Olive, D., Harris, D., Poggi, A., Moretta, L. and Moretta, A. (1986). Signal transducing mechanisms involved in human T cell activation via surface T44 molecules. Comparison with signals transduced via the T cell receptor complex. *Eur. J. Immunol.*, **16**, 1639–42
53. Van Lier, R. A. W., Brouwer, M., de Groot, E., Kramer, I. J., Aarden, L. A. and Verhoeven, A. J. (1991). CD3/T cell receptor and CD28 use distinct intracellular signalling pathways. *Eur. J. Immunol.* (In press)
54. Hofmann, B., Moller, J., Langhoff, E., Damgård Jakobsen, K., Odum, N., Dickmeiss, E., Ryder, L. P., Thastrup, O., Scharff, O, Foder, B., Platz, P., Petersen, C., Mathiesen, L., Hartvig Jensen, T., Skinhoj, P. and Svejgaard, A. (1989). Stimulation of AIDS lymphocytes with calcium ionophore (A23187) and phorbol ester (PMA): Studies of cytoplasmic free Ca, IL-2 receptor expression, IL-2 production, and proliferation. *Cell. Immunol.*, **119**, 14–21

55. Morimoto, C., Letvin, N. L., Boyd, A. W., Hagan, M., Brown, H. M., Kornacki, M. M. and Schlossman, S. F. (1985). The isolation and characterization of the human helper inducer T cell subset. *J. Immunol.*, **134**, 3762–9
56. Morimoto, C. N., Letvin, N. L., Distaso, J. A., Aldrich, W. R. and Schlossman, S. F. (1985). The isolation and characterization of the human suppressor inducer T cell subset. *J. Immunol.*, **134**, 1508–15
57. White, J., Herman, A., Pullen, A. M., Kubo, R., Kappler, J. W. and Marrack, P. (1989). The Vβ-specific superantigen staphylococcal enterotoxin B: stimulation of mature T cells and clonal deletion in neonatal mice. *Cell*, **56**, 27–35
58. Sanders, M. E., Makgoba, M. W., Sharrow, S. O., Stephany, D., Springer, T. A., Young, H. A. and Shaw, S. (1988). Human memory T lymphocytes express increased levels of three cell adhesion molecules (LFA-3, CD2, and LFA-1) and three other molecules (UCHL-1, CDw29 and Pgp-1) and have enhanced IFN-gamma production. *J. Immunol.*, **140**, 1401–7
59. Sanders, M. E., Makgoba, M. W., June, C. H., Young, H. A. and Shaw, S. (1989). Enhanced responsiveness of human T cells to CD2 and CD3 receptor mediated activation. *Eur. J. Immunol.*, **19**, 803–8
60. Merkenschlager, M., Terry, L., Edwards, R. and Beverley, P. C. L. (1988). Limiting dilution analysis of proliferative responses in human lymphocyte populations defined by the monoclonal antibody UCHL1: Implications for differential CD45 expression in T cell memory formation. *Eur. J. Immunol.*, **18**, 1653–61
61. Tedder, T. F., Clement, L. T. and Cooper, M. D. (1985). Human lymphocyte differentiation antigens HB-10 and HB-11: II Differential production of B-cell growth and differentiation factors by distinct helper T cell subpopulations. *J. Immunol.*, **134**, 2989–94
62. Sanders, M. E., Makgoba, M. W. and Shaw, S. (1988). Human naive and memory T cells: reinterpretation of helper-inducer and suppressor–inducer subsets. *Immunol. Today*, **9**, 195–8
63. Fletcher, M. A., Azen, S. P., Adelsberg, B., Gjerset, G., Hassett, J., Kaplan, J., Niland, J. C., Odom Maryon, T., Parker, J. W., Stites, D. P., Mosley, J. W. and Transfusion Safety Study Group (1989). Immunophenotyping in a multicentre study: the transfusion safety study experience. *Clin. Immunol. Immunopathol.*, **52**, 38–47
64. Giorgi, J. V., Fahey, J. L., Smith, D. C., Hultin, L. E., Cheng, H. L., Mitsuyasu, R. T. and Detels, R. (1987). Early effects of HIV on CD4 lymphocytes *in vivo*. *J. Immunol.*, **138**, 3725–30
65. De Martini, R. M., Turner, R. R., Formenti, S. C., Boone, D. C., Bishop, P. C., Levine, A. M. and Parker, J. W. (1988). Peripheral blood mononuclear cell abnormalities and their relationship to clinical course in homosexual men with HIV infection. *Clin. Immunol. Immunopathol.*, **46**, 258–71
66. De Paoli, P., Battistin, S., Crovatto, M., Modolo, M. L., Carbone, A., Tirelli, U. and Santini, G. (1988). Immunologic abnormalities related to antigenaemia during HIV-1 infection. *Clin. Exp. Immunol.*, **74**, 317–20
67. De Paoli, P., Carbone, A., Battistin, S., Crovatto, M., Arrighini, N. and Santini, G. (1987). Selective depletion of the OKT4+ 4B4+ subset in lymph nodes from HIV+ patients. *Immunol. Lett.*, **16**, 71–3
68. Gruters, R. A., Terpstra, F. G., De Goede, R. E. Y., Mulder, J. W., De Wolf, F., Schellekens, P. T. A., Van Lier, R. A. W., Tersmette, M. and Miedema, F. (1991). Immunological and virological markers in individuals progressing from seroconversion to AIDS. *AIDS*, **5**, 837–844
69. Gallatin, W. M., Gale, M. J., Hoffman, P. A., Willerford, D. M., Draves, K. E., Beneviste, R. E., Morton, W. R. and Clark, E. A. (1989). Selective replication of simian immunodeficiency virus in a subset of CD4+ lymphocytes. *Proc. Natl. Acad. Sci. USA*, **86**, 3301–5
70. Gowda, S. D., Stein, B. S., Mohagheghpour, N., Benike, C. J. and Engleman, E. G. (1989). Evidence that T cell activation is required for HIV-1 entry in CD4+ lymphocytes. *J. Immunol.*, **142**, 773–80
71. Schnittman, S. M., Lane, H. C., Greenhouse, J., Justement, J. S., Baseler, M. and Fauci, A. S. (1990). Preferential infection of CD4+ memory T cells by human immunodeficiency virus type 1: Evidence for a role in the selective T-cell functional defects observed in infected individuals. *Proc. Natl. Acad. Sci. USA*, **87**, 6058–62
72. Cayota, A., Vuillier, F., Scott-Algara, D. and Dighiero, G. (1990). Preferential replication of HIV-1 in memory CD4+ subpopulation. *Lancet*, **336**, 941
73. Siliciano, R. F., Lawton, T., Knall, C., Karr, R. W., Berman, P., Gregory, T. and Reinherz, E. L. (1988). Analysis of host-virus interactions in AIDS with anti-gp120 T cell clones:

Effect of HIV sequence variation and a mechanism for CD4+ cell depletion. *Cell*, **54**, 561–75

74. Lanzavecchia, A., Roosnek, E., Gregory, T., Berman, P. and Abrignani, S. (1988). T cells can present antigen such as HIV gp120 targeted to their own surface molecules. *Nature*, **334**, 530–2
75. Belsito, D. V., Sanchez, M. R., Baer, R. L., Valentine, F. and Thorbecke, G. J. (1984). Reduced Langerhans' cell Ia antigen and ATPase activity in patients with the acquired immunodeficiency syndrome. *N. Engl. J. Med.*, **310**, 1279–82
76. Petit, A. J. C., Terpstra, F. G. and Miedema, F. (1987). HIV infection down-regulates HLA-class II expression and induces differentiation in promonocytic U937 cells. *J. Clin. Invest.*, **79**, 1883–9
77. Petit, A. J. C., Tersmette, M., Terpstra, F. G., De Goede, R. E. Y., Van Lier, R. A. W. and Miedema, F. (1988). Decreased accessory cell function by human monocytic cells after infection with HIV. *J. Immunol.*, **140**, 1485–9
78. Lunardi-Iskandar, Y., Nugeyre, M. T., Georgoulias, V., Barŕ-Sinoussi, F., Jasmin, C. and Chermann, J. C. (1989). Replication of the human immunodeficiency virus 1 and impaired differentiation of T cells after in vitro infection of bone marrow immature T cells. *J. Clin. Invest.*, **83**, 610–15
79. Donahue, R. E., Johnson, M. M., Zou, L. I., Clark, S. C. and Groopman, J. E. (1987). Suppression of in vivo hematopoiesis following human immunodeficiency virus infection. *Nature*, **326**, 200–3
80. Folks, T. M., Kessler, S. W., Orenstein, J. M., Justement, J. S., Jaffe, E. S. and Fauci, A. S. (1988). Infection and replication of HIV-1 in purified progenitor cells of normal human bone marrow. *Science*, **242**, 919–22
81. Bagnara, G. P., Zauli, G., Giovannini, M., Re, M. C., Furlini, G. and La Placa, M. (1990). Early loss of circulating hemopoietic progenitors in HIV-1-infected subjects. *Exp. Hematol.*, **18**, 426–30
82. Hofmann, B., Jakobsen, K. D., Odum, N., Dickmeiss, E., Platz, P., Ryder, L. P., Pederson, C., Mathiesen, L., Bygbjerg, I., Faber, V. and Svejgaard, A. (1989). HIV-induced immunodeficiency. Relatively preserved phytohemagglutinin as opposed to decreased pokeweed mitogen responses may be due to possibly preserved responses via CD2/phytohemagglutinin pathway. *J. Immunol.*, **142**, 1874–80
83. Schellekens, P. T. A., Roos, M. T. L., De Wolf, F., Lange, J. M. A. and Miedema, F. (1990). Low T-cell responsiveness to activation via CD3/TCR is a prognostic marker for AIDS in HIV-1 infected men. *J. Clin. Immunol.*, **10**, 121–7
84. Joly, P., Guillon, J.-M., Mayaud, C., Plata, F., Theodorou, I., Denis, M., Debre, P. and Autran, B. (1989). Cell-mediated suppression of HIV-specific cytotoxic T lymphocytes. *J. Immunol.*, **143**, 2193–201
85. Stites, D. P., Moss, A. R., Bacchetti, P., Osmond, D., McHugh, T. M., Wang, Y. J., Hebert, S. and Colfer, B. (1989). Lymphocyte subset analysis to predict progression to AIDS in a cohort of homosexual men in San Francisco. *Clin. Immunol. Immunopathol.*, **52**, 96–103
86. Pantaleo, G., Koenig, S., Baseler, M., Lane, H. C. and Fauci, A. S. (1990). Defective clonogenic potential of $CD8^+$ T lymphocytes in patients with AIDS: Expansion in vivo of a nonclonogenic $CD3^+CD8^+DR^+CD25^-$ T cell population. *J. Immunol.*, **144**, 1696–704
87. Pantaleo, G., De Maria, A., Koenig, S., Butini, L., Moss, B., Baseler, M., Lane, H. C. and Fauci, A. S. (1990). $CD8^+$ T lymphocytes of patients with AIDS maintain normal broad cytolytic function despite the loss of human immunodeficiency virus-specific cytotoxicity. *Proc. Natl. Acad. Sci. USA*, **87**, 4818–22
88. Leroy, E., Calvo, C. F., Divine, M., Gourdin, M. F., Beaujean, F., Aribia, M. H. B., Mishal, Z., Vernant, J. P., Farcet, J. P. and Senik, A. (1986). Persistence of $T8^+/HNK^+$ suppressor lymphocytes in the blood of long-term surviving patients after allogeneic bone marrow transplantation. *J. Immunol.*, **137**, 2180–9
89. Viscidi, R. P., Mayur, K., Lederman, H. M. and Frankel, A. D. (1989). Inhibition of antigen-induced lymphocyte proliferation by Tat protein from HIV-1. *Science*, **246**, 1606–8
90. Frankel, A. D. and Pabo, C. O. (1988). Cellular uptake of the tat protein from human immunodeficiency virus. *Cell*, **55**, 1189–93
91. Diamond, D. C., Sleckman, B. P., Gregory, T., Lasky, L. A., Greenstein, J. L. and Burakoff, S. J. (1988). Inhibition of $CD4^+$ T cell function by the HIV envelope protein, gp120. *J. Immunol.*, **141**, 3715–17

92. Weinhold, K. J., Lyerley, H. K., Stanley, S. D., Austin, A. A., Matthews, T. J. and Bolognesi, D. P. (1989). HIV-1 GP120-mediated immune suppression and lymphocyte destruction in the absence of viral infection. *J. Immunol.*, **142**, 3091–7
93. Chirmule, N., Kalayanaraman, V. S., Oyaizu, N., Slade, H. B. and Pahwa, S. (1990). Inhibition of functional properties of tetanus-specific T-cell clones by envelope glycoprotein gp120 of human immunodeficiency virus. *Blood*, **75**, 152–9
94. Smith, C. A., Williams, G. T., Kingston, R., Jenkinson, E. J. and Owen, J. J. T. (1989). Antibodies to CD3/T-cell receptor complex induce death by apoptosis in immature T cells in thymic cultures. *Nature*, **337**, 181–4
95. Newell, M. K., Haughn, L. J., Maroun, C. R. and Julius, M. H. (1990). Death of mature T cells by separate ligation of CD4 and the T cell receptor for antigen. *Nature*, **347**, 286–8
96. De Wolf, F., Lange, J. M. A., Houweling, J. T. M., Coutinho, R. A., Schellekens, P. T., Van der Noordaa, J. and Goudsmit, J. (1988). Numbers of CD4+ cells and the levels of core antigens of and antibodies to the human immunodeficiency virus as predictors of AIDS among seropositive homosexual men. *J. Infect. Dis.*, **158**, 615–22
97. Masur, H., Ognibene, F. P., Yarchoan, R., Shelhamer, J. H., Baird, B. F., Travis, W., Suffredini, A. F., Deyton, L., Kovacs, J. A., Falloon, J., Davey, R., Polis, M., Metcalf, J., Baseler, M., Wesley, R., Gill, V. J., Fauci, A. S. and Lane, H. C. (1989). CD4 counts as predictors of opportunistic pneumonias in human immunodeficiency virus (HIV) infection. *Ann. Intern. Med.*, **111**, 223–31
98. Moss, A. R., Bachetti, P., Osmond, D., Krampf, W., Chaisson, R. E., Stites, D., Wilber, J., Allain, J. P. and Carlson, J. (1988). Seropositivity of HIV and the development of AIDS or AIDS-related conditions: three year follow-up of the San Francisco General Hospital cohort. *Br. Med. J.*, **269**, 745–50
99. Gruters, R. A., Terpstra, F. G., Lange, J. M. A., Roos, M. T. L., Harkema, T., Mulder, J. W., De Wolf, F., Schellekens, P. T. A. and Miedema, F. (1991). Differences in clinical course in zidovudine-treated asymptomatic HIV-infected men associated with T-cell function at intake. *AIDS*, **5**, 43–47
100. Bloemena, E., Van Oers, R. H. J., Weinreich, S., Stilma-Meinesz, A. P., Schellekens, P. T. A. and Van Lier, R. A. W. (1989). The influence of cyclosporin A on the alternative pathways of human T cell activation *in vitro*. *Eur. J. Immunol.*, **19**, 943–6
101. De Wolf, F., Goudsmit, J., Paul, D. A., Lange, J. M. A., Hooijkaas, C., Schellekens, P. T. A., Coutinho, R. A. and Van der Noordaa, J. (1987). Risk of AIDS related complex and AIDS in homosexual men with persistent HIV antigenaemia. *Br. Med. J.*, **295**, 569–72

6
Monitoring of disease progression of HIV infection

A. G. BIRD

INTRODUCTION

The CD4 T lymphocyte is one of the central targets for HIV infection. It is the selective deletion and depletion of this population that appears largely responsible for the increasing range and severity of opportunistic infections and tumours that characterize the later stages of the natural history of this disease. Decline over time of CD4 counts in patient populations has been a consistent feature in longitudinally studied cohorts of HIV patients in most series[1–7] with few exceptions[8]. In most studies, however, the use of CD4 counts has been examined alongside a variety of other available serum or cell markers to identify groups of patients at increased risk of progression, and most have assessed the predictive value of a single CD4 count on subsequent progress.

Few studies have attempted to examine the power of single CD4 counts or sequential trends to predict outcome or treatment response in individual patients. Such analysis becomes increasingly important now that specific antiviral therapy is being applied earlier in the natural history of disease. Moreover, the increasing logistical difficulties involved in the evaluation of treatment response on the basis of disease progression endpoints in a disease with such an exceptionally long and varied natural history is forcing the scrutiny of surrogate markers of disease progression against which therapeutic response can be measured.

In the assessment of primary immunodeficiency states it is axiomatic to investigate the function of an immunological compartment or effector system in the diagnosis and characterization of individual disorders, rather than the mere absence or presence of a cell population. By analogy in the early stages of HIV infection the early and subtle levels of immunodeficiency will probably be revealed only by functional analyses of the cellular immune system. Dr

Gruters and Dr Miedema, in Chapter 5, discussed the potential of some of the more promising of these assays in detail. However, at the present time the large scale of the clinical problem, the time-consuming and biohazard constraints of the techniques involved, and difficulties in the standardization and quality control of assays means that it is unlikely that functional assessment will be widely or routinely adopted in the foreseeable future.

Even lymphocyte surface marker analysis has until recently remained largely a research tool. Until the arrival of HIV immunodeficiency the quantitative assessment of lymphocyte populations was not required for the diagnosis of any condition other than the rare primary immunodeficiencies of the neonate. Therefore little attention had been directed at standardization of methodologies, internal and external quality control of the investigations required for the use of comparative data between centres for the establishment of normal ranges and the evaluation of multicentre clinical trials.

This chapter will deal with the current status of lymphocyte surface marker analysis and other immunological markers of disease progression in HIV infection.

DEVELOPMENTS IN METHODOLOGY

Three major developments have allowed the accurate quantitation of lymphocyte subpopulations to emerge as a useful clinical investigation.

The first was the production by cell fusion technology of a panel of specific and internationally available monoclonal antibodies that allowed the detection with ease of total and T cell subpopulation factors within lymphoid cell preparations.

The availability of excellent specific antibodies virtually coincided with the introduction and subsequent simplification of laser-based flow cytometry systems for the rapid identification and enumeration of cell populations bearing multiple defined parameters. The sophistication and accessibility of the software programs for the analysis of data generated have undergone rapid development. The introduction of flow cytometry has been a major factor in increasing the precision of counting, since it permits the enumeration of thousands, rather than the hundreds, of cells that were assessed previously by cell microscopy.

Finally, the availability of new fluorochromes which allow dual antigen detection following single-wavelength excitation has permitted the introduction of whole-blood analysis techniques for identification of blood lymphoid populations. This latter technique avoids the need for prior purification and separation of mononuclear cells, and thus the possibility of selective cell loss inherent in buoyant density separation techniques. In addition, the availability of whole-blood staining with directly conjugated monoclonal antibodies allows considerable savings in sample preparative time, and minimizes the number of manipulations required on biohazard samples.

It remains an intriguing fact that the arrival and convergence of these new technologies coincided exactly with the first clinical reports of AIDS. HIV infection remains the only condition in which the accurate enumeration of lymphocyte subpopulations is an essential requirement for diagnosis or monitoring of human disease on any scale, and continues to provide an impetus for new developments.

LYMPHOCYTE SUBPOPULATION CHANGES AT DIFFERENT STAGES OF HIV DISEASE

A number of comprehensive natural history cohort studies have now allowed very accurate descriptions of the changes in the distribution of individual lymphocyte subpopulations in HIV infection at different stages of the disease in the various population groups at risk of infection[1–7]. Such natural history studies are now more difficult to sustain or complete, because of the introduction of therapeutic approaches which may have profound short-term effects on clinical outcome.

Reviewed here are the available natural history data for risk groups so far. These will now form essential baselines against which all subsequent studies incorporating improvements in management will have to be compared.

ACUTE SEROCONVERSION ILLNESS

Studies performed at this crucial stage in the initiation of infection are few in number, and for obvious reasons small in scale. The reductions in rate of transmission that have resulted from awareness of risk and action on the mode of transmission have resulted in low levels of subsequent seroconversion in HIV seronegative cohorts under longitudinal study.

A number of small studies do, however, provide valuable information about the acute changes in lymphocyte populations that occur following HIV exposure. They demonstrate that, in common with other lymphotropic virus infections such as Epstein–Barr virus (EBV) or cytomegalovirus (CMV), HIV produces dramatic acute changes in lymphocyte subpopulations. However, in the herpes virus infections, acute immunological disturbance is later followed by a return to immunological normality as productive virus infection is brought under control by specific host immune responses. In contrast, in HIV infection return to pre-exposure lymphoid population distributions is not seen.

Careful sequential studies by a number of groups have confirmed a consistent pattern of lymphocyte subpopulation changes during the phase of acute HIV infection and seroconversion. In different populations at risk of infection there is little evidence that these major disturbances in lymphocyte populations precede HIV exposure in the absence of other acute and chronic viral infections. Thus in homosexual men, pre-exposure CD4 and CD8 counts are comparable between those in cohorts who subsequently HIV seroconvert and those that remain seronegative[9]. Immediately after exposure all studies agree that acute and dramatic changes in populations are seen[9–11]. In the first 2 weeks of illness, lymphopenia associated with reductions in both CD8 and CD4 populations are observed in association with the appearance of small numbers of 'atypical' activated lymphocytes in the peripheral blood film. Over the next 2 weeks, to the end of the first month of a seroconversion illness, increasing numbers of CD8 lymphocytes, many bearing DR class II major histocompatibility complex (MHC) in co-association, are seen in the blood together with levels of CD4 cells which remain depressed[10]. This pattern of change is directly analogous to the findings in other acute viral infections with lymphotropic viruses including acute EBV[12] and CMV[13] infections. The appearance of activated CD8 cells often coincides with the disappearance of free p24 antigen from the serum of acute seroconverting individuals. It is probable that the activated CD8 cell population includes viral-specific cytotoxic (CTL) cells which may bring the early phase of HIV replication to an end. Once again there is a close analogy with EBV infection in which the activated CD8 population contains ciral-specific CTL[14] during the acute EBV seroconversion illness.

Over the next 4 months there is a decline in the numbers of activated CD8 T cells. However, these do not return to pre-HIV exposure levels in contrast to the gradual normalization seen in other acute viral infections. The persistent elevation of the CD8 population in addition to the consistent ability to isolate virus from such individuals is an indication that HIV infection remains continuously productive in such individuals following seroconversion. Studies disagree about the levels of CD4 cells found in the first few months post-infection. Cooper argues that counts return to pre-exposure levels[9], but two other studies suggest that persistent CD4 lymphopenia is the result of HIV infection in association with seroconversion illness[10,11]. Recent studies have suggested that particularly severe or prolonged seroconversion illness is associated with more rapid progression to symptomatic immunodeficiency[15]. Since it is such cases that are more likely to present for such sequential study it is probable that the acute prolongation of CD4 depletion identifies a group of patients with more severe initial (and eventual) disease, and probably represents a subgroup with greater initial HIV replication and CD4 depletion.

In summary a clear pattern emerges from these studies. An acute seroconversion illness is associated with a fall in CD4 cells and a rise in CD8 class II positive T cells. This pattern is preserved following clinical recovery from the acute features of the illness. Although in some cases there is a partial return to normality this is incomplete, and features associated with HIV infection are retained thereafter even through the subsequent asymptomatic stages of the disease which are principally characterized by an elevation of the CD8 population.

LYMPHOCYTE SURFACE MARKER TRENDS DURING ASYMPTOMATIC DISEASE

The asymptomatic phase of HIV infection may last for many years. Sequential lymphocyte surface marker analysis on patient cohorts in the early stages of disease indicate that there is an overall linear fall in CD4 count throughout this period[4]. The rate of loss of cells within cohorts is of the order of 60–100

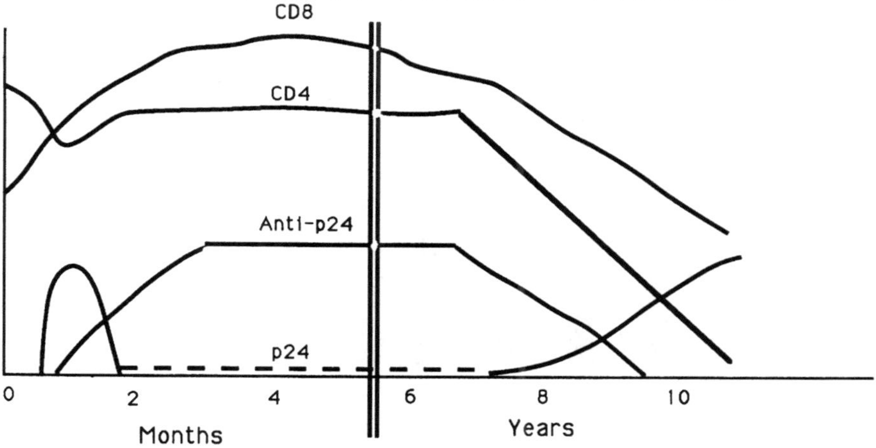

Figure 6.1 Schematic natural history of HIV infection. This diagram identifies the dynamic changes immediately following HIV seroconversion and again in the later stages of disease

cells/mm^3 per year. This overall trend is a composite of the trend within individual patients which represents a more complex picture. At any stage of disease a proportion of patients (<25%) will display a stable or even improving CD4 count trend with time, whereas another minority will show rates of decline that are much more rapid than the mean. Tersmette *et al.* have claimed to relate the slope of CD4 decline within individual patient populations to the biological properties of individual viral isolates. Syncytia-inducing isolates were associated with steep decline and early development of symptomatic disease, whereas slowly replicating non-syncytia-forming strains were associated with more stable trends and low rates of short-term progression[16] (see also Chapter 2). Other groups have confirmed the linearity of CD4 count fall, variability of slope and adverse prognosis associated with steeper slopes[2,6], although not all accept the hypothesis that rate in individual patients is attributable to behaviour of different viral isolates.

Since the estimations of individual CD4 counts are subject to considerable biological variation and a smaller degree of interassay variability it is essential to assess a series of results if reliable trends are to be observed. Single estimations or pairs of results taken months or years apart provide inadequate data upon which to base assessments in either patient cohorts or more particularly in individual patients. In individual subjects serial counts can be plotted as mathematical slopes. Philips *et al.* have successfully used the root mean-square error method to plot slopes from time of seroconversion in individual patients to predict incubation time to AIDS in individual HIV-infected haemophiliacs[4,17]. Such an approach has allowed extremely impressive correlations between predicted and observed AIDS progressions and non-progressions in individual cases, validating their linear model of CD4 decline throughout all stages of disease. The use of CD4 count decline trends also allows the separation of progression rates in populations of older and younger patients[4]. Trend analysis clearly indicates more rapid progression rates in haemophiliacs aged over 25 to those below 25, and has been confirmed

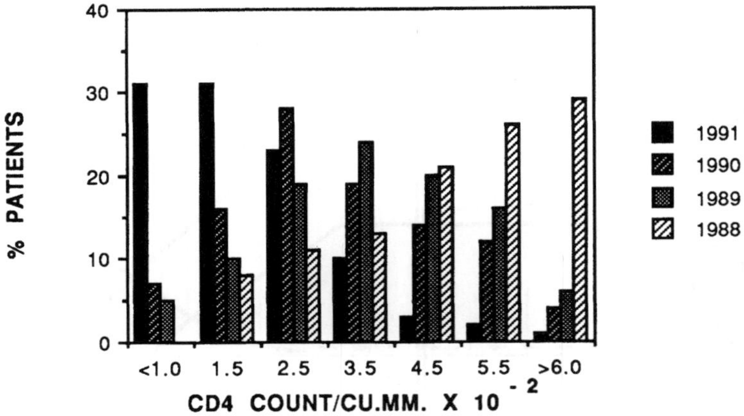

Figure 6.2 The distribution of CD4 counts in a population of 130 Edinburgh HIV-infected drug users followed up annually between 1988 and 1991. Available epidemiology suggests that the majority of individuals under study were infected between 1983 and 1984

in other studies examining clinical progression rates to AIDS[18].

Other lymphocyte markers provide less valuable information during this stage of disease. CD8 counts present a more complex picture. In the early asymptomatic stages there is a tendency for CD8 cells to continue to rise whilst CD4 counts are stable or fall, widening the discrepancy between the two populations and lowering the CD4/8 ratio. On progression to symptoms the CD8 count may begin to fall again[19], but this is variable between patients and can be masked by fluctuations and spikes of CD8 cells which may be related to subclinical reactivations of herpes virus infections in some cases[1]. The lability of the CD8 count makes it an unreliable marker for the staging of HIV disease. It is also the major reason why the CD4/8 ratio is an inherently meaningless assessment of disease progression in individual patients.

SYMPTOMATIC HIV DISEASE AND AIDS

As CD4 counts in individual patients fall to progressively lower levels so the proportion of individuals who present with symptoms of opportunistic infections rises steadily. Some studies have reported that the CD4 trend may enter a phase of accelerated and rapid decline immediately prior to the development of AIDS[2,19], although other cohorts have failed to confirm this trend and report linear falls throughout the natural history[4]. What is certain is that the rate of CD4 decline is variable between individuals, and the level at which an AIDS-defining infection or tumour occurs is also variable.

There is an approximate hierarchy of opportunistic infections which present at different stages of the accumulating immunodeficiency. Herpes zoster is an early feature of clinical immunodeficiency occurring on average 5 years

Table 6.1 Incidence of AIDS in cohort studies following identification of low CD4 count

Basic group	*CD4 threshold*	*AIDS incidence (%)*		*Reference*
		24 months	*33–36 months*	
Homosexual/bisexual	<200		87	3
	201–400		46	
	>400		16	
Homosexual/bisexual	<242		68	6
	243–345		40	
	346–490		23	
	>490		11	
Homosexual/bisexual	>600		6	7
	300–600		22	
	<300		89	
IDU	<200		100	20
	201–500		51	
	>500		22	
Haemophiliacs	<200	67		21

prior to development of AIDS. A zoster presentation is so early and variable that it lacks predictive power in individual patients[20]. Oral candida and oral hairy leukoplakia occur later in the natural history, and are usually but not invariably associated with overt reductions in CD4 counts. These generally fall below 300/mm^3, particularly if oral manifestations are associated with constitutional symptoms.

The most frequent major opportunistic infection, *Pneumocystis* pneumonia, is uncommon in adults until advanced immunodeficiency. Two longitudinal studies have clearly demonstrated that *Pneumocystis* pneumonia is very uncommon before the CD4 count has persistently fallen below 200/mm^3 or 20% of total lymphocytes[23,24]. These studies have resulted in general recommendations that primary prophylaxis for PCP should be considered in patients progressing to this stage of disease[25].

Exceptions to this observation occur, but are uncommon in patients who have been regularly followed up. Such occasional examples are usually in individuals who still show low CD4% counts (<20%) but who do not demonstrate the lymphopenia which is the usual feature of later-stage disease. Such exceptions may indeed show a mild lymphocytosis which is reflected by low normal CD4 counts but pathologically elevated levels of CD8 cells, many of which bear activation markers.

In contrast, Kaposi's sarcoma (KS) may present at a relatively early stage of immunodeficiency in HIV-infected homosexual males. In one prospective actuarial study[7] five out of 10 patients presenting with KS had CD4 counts >200/mm^3 at presentation, whereas none of 16 patients presenting with a range of opportunistic infections had CD4 counts of >200/mm^3. In this study the mean CD4 count for presentation with AIDS and an opportunistic infection was 73/mm^3, in contrast to 245/mm^3 when KS was the indicator presentation. Therefore, the nature of the risk groups and the range of infections or tumours anticipated as presentation features of AIDS will determine the characteristics of the CD4 profiles at which AIDS will present in individual cohorts. Evidence suggests that KS presenting in HIV-infected subjects with CD4 counts $>300/mm^3$ has a more indolent course and is associated with a good 12-month survival in comparison to its presentation in patients with very low ($<100/mm^3$) CD4 counts[26].

MARKERS OF CELLULAR ACTIVATION

HIV infection is characterized by two major types of immunological abnormality, the progressive CD4 depletion and associated immunodeficiency and evidence of chronic cellular immune activation. The two features coexist in the later stages of the disease, but in the earlier asymptomatic phase of disease immune activation is often the most striking initial immune abnormality. Since such activation is a feature of the very earliest stages of the disease before immunodeficiency or secondary infections are apparent, this suggests that the activation is a primary feature of HIV infection rather than secondary to the acquired immunodeficiency. In view of the recognized requirement of cellular activation for the upregulation of HIV replication it remains possible that the high levels of immune activation may play a role in sustaining HIV replication and hastening the self-destructive and accumulating immunodeficiency.

Two major examples of immune activation have been extensively examined in HIV infection. The first is the appearance of activation markers on the surface of lymphoid cells assessed by immunofluorescence flow cytometry. The second approach has been to quantitate released products from activated cells in serum. β_2-Microglobulin, neopterin and soluble interleukin-2 receptors have received particular attention.

Cell activation markers

Activation of lymphocytes, most especially $CD8^+$ T cells, is a consistent feature of the early phase of many early viral infections. However, in HIV infection activation is a persistent feature throughout all stages of the disease. Activated class II bearing T cells appear in elevated numbers within the first weeks of symptoms in patients with a seroconversion illness[10] and persist at elevated levels in most patients thereafter. Other markers of activation including CD38 expression on T cells also appear early and persist throughout infection. Sequential studies have indicated that levels of activated T cells rise throughout the asymptomatic phase of disease in both percentage and absolute numbers, and exceptionally high levels often precede the final deterioration in CD4 count and the appearance of opportunistic infections[19,26]. Class II DR bearing T cells often fall after the development of symptomatic disease, whereas the proportion of $CD38^+$ T cells continues to rise even in the final stages of HIV disease. In multivariate analysis on the San Francisco General cohort, the addition of activated DR+ T cells significantly improves the power of a model which also includes the β_2-microglobulin, CD4 count and p24 antigen positivity[27] to predict disease progression.

Serum markers of cellular activation

These markers have been receiving increasing attention, principally because of the simplicity of their measurement and since they offer the opportunity to retrospectively examine these markers in stored serum samples. Two markers have been extensively evaluated, β_2-microglobulin (β_2M) and neopterin. β_2M is the light chain of class I MHC antigens and is released from activated lymphocytes and other cells. High levels of β_2M are seen in lymphoproliferative diseases, autoimmune diseases and acute viral infections, particularly primary EBV infection. Elevated serum levels are also associated with renal failure, in which there is failure of excretion of the low molecular weight protein. In HIV infection the very high levels which are frequently seen represent the excessive degrees of lymphocyte activation in both B and T lymphocyte compartments which is a consistent feature throughout HIV infection. Numerous studies have indicated that highest levels of β_2M are associated with the later stages of HIV infection. In the early stages of disease, high levels are predictive of those patients at high risk of short-term progression[3,11,28]. These studies have convincingly demonstrated that serum β_2M levels reflect an independent progression marker when assessed alongside low CD4 counts[3,6,29]. Equally significantly, low levels of β_2M, when associated with normal levels of CD4 cells, identify a subgroup of HIV-infected patients with very low rates of disease progression. In one study of a population-based cohort in San Francisco, patients with elevated β_2M levels and low CD4 counts were associated with an 18.4 times risk of short-term progression when compared to a group of patients with normal values of both parameters[29]. One study has suggested that the levels of β_2M in individual patients correlates with survival in patients treated with zidovudine, and indicated that levels of this parameter fall after successful antiviral therapy[30]. This report suggests that β_2M has potential as a surrogate marker to identify early benefit from anti-retroviral therapy in individual patients although larger studies are required to confirm this preliminary finding.

β_2M and neopterin levels are strongly correlated in HIV infection. Although they reflect activation of different cell types, their concordance means that they essentially provide similar information, and measurement of one or the other will suffice. Since levels of the former also correlate with levels of soluble interleukin-2 receptors or activated T cells there is probably little benefit from additional inclusion of the latter in a monitoring panel[6], particularly since the latter assays are less well standardized and more expensive to perform. One advantage of the inclusion of immune activation markers in a monitoring panel is their ability to predict CD4 T cell levels in patient cohorts 2–3 years in advance. Presentation β_2M levels have been shown to be highly correlated with CD4 count levels 2–3 years later[11]. β_2M may therefore be valuable in selecting asymptomatic patients at high risk of short-term progression for clinical trial, and also to plan follow-up requirements in clinics assessing asymptomatic subjects.

It is important to recognize that immune activation markers probably represent and reflect activation by HIV itself, and thus reflect viral activity rather than the degree of immunodeficiency that is responsible for the majority of the clinical manifestations of HIV-associated disease. It is probably for this reason that in follow-up the CD4 count and activation markers together provide cumulative information.

Neopterin is a metabolite of guanosine triphosphate and is synthesized by macrophages when stimulated by γ-interferon released from activated T cells. Serum and urine neopterin levels have been shown to be consistently elevated in HIV-infected patients and correlate with disease stage[31,32]. In a study using stepwise proportional hazard methodology to determine the relative importance of a number of parameters to predict disease progression, the serum neopterin level emerged as a strong predictor of AIDS progression and slightly superior to the β_2M over a 4-year follow-up period[6]. Both markers appeared to predict CD4 decline and symptomatic disease at least 2–3 years before progression, suggesting that they may have particular value in identifying patients at medium-term risk of progression. Both markers are strongly correlated; thus measurement of one can substitute for the other, but both operate independently from the CD4 count as progression markers in patient cohorts. In combination they offer substantially greater prognostic value than either the CD4 count or an activation marker used alone. These studies suggest the dual importance of both the immunodeficiency and immune activation states in predicting prognosis, and suggest that one may predispose the development of the other.

These serological tests have the dual advantages of both being relatively inexpensive and easy to standardize and can also be performed on archived serum samples allowing retrospective analysis. The rapid turnover and renal clearance of these markers also suggests that they may offer sensitive and early indicators of successful therapy. It is, however, important that normal ranges are defined for individual HIV seronegative population controls. Although it has been shown that HIV negative homosexual males have a normal range of β_2M equivalent to age-matched heterosexual HIV negative adults[29], seronegative drug users have elevated β_2M levels when compared to normal population controls (personal observations) which may diminish the predictive power of the marker in the assessment of disease progression in infected drug users.

Serum immunoglobulins

Polyclonal B cell activation and serum hypergammaglobulinaemia is an early and consistent feature in patients with HIV infection[33]. These changes are reflected in the appearance of increased numbers of activated and spontaneously immunoglobulin secreting cells in the circulation. Although elevated IgM and IgG levels can be seen at all stages of infection, their elevation is inconsistent and can be influenced by other factors, particularly coexisting viral hepatitis with which HIV is frequently associated. Elevations of IgM and IgG, therefore, have low sensitivity and specificity in patient assessment. Serum IgA levels rise late in the natural history of HIV infection and are frequently found in patients with AIDS[34]; thus high IgA levels are associated with poor short-term prognosis. However, levels rise after the development of symptoms in many cases, making them of little value in the assessment of progression likelihood in individual asymptomatic patients.

Hypergammaglobulinaemia is probably a reflection of the overall immune activation that characterizes the earlier stages of HIV disease and, therefore, parallels other activation markers although less reliable. When summated with other markers which included $CD4^+$ T cells, serum neopterin, and p24 antigenaemia, one study showed that the combination marginally increased prognostic information over the use of single markers[26]. Serum immunoglobulin measurement is of very much greater value in the routine assessment of the HIV-infected child (see later section).

HIV p24 (core) antigen and antibody

The detection of HIV p24 antigen and the loss of p24 antibody reflects a high rate of viral replication and thus represents active HIV disease. The appearance of p24 antigen and disappearance of antibody has been shown to indicate poor prognosis in a number of prospective studies[3,5,8,21,35]. Moreover, the early appearance of p24 antigen after seroconversion will identify a subgroup of patients with more rapid CD4 count fall and early disease progression[36]. When directly compared in longitudinal studies, CD4 counts and p24 antigen perform as independent and complementary predictive markers of AIDS development[3,5,21]; p24 antigenaemia and loss of antibody have high specificity but low sensitivity in the identification of AIDS progression, the latter reflected by the fact that only about half of patients who eventually progress will ever show the marker. It seems that p24 antigenaemia preferentially identifies a subgroup of HIV-infected patients who produce a low initial antibody response to p24 and develop AIDS within a relatively short period following infection[5,36], whereas patients never manifesting antigenaemia generally display longer incubation times.

The reliability of p24 antigen to reflect viral replication rates must inevitably be lessened by the consideration that detection of antigenaemia can result from either enhanced viral replication or decreased specific antibody formation. Balanced antigen and antibody production will induce immune complex formation and the subsequent removal of complexes from the circulation, further limiting the reliability of the marker. More recently described methods for the detection of plasma viraemia[37] limiting dilution polymerase chain reaction quantitation of virally infected cells[38] or biological characterization of viral isolates (see Chapter 2) hold more promise for the direct assessment of levels of viral infection and replication.

PROGRESSION MARKERS IN CHILDREN

The principal non-specific immunological laboratory markers that have proved of value in the assessment and monitoring of adult infection have proved much less useful in children. Firstly, the normal ranges for lymphoid markers in children are much higher than in adults, particularly below the age of 1 year. Individual results must therefore be related to age-matched control ranges generated locally. Even when correcting for age-related normal ranges it is apparent that the fall in CD4 count is a late feature in paediatric HIV disease. Counts often fall to unequivocally low levels only after development of established growth retardation or opportunistic infections have already drawn clinical attention to underlying HIV infection. CD8 counts are often elevated early in paediatric infection, but this change lacks specificity. As in adults, CD8 elevation is a non-specific finding; it will not reliably indicate HIV infection or progression of disease when this would be most useful in the early stages of disease in infants of uncertain HIV status below 18 months of age.

The recently published update to the European Collaborative Study of children born to HIV-infected mothers[39] clearly identified that of those children who will lose maternal antibody, and thus are presumed HIV uninfected, 97.5% will have done so by 18 months. This indicates that peristence of specific IgG antibody beyond that time is strongly indicative of vertically acquired infection. In these children elevated immunoglobulins at 6 months has emerged as a reliably early marker of vertically acquired HIV infection. Elevated levels currently identify 77% of children subsequently shown to be HIV infected with an estimated false-positive rate of only 3%[39]. Addition of lymphocyte subpopulation markers added little additional information in this study. It remains possible that, as in adults, the assessment of CD4 trends in individual children will prove a more sensitive indicator of early disease progression, but large-scale longitudinal studies are lacking. Such prospective studies will need to be multicentre to evaluate this.

Studies which have examined the prognostic value of the CD4 count have indicated that low CD4 counts fail to accurately identify a substantial proportion of children at risk of subsequent development of opportunistic infections. Not even the inclusion of lymphocyte proliferation assays greatly facilitates the discrimination of those with immunodeficiency from those without. In general, however, those children with low CD4 counts and poor lymphocyte proliferations responses have much poorer immediate outcomes and short-term prognosis[40].

Pneumocystis carinii pneumonia is the most common AIDS-defining illness in children, and is responsible for 70% of paediatric cases reported to Centres for Disease Control in the USA. PCP also carries a very high mortality rate in children even when new diagnostic and therapeutic advances have been employed. In one recent retrospective study[41] of 22 children 36% had a CD4 count of >450 cells/mm^3 at the time of PCP diagnosis and 27% had a count >1000/mm^3. A larger study has confirmed this finding, reporting that only 10 of 21 perinatally infected children presenting with PCP had CD4 counts <500/mm^3. However, CD4 counts <1500/mm^3 in HIV-infected children below the age of 1 year identified the majority who developed PCP but included only a small proportion of infants who did not develop the complication[42]. Although the risk of developing PCP can be established only by prospective studies, the high mortality associated with PCP in children, and the success of primary PCP prophylaxis in adults, has recently led the

Centers for Disease Control to issue guidelines. These recommend that prophylaxis be offered to children below 1 year with CD4 counts $<1500/mm^3$, between 1 and 2 years with counts $<750/mm^3$ and from 2–5 years with counts $<500/mm^3$. This recommendation takes into account the higher normal ranges for lymphocyte populations seen in normal infants. A CD4% <20% is also regarded as abnormally low, and is seen as an indication for prophylaxis regardless of CD4 count[43].

The poor correlation between very low CD4 counts and PCP infection in children may reflect the severe functional inability of HIV-infected children to mount primary immune responses following initial exposure to PCP at a stage of disease when global CD4 depletion has not yet occurred. A compelling implication of these observations for potentially vertically infected children is that improved methods for the reliable early identification of HIV infection and more discriminating laboratory assessments of immunodeficiency are required to improve prophylaxis and clinical management of opportunistic infections in this age group. Such infections are currently associated with a very high mortality rate, particularly in HIV-infected children below the age of 1 year.

Studies using other cellular or serum markers of immune activation are even less complete in children, and have not been followed prospectively to evaluate crucial questions regarding their value as progression markers or surrogate indicators of HIV infection in children below the age of 18 months. In one retrospective study of reasonable size[44], approximately 60% of children with indeterminate serology had β_2M and neopterin levels within the age-matched normal range, whereas the remainder had elevated levels. Whether these children with elevated levels represent the infected children will require adequate longitudinal studies; these are urgently required.

METHODOLOGICAL AND BIOLOGICAL INFLUENCES ON THE STABILITY OF CD4 COUNTS

Awareness of the biological and technical variables which can influence the measurement of lymphocyte surface markers are essential if they are to be used as laboratory indicators of disease staging or progression in individual patients. A number of factors can influence the stability of CD4 counts, and together these variables can result in variation of 20% or greater between individual counts in HIV-infected patients whose underlying CD4 count trend is otherwise stable. If CD4 counts are to be used as indicators for clinical intervention or trial assessment it is essential that these factors which produce variation are understood. Some, but not all, of these can be minimized by standardization of laboratory techniques.

Considerations of methodology

A number of methodological factors can influence individual counts. Many of these can be reduced by use of standardized protocols. Quality control schemes are valuable for identifying variation both with and between laboratories.

Many early methods for staining lymphoid populations employed an initial lymphocyte separation stage. This may lead to selective loss of individual cell populations and double-layer fluorescent techniques, then used, are prone to problems of non-specific antibody binding, particularly to monocytes. However, the greatest single potential variable in early methodologies resulted when visual microscopic assessment was used of a limited number (usually only 100–200) of cells. For statistical reasons alone the confidence limits of such techniques are unacceptably wide. The inaccuracy and imprecision are further compounded if the observer is inexperienced in distinguishing individual cell types or fluorescent thresholds. The increasing use of flow cytometry has minimized most of these variables, provided that the instrument is appropriately set up and operated. Flow cytometry allows the assessment of much larger numbers of cells, and whole-blood fluorescence techniques eliminate potential selective cell loss. Cytometry permits very accurate gating of the lymphocyte population, which minimizes monocyte contamination of the lymphoid cells enumerated.

Delay in analysis of samples and fluctuations in temperature during transit may influence evaluated results[45,46]. Recent studies suggest that, provided the samples are prepared within 24 hours of venesection and transported in anticoagulant at an ambient temperature of 22°C, the lymphocyte subpopulation results are relatively stable[47]. Deviation from this protocol will significantly affect results of subpopulations of lymphocytes, but delays in analysis of more than 6 hours have much more marked effects on total white cell counts performed using automated haematology counters. Beyond 6 hours automated white cell counters will begin to reject samples because of cell degeneration[48]. This may be one explanation why, in many hands, subpopulations percentages are more consistent than absolute numbers for sequential monitoring of HIV-infected subjects[49]. However, CD4 percentages can be influenced by either a fall in CD4 or a rise in CD8. The CD8 proportion can be influenced by other intercurrent events, particularly infections; therefore the absolute count is a more reliable biological marker overall if trends are to be analysed despite the slightly greater inherent variability between single measurements[17].

Biological variation

In addition to methodological variations a number of biological causes of variability which operate independently of the natural history of HIV infection need to be considered.

The most important cause of acute variation in lymphocyte surface marker trends results from analysis during acute intercurrent infection. Acute sepsis has been documented to produce marked transient changes in lymphocyte subpopulations even in the absence of HIV infection[50]. Experience suggests that acute bacterial sepsis will produce similar acute transient changes in HIV-infected subjects. If CD4 counts are to be used to stage patients clinically they must not be assessed during an acute exacerbation of disease or during an irrelevant intercurrent infection. This consideration emphasizes the need for clinical follow-up and baseline monitoring during the long asymptomatic phase of HIV infection against which therapy or clinical trials can be assessed.

A further cause of clinical variability is diurnal variation in lymphocyte counts. Total white cell counts and the derived lymphocyte subpopulation values are subject to predictable and marked variation[51]. Peak CD4 counts in normal individuals are found at 2300 hours and trough levels at 1100 hours. Counts are inversely correlated with plasma cortisol levels. Diurnal effects are substantial and counts may vary by as much as 50% between 1600 and 1700 hours. Limited studies suggest that, in HIV-infected subjects with normal or moderately reduced CD4 counts, such variations can also be demonstrated and can result in apparent but spurious immunological deterioration if sequential samples are taken during clinic attendances at different times of day. Diurnal variation is a much more marked feature in early stages of HIV disease when CD4 counts are relatively normal than they are in the later stages of CD4 depletion.

Individual clinicians should be aware of this substantial source of individual variation, and either attempt to limit its effects by synchronizing clinic visits or to discount for its possible effects when assessing results from uneven timing.

To further complicate the picture, two groups have described variation in lymphocyte markers at different times of year (circannual) amongst normal volunteer donors[52,53]. Circannual variation produces accentuation or flattening of individual diurnal variation depending on the time of year, as well as significant changes in absolute values from month to month at the same time of day. In one study the mean CD4 count rose by 40% from June to November in one individual. This pattern was reproducible year on year[17].

Overall these various factors combine to produce significant levels of variability between individual CD4 counts in many patients with even stable HIV disease. This consideration does not invalidate the use of these counts in the assessment of individual patients, but indicates that trends should be assessed over a period of time when lymphocyte counts have been measured uninfluenced by acute clinical events. Serial counts eliminate much of the background variability, and will permit the more accurate determination of thresholds at which prophylactic or antiviral therapy should be introduced. Individual counts should be interpreted with care, particularly the attachment of undue significance to a last CD4 which appears to demonstrate a falling trend. It is advisable to produce graphic plots of sequential results from individual patients so that overall trends can be visually assessed.

ASSESSMENT OF SPECIFIC THERAPY IN HIV DISEASE

The pressure to develop and evaluate specific and effective therapy against HIV infection has been intense and mounting since the scale and severity of the HIV epidemic has become fully apparent. Initial trials evaluating the therapeutic effects of zidovudine and other candidate antiretroviral agents were directed at patients with advanced symptomatic disease, and the endpoint of such early trials was prolongation of patient survival. Although such trials provided limited evidence of therapeutic efficacy they raised a series of new questions and concerns. In particular, there were doubts expressed about how sustained were the clinical and antiviral responses observed in the cases of late-stage immunodeficiency, and such concern was reinforced by the observations of drug resistance observed *in vitro* in patients receiving zidovudine for 6 months or longer[54]. Trial development has been driven by the dual and conflicting requirements of more rapid endpoints for drug effectiveness and the need to assess the influence of therapy in early stages of disease when chosen endpoints are extended. This has resulted in the search for earlier indicators of disease progression during the asymptomatic phase of HIV disease.

A second generation of trials have examined the effects of different doses of zidovudine to slow short-term disease progression in early symptomatic or asymptomatic HIV-infected patients[55,56]. In two recent published trials, early benefit was apparent in patients with CD4 counts below 500/mm^3. In addition to slowing progression, the short-term effects of the drug were observed as a slowing of the rate of fall in CD4 counts observed when compared to placebo arm patients which represented the natural history of the untreated disease. These trials have raised hopes that surrogate markers such as CD4 progression endpoints could be used on earlier assessments of drug efficacy or dosage requirements. Indeed a continuation of the existing asymptomatic zidovudine trial for patients entered with CD4 counts >500/mm^3 will terminate for individual patients once this threshold is reached, since zidovudine has already been shown to be effective in delaying short-term clinical progression in patients with counts below this threshold entered to this trial[56].

The potential ability of surrogate markers to yield earlier information about efficacy or dosage is fuelling interest in the potential of such markers in future HIV clinical trials. It is also creating intense pressure for such markers to be used as endpoints for therapeutic intervention in the management of patients not entered into such clinical trials. For example, as a consequence of the trial results already discussed, zidovudine was relicensed in the USA and Australia for use in all asymptomatic HIV-infected individuals with CD4 counts <500/mm^3. This change in approach was introduced even though it was acknowledged that such universal therapy might include many patients only recently infected, and with many years of asymptomatic disease ahead. Such concerns resulted in the introduction of a European licence for zidovudine therapy in asymptomatic individuals whose CD4 counts were <500/mm^3 and whose counts were 'rapidly falling'. Since the characteristics of a rapidly falling count were not defined, the criteria for the use of surrogate markers for therapeutic intervention could be viewed as having made an uncertain or even shaky debut.

Confidence is not enhanced by the fact that few studies have so far examined the relationship between trials using surrogate markers and endpoints and eventual survival in individual patients. Such information is an essential baseline if the transition is to be made from a clinical to a laboratory endpoint, since it is entirely feasible for a therapy to stabilize or improve an individual surrogate marker and yet exert no or even adverse influences on long-term survival. For example, one possibility is that antiretroviral therapy might be effective in the short or medium term on the systemic immunosuppressive effects of HIV, and yet exert little influence on the progression of HIV-induced central nervous system damage. One eventual therapeutic outcome could be retained immunocompetence, and thus freedom from opportunistic infections despite progressive HIV neurological disease. If the natural history of the latter were unaffected it might be possible for surrogate immunological markers to demonstrate sustained improvement, but for overall survival (and morbidity) to be much less significantly affected.

There is therefore an urgent requirement for studies which relate surrogate markers to natural history in individual patients. Analysis of the placebo control arms of double-blind studies will provide important natural history data of this type. Analysis of large data sets will be required to confirm the trends observed in small natural history studies such as those reported for untreated haemophiliacs[17]. So far, only one published study has related prognostic value of laboratory markers to eventual survival in individual patients receiving zidovudine[30]. This study was small, but within this limitation did suggest that both CD4 lymphocyte count estimated 8–12 weeks after commencing therapy and a decrease in serum β_2M correlated with individual survival. If such trends are borne out by more extensive studies these markers may have validity as surrogate endpoints for future trials.

A further feature in the monitoring of specific therapy is the need for an increased awareness of an extended range of complications consequent upon the prolongation of a stage of severe immunodeficiency. One example of what will probably emerge as a range of new features is the recent report of a high prevalence of high-grade non-Hodgkin's lymphoma in patients on zidovudine therapy. These patients had survived with very low CD4 counts for prolonged periods of time[57].

The occurrence of non-Hodgkin's lymphoma in primary or secondary immunodeficiency states associated with T cell impairment has been well recognized and has more recently been described in association with HIV infection. However, this recent review of HIV-infected patients, many of whom were some of the earliest recipients of zidovudine, revealed an unexpectedly high late incidence of non-Hodgkin's lymphomas in long-term survivors with prolonged reduction of CD4 counts. Non-Hodgkin's lymphoma developed in eight out of 55 patients, producing an estimated probability of developing lymphoma after 36 months of therapy of 46.4%. It remains possible that this figure may increase further with time. Patients who developed lymphoma had received antiretroviral therapy for a mean of 24 months and the mean CD4 count at the time of lymphoma presentation was 26 cells/mm^3. Patients who developed lymphomas had sustained CD4 counts <100/mm^3 for a median duration of 18 months. Although other possibilities have not been excluded it is likely that the prolonged severe T cell immunodeficiency sustained by these patients is the crucial factor in the high incidence of lymphoma observed.

The broadening spectrum of clinical disease associated with the prolongation of survival resulting from partially effective therapy indicates the importance of continued clinical and laboratory assessment of these patients, and the development of more selective methods for defining specific immunodeficiency.

CONCLUSIONS AND FUTURE PROSPECTS

Lymphocyte surface marker analysis offers additional information which, when combined with clinical features, should result in improvements in the classification and staging of HIV disease. Although it is possible that markers of cell activation or the identification of further subdivisions of lymphocyte subpopulations may extend the power of immunological investigation in such classification, at the present time the absolute CD4 count, combined with a serum marker of immune activation, remain the most reliable parameters for immunological staging. Future assessment will be complicated by the increasing trend towards early therapeutic intervention in disease which will compromise the assessment of natural history.

Nevertheless, immunological markers are likely to play an increasing role in clinical decision-making and the evaluation of clinical trial endpoints. This will require improved methods of standardization in laboratory techniques and the introduction of external and internal quality control for these investigations. In the assessment of HIV disease the laboratory quantitation of lymphocyte subpopulations is the cornerstone of laboratory monitoring, and is unlikely to be displaced from this position in the foreseeable future.

References

1. Goedert, J. J., Biggar, R. J., Melbye, M., Mann, D. L., Wilson, S., Gail, M. H., Grossman, R. J., Digioia, R. A., Sanchez, W. C., Weiss, S. H. and Blattner, W. A. (1987). Effect of T4 count and cofactors on the incidence of AIDS in homosexual men infected with human immunodeficiency virus. *J. Am. Med. Assoc.*, **257**, 331–4
2. Eyster, M. E., Ballard, J. O., Gail, M. H., Drummond, J. E. and Goedert, J. J. (1987). Natural History of immunodeficiency virus infection in haemophiliacs effects: of T cell subsets, platelet counts and age. *Ann. Intern. Med.*, **107**, 1–6
3. Moss, A. R., Bacchetti, P., Osmond, D., Krampf, W., Chaisson, R. E., Stites, D., Wilber, J., Allain, J. P. and Carlson, J. (1988). Seropositivity from HIV and the development of AIDS or AIDS related condition: three year follow up of the San Francisco General Hospital cohort. *Br. Med. J.*, **296**, 745–9
4. Philips, A., Lee, C. A., Elford, J., Janossy, G., Bofill, M., Timms, A. and Kernoff, P. B. A. (1989). Prediction of progression to AIDS by analysis of CD4 lymphocyte counts in a haemophiliac cohort. *AIDS*, **3**, 737–41
5. De Wolf, F., Lange, J. M. A., Houweling, J. T. M., Mulder, J. W., Beemster, J., Schellekens, P. T., Coutinho, R. A., Van der Noordaa, J. and Goudsmit, J. (1989). Appearance of predictors of disease progression in relationship to the development of AIDS. *AIDS*, **3**, 563–9
6. Fahey, J. L., Taylor, J. M. G., Detels, R., Hofman, B., Melmed, R., Nishanian, P. and Giorgi, J. V. (1990). The prognostic value of cellular and serologic markers in infection with human immunodeficiency virus type I, *N. Engl. J. Med.*, **322**, 166–72
7. Venet, A., Tourani, J. M., Beldjord, K., Eme, D., Even, P. and Andrieu, J. M. (1990). Actuarial rate of clinical and biological progression in a cohort of 250 HIV seropositive subjects. *Clin. Exp. Immunol.*, **80**, 151–5
8. Weber, J. N., Wadsworth, J., Rogers, L. A., Moshtael, O., Scott, K., McManus, T., Berrie, E., Jeffries, O. J., Harris, J. R. W. and Pinching, A. J. (1986). Three year prospective study of HTLVIII/LAV infection in homosexual men. *Lancet*, **1**, 1179–82
9. Cooper, D. A., Tindall, B., Wilson, E. J., Imrie, A. A. and Penny, R. (1988). Characterization of T lymphocyte responses during primary infection with human immunodeficiency virus. *J. Infect. Dis.*, **157**, 889–96
10. Gaines, H., Von Sydow, M. A. E., Von Stedingk, L., Biberfeld, G., Böttiger, B., Hanson, L. O., Lundbergh, P., Sönnerborg, A. B., Wasserman, J. and Strannegard, Ö. O. (1990). Immunological changes in primary HIV-1 infection. *AIDS*, **4**, 995–9

11. Hofman, B., Wang, Y., Cumberland, W. G., Detels, R., Bozergmehri, M. and Fahey, J. L. (1990). Serum beta 2 microglobulin level increases in HIV infection: relation to seroconversion, CD4 T cell fall and prognosis. *AIDS*, **4**, 207–14
12. De Waele, M., Thielemans, C. and Van Camp, B. K. G. (1981). Characterization of immunoregulatory T cells in EBV-induced infectious mononucleosis by monoclonal antibodies. *N. Engl. J. Med.*, **304**, 460–2
13. Carney, W. P., Rubin, R. H., Hoffmann, R. A., Hansen, W. P., Healey, K. and Hirsch, M. S. (1981). Analysis of T lymphocyte subsets in cytomegalovirus mononucleosis. *J. Immunol.*, **126**, 2114–16
14. Svedmyr, E. and Jondal, M. (1975). Cytotoxic effector cells specific for B cell lines transformed by Epstein–Barr virus are present in patients with infectious mononucleosis. *Proc. Natl. Acad. Sci. USA*, **72**, 1622–6
15. Pedersen, C., Lindhardt, B., Jensen, B. L., Lauritzen, E., Gerstoft, J. and Dickmeiss, E. (1989). Clinical course of primary HIV infection: consequences for the subsequent course of the infection. Vth International AIDS Conference, Montreal, Abstract TAO 30
16. Tersmette, M., Lange, J. M. A., De Goede, R. E. Y., De Wolf, F., Eeftink-Schattenkerk, J. K. M., Schellekens, P. T. A., Coutinho, R. A., Huisman, J. G., Goudsmit, J. and Miedema, F. (1989). Association between biological properties of human immunodeficiency virus variants and risk for AIDS and mortality. *Lancet*, **1**, 983–5
17. Philips, A. N., Lee, C. A., Elford, J., Janossy, G., Timms, A., Bofill, M. and Kernoff, P. B. A. (1991). Serial CD4 lymphocyte counts and development of AIDS. *Lancet*, **337**, 389–92
18. Darby, S. C., Rizza, C. R., Doll, R., Spooner, R. J. D., Stratton, I. M. and Thakrar, B. (1989). Seropositivity for HIV and incidence of AIDS and AIDS related complex in UK haemophiliacs; report on behalf of directors of Haemophilia Centres in the UK. *Br. Med. J.*, **298**, 1064–8
19. Giorgi, J. V. and Detels, R. (1989). T-cell subset alterations in HIV infected homosexual men. NIAID multicentre AIDS cohort study. *Clin. Immunol. Immunopathol.*, **52**, 10–18
20. Fernandez-Cruz, E., Desco, M., Montes, M. G., Longo, N., Gonzalezx, B. and Zabay, J. M. (1990). Immunological and serological markers predictive of progression to AIDS in a cohort of HIV infected drug users. *AIDS*, **4**, 987–94
21. Eyster, M. E., Ballard, J. O., Gail, M. H., Drummond, J. E. and Goedert, J. J. (1989). Predictive markers for the acquired immunodeficiency syndrome (AIDS) in haemophiliacs: Persistance of p24 antigen and low T4 cell count. *Ann. Intern. Med.*, **110**, 963–9
22. Mellbye, M., Goedert, J. J., Grossman, R. J., Eyster, M. E. and Biggar, R. E. (1987). Risk of AIDS after herpes zoster. *Lancet*, **1**, 728–30
23. Masur, H., Ognibene, F. P., Yarchoan, R. *et al.* (1989). CD4 counts as predictors of opportunistic pneumonias in human immunodeficiency virus (HIV) infection. *Ann. Intern. Med.*, **III**, 223–31
24. Phair, J., Munoz, A., Detels, R., Kaslow, R., Rinaldo, C. and Saah, A. (1990). The risk of *Pneumocystis carinii* pneumonia among men infected with human immunodeficiency virus type 1. *N. Engl. J. Med.*, **322**, 161–5
25. Centres for Disease Control (1989). Guidelines for prophylaxis against *Pneumocystis carinii* pneumonia for persons infected with human immunodeficiency virus. *Morbid. Mortal. Weekly Rep.*, **38** (Suppl. S-5), 1–9
26. Fahey, J. L., Prince, H., Weaver, M., Groopman, J., Visscher, B., Schwartz, K. and Detels, R. (1984). Quantitative changes in T helper or T suppressor/cytotoxic lymphocyte subsets that distinguish acquired immune deficiency syndrome from other immune subset disorders. *Am. J. Med.*, **78**, 95–100
27. Stites, D. P., Moss, A. R., Bachetti, P., Osmond, D., McHugh, T. M., Wang, Y. J., Herbert, S. and Colfer, B. (1989). Lymphocyte subset analysis to predict progression to AIDS in a cohort of homosexual men in San Francisco. *Clin. Immunol. Immunopathol.*, **52**, 96–103
28. Lacey, C. N., Forbes, M. A., Waugh, M. A., Cooper, E. H., Hambling, M. H. (1987). Serum B_2 microglobulin and human immunodeficiency virus infection. *AIDS*, **1**, 123–7
29. Anderson, R. E., Lang, W., Shiboski, S., Royce, R., Jewell, N. and Winkelstein, W. (1990). Use of B_2 microglobulin level and CD4 count to predict development of acquired immunodeficiency syndrome in patients with human immunodeficiency virus infection. *Arch. Intern. Med.*, **150**, 73–7
30. Jacobsen, M. A., Bacchetti, P., Kolokathis, A., Chaisson, R. E., Szabo, S., Polsky, B., Valainis,

G. T., Mildvan, D., Abrams, D., Wilber, J., Winger, E., Sachs, H. S., Hendrickson, C. and Mosos, A. (1991). Surrogate markers for survival in patients with AIDS and AIDS related complex treated with zidovudine. *Br. Med. J.*, **302**, 73–8

31. Fuchs, D., Hansen, A., Reibnegger, G., Werne, E. R., Dierich, M. P. and Wachter, H. (1988). Neopterin as a marker for activated cell-mediated immunity: application in HIV infection. *Immunol. Today*, **9**, 150–5
32. Melmed, R. N., Taylor, J. M., Detels, R., Bozorgmehri, M. and Fahey, J. L. (1989). Serum neopterin changes in HIV infected subjects: indicator of significant immunopathology, CD4 T cell change and the development of AIDS. *J. AIDS*, **2**, 70–6
33. Lane, H. C., Masur, H., Edgar, L. C., Whalen, G., Rook, A. H. and Fauci, A. S. (1983). Abnormalities of B cell activation and immunoregulation in patients with the acquired immunodeficiency syndrome. *N. Engl. J. Med.*, **309**, 453–8
34. Munoz, A., Carey, W. and Saah, A. J. (1988). Predictors of decline in CD4 lymphocytes in a cohort of homosexual men infected with human immunodeficiency virus. *J. AIDS*, **1**, 396–404
35. Lange, J. M. A., Paul, D. A. and Huisman, H. G. (1986). Persistent HIV antigenaemia and decline of HIV core antibodies associated with the transition to AIDS. *Br. Med. J.*, **293**, 1459–62
36. Cheinsong-Popov, R., Panagiotidi, C., Bowcock, S., Aronstam, A., Wadsworth, J. and Weber, J. (1991). Relation between humoral responses to HIV gag and env proteins at seroconversion and clinical outcome of HIV infection. *Br. Med. J.*, **302**, 23–6
37. Ho, D. D., Moudgil, T. and Alam, M. (1989). Quantitation of the human immunodeficiency virus type 1 in the blood of infected persons. *N. Engl. J. Med.*, **321**, 1621–5
38. Balfe, P., Simmonds, P., Ludlam, C. A., Bishop, J. O. and Leigh-Brown, A. J. (1990). Concurrent evolution of human immunodeficiency virus type 1 in patients infected from the same source. *J. Virol.*, **64**, 6221–33
39. European Collaborative Study (1991). Children born to women with HIV-1 infection: natural history and risk of transmission. *Lancet*, **337**, 253–60
40. Bernstein, L. J., Bye, M. R. and Rubinstein, A. (1989). Prognostic factors and life expectancy in children with acquired immunodeficiency syndrome and *pneumocystis carinii* pneumonia. *Am. J. Dis. Child.*, **143**, 775–8
41. Leibovitz, E., Rigaud, M., Pollack, H., Lawrence, R., Chandwani, S., Krasinski, K. and Berkowsky, W. (1990). *Pneumocystis carinii* pneumonia in infants infected with the human immunodeficiency virus with more than 450 CD4 T lymphocytes per cubic millimeter. *N. Engl. J. Med.*, **323**, 531–3
42. Kovacs, A., Frederick, T., Church, J., Eller, A., Oxtoby, M., Mascola, L. (1991). CD4 T lymphocyte counts and *pneumocystis carinii* pneumonia in paediatric HIV infection. *J. Am. Med. Assoc.*, **265**, 1698–703
43. CDC (1991). CDC Guidelines for prophylaxis against *pneumocystis carinii* pneumonia for children infected with human immunodeficiency virus. *J. Am. Med. Assoc.*, **265**, 1637–44
44. Chan, M. M., Campos, J. M., Josephs, S. and Rifae, N. (1990). B_2 microglobulin and neopterin: predictive markers for human immunodeficiency versus infection type 1 in children. *J. Clin. Microbiol.*, **28**, 2215–19
45. Grunow, J. E., Lubet, R. A., Ferguson, M. J. and Goulden, M. E. (1976). Preferential decrease in thymus dependent lymphocytes during storage at 4°C in anticoagulant. *Tranfusion*, **16**, 610–15
46. Weiben, B. J., Debell, R. and Valem, C. R. (1983). Acquired immunodeficiency of blood stored overnight. *N. Engl. J. Med.*, **309**, 793
47. Paxton, H., Kidd, P., Landay, A., Giorgi, J., Flomenberg, N., Walker, E., Valentine, F., Fahey, J. and Gelman, R. (1989). Results of the flow cytometry ACTG quality control programme. Analysis and findings. *Clin. Immunol. Immunopathol.*, **52**, 68–84
48. Landay, A. L. and Muirhead, R. A. (1989). Procedural guidelines for performing immunophenotyping by flow cytometry. *Clin. Immunol. Immunopathol.*, **52**, 48–60
49. Taylor, J. M. G., Fahey, J. L., Detels, R. and Giorgi, J. V. (1989). CD4 percentage CD4 number and CD4:CD8 ratio in HIV infection: which to choose and how to use. *J. AIDS*, **2**, 114–24
50. Williams, R. C., Koster, F. T. and Kilpatrick, K. A. (1983). Alterations in lymphocyte cell surface markers during various human infections. *Ann. J. Med.*, **74**, 807–16
51. Ritchie, A. W. S., Oswald, I., Micklem, H. S., Boyd, J. E., Elton, R. A., Jazwinska, E. and James, K. (1983). Circadian variation of lymphocyte subpopulations: a study with monoclonal antibodies. *Br. Med. J.*, **286**, 1773–5

52. Abo, T., Miller, C. A. and Cloud, G. A. (1985). Annual stability in levels of lymphocyte subpopulations identified by monoclonal antibodies in blood of healthy individuals. *J. Clin. Immunol.*, **5**, 13–20
53. Levi, F. A., Canon, C., Touitou, Y., Reinberg, A. and Mathe, G. (1988). Seasonal modulation of the circadian time structure of circulating and natural killer lymphocyte subsets from healthy subjects. *J. Clin. Invest.*, **81**, 407–13
54. Larder, B. A., Darby, G. and Richmann, D. D. (1989). HIV with reduced sensitivity to zidovudine (AZT) isolated during prolonged therapy. *Science*, **243**, 1731–4
55. Fishl, M. D., Richmann, D. D., Hansen, N. *et al.* (1990). The safety and efficiency of Zidovudine (AZT) in patients with mildly symptomatic human immunodeficiency virus type 1 (HIV) infection. A double-blind placebo controlled trial. *Ann. Intern. Med.*, **112**, 727–37
56. Volberding, P. A., Lagakos, S. W., Koch, M. A. *et al.* (1990). Zidovudine in asymptomatic human immunodeficiency virus infection: a controlled trial in patients with fewer than 500 CD4 positive cells per cubic millimeter. *N. Engl. J. Med.*, **322**, 941–9
57. Pluda, J. M., Yarchoan, R., Jaffe, E. S., Feuerstein, I. M., Solomon, D., Steinberg, S. M., Wyvill, K. M., Raubitschek, A., Katz, D. and Broder, S. (1990). Development of non-Hodgkin's lymphoma in a cohort of patients with severe human immunodeficiency virus (HIV) infection on long-term antiretroviral therapy. *Ann. Intern. Med.*, **113**, 276–82

7

Mycobacterial immunity and mycobacterial disease in relation to HIV infection

D. S. KUMARARATNE, A. PITHIE, E. O. E. BASSI and R. BARTLETT

GENERAL INTRODUCTION

Mycobacterium tuberculosis is an obligatory parasite with no free-living (saprophytic) forms. It has the capacity to survive and multiply within mononuclear phagocytes (i.e. monocytes and macrophages), as well as survive extracellularly. Unlike pyogenic bacterial pathogens, mycobacteria multiply slowly with a generation time of 12–24 h. In consequence, tuberculosis is a chronic disease which is slow to develop and progress (cf. meningococcal septicaemia). The tubercle bacillus is well adapted to be a successful parasite in the human host and can survive for many years within an infected host. Factors which contribute to the prolonged *in vivo* survival of *M. tuberculosis* are summarized in Table 7.1.

It is estimated by the World Health Organization that 1 billion individuals (20% of the world population) are infected with *M. tuberculosis*. However, of those who become infected, no more than 20% develop clinically apparent disease, within their lifetime[1]. Hence the large majority of infected individuals are capable of controlling the infection, i.e. exhibit immunity. However, in many infected individuals the organisms persist and retain the potential to become reactivated and cause progressive disease, even years after the initial infection. Skin test surveys suggest that in many developing countries 50% of the adult population have been exposed to *M. tuberculosis*. Reactivation, progressive primary disease and secondary exogenous infection result in 8–10 million new cases of tuberculosis each year, with 2–3 million deaths[1].

Conservative estimates suggest that at least 5 million individuals are infected with the HIV virus. Clinical experience with other immunocompromised patients, such as tissue transplantation recipients and those receiving cytotoxic drug therapy, would suggest that HIV infection might predispose to

Table 7.1 Factors contributing to intracellular survival of Mycobacteria

1.	Outer glycopeptidolipid layer of the mycobacterial cell wall conferring resistance to active oxygen radicals and other microbiocidal mechanisms. (These GPLs can form a capsule-like zone, visible by EM, surrounding intracellular mycobacterial species including *M. avium.*[a])
2.	Superoxide dismutase – inactivates reactive oxygen intermediates
3.	Prevention of phagosyme–lysosome fusion* following phagocytosis of mycobacteria
4.	Ability to develop dormant forms which have low metabolic activity and can persist *in-vivo* (?intracellularly) for many years[b]
5.	Inhibition of T-cell responses by mycobacterial cell wall components[c,d]; e.g. lipoarabinomannan stimulates (?)suppressor T-cell function

* This is unlikely to be a major mechanism of bacterial survival within phagocytes as reversal of this process by opsonizing mycobacteria with antibody and complement does not result in increased bacterial killing

[a] Brennan, P. J. (1989) *Rev. Infect. Dis.* **11**, S420–30

[b] Toman, K. (1981) *Int. J. Leprosy*, **49**, 205

[c] Ivanyi, J. (1986) *Clin. Immunol. Allergy*, **6**, 127–57

[d] Ellner, J. J. and Wallis, R. S. (1989) *Rev. Infect. Dis.*, **11**, S455–9

tuberculosis. There is now considerable epidemiological evidence, from developed and developing countries, to support this belief.

NATURAL HISTORY AND PATHOLOGY OF TUBERCULOSIS

The most important mode of infection (see ref. 8 for discussion of other modes of infection) is the inhalation of droplet nuclei small enough to reach the alveolar spaces. Larger particles settle in proximal airways and are eliminated by mucociliary clearance and swallowing, following which they are presumably destroyed by gastric acid[2,3].

The probability of infection depends on the density of infected droplet nuclei in the air[4], and hence is increased by overcrowding, especially in poorly ventilated surroundings[5]. Experimental evidence indicates that strains of tubercle bacilli vary in their virulence for rabbits[6], and guinea pigs[7]. For example, Asian strains of *M. tuberculosis* are less virulent to guinea pigs than are European strains[7]. While virulence in animal species cannot be equated with capacity to cause disease in humans, it is plausible that strains of *M. tuberculosis* may vary in their virulence for humans. Work by Riley[4] showed that human infection can result from very small inocula of tubercle bacilli (one to three bacilli) reaching alveolar spaces. Effective chemotherapy rapidly renders even sputum-positive patients non-infectious within 1–2 weeks[8,9].

Entry of tubercle bacilli into the lung alveoli induces an inflammatory response with initial accumulation of neutrophils[10,11], followed by an influx of monocytes. Recent evidence suggests that neutrophils have a modest capacity to kill virulent tubercle bacilli (H37Rv) by a mechanism independent of toxic oxygen-radical generation. This capacity is exhibited by neutrophils of patients with chronic granulomatous disease, and may be an extracellular process as it is not diminished by lack of serum, or treatment of neutrophils with 2-deoxyglucose, both of which reduce phagocytosis[12]. Nevertheless neutrophils are unlikely to be a major component of antimycobacterial immunity as there is no evidence that neutropenic patients have an increased susceptibility to mycobacterial infections.

Tubercle bacilli become coated with C3b generated via the alternative pathway following which, binding to complement receptors CR3 and CR1 mediates uptake by mononuclear phagocytes[13]. Complement receptors are also important for the uptake of other mycobacteria into phagocytic cells. CR1 mediate the uptake of *M. leprae*[14], and C3 is required for the entry of MAI into phagocytes[15]. The bacteria multiply within monocytes and macrophages, which develop pale foamy cytoplasm, rich in lipid and aggregate together as 'epithelioid' cells forming granulomatous lesions or tubercles. Recent evidence indicates that granuloma formation depends on the local synthesis of a cytokine called tumour necrosis factor-α (TNFα) by infected macrophages. Treatment of BCG-infected mice with rabbit anti-TNFα antibody prevents the formation of epithelioid granulomata and causes the dissolution of previously formed granulomata. This is associated with an increase in the number of viable BCG bacilli isolated from the livers of anti-TNF treated mice[16]. The accumulated epithelioid cells are surrounded by a cuff of lymphocytes which induce fibroblasts to produce collagen under the influence of cytokines[17]. The lymphocyte component of a tubercle comprises mainly CD4-positive T cells, but as in granulomata of tuberculoid leprosy CD8-bearing T lymphocytes are also found. Multinucleated giant cells (Langhans cells) derived from fused mononuclear cells and eosinophilic (caseous) necrosis occurring at the centre of lesions are also features of tuberculous granulomata.

Infection of a naive individual with tubercle bacilli results in primary tuberculosis. The primary, or Ghon focus, usually occurs as a subpleural lesion in any lung zone. From here, tubercle bacilli spread via lymphatics to hilar lymph nodes and seed via the blood stream to other pulmonary and extrapulmonary sites. Experimental studies have shown that radiolabelled BCG reach the lymph nodes and blood stream within hours of reaching the lung[18].

Most primary lesions heal spontaneously due to containment of the mycobacterial infection by host defence mechanisms (see later). Healing of tuberculous lesions does not result in sterilization of the infected tissues. Tubercle bacilli can become metabolically inactive and remain dormant for prolonged periods (months or years). Most 'persistent' bacilli are probably intracellular or contained within the centre of closed caseous lesions. The best evidence for the existence of persistent forms comes from the work of McCune and Tompsett[19] and Grosset[20] on experimental chemotherapy of tuberculosis, in small rodents. After prolonged periods of chemotherapy with isoniazid (INAH) and rifampicin no tubercle bacilli could be cultured from the tissues of experimentally infected mice. However, when the duration of treatment was less than 9 months, up to 20% of the mice relapsed with fully drug-sensitive organisms. A high percentage of relapses could also be induced by corticosteroid treatment of mice which had been given 1 year of chemotherapy with INAH and rifampicin, indicating that even highly effective drug therapy in the mouse results in latency rather than complete bacterial elimination. Anti-mycobacterial chemotherapeutic agents are generally

Table 7.2 Risk factors for reactivation of tuberculosis

Protein–calorie malnutrition
Alcoholism
Drug addiction
Poor socioeconomic status
Old age
Intercurrent infection (e.g. measles)
Impairment of T cell function (e.g. HIV, immunosuppression therapy following organ transplantion)
Genetic factors

ineffective against dormant bacilli. These are killed only when they undergo intermittent bursts of metabolic activity or cell division (see refs 21 and 22 for reviews).

In a proportion of infected individuals the 'healed' foci established during a primary infection may become reactivated and give rise to progressive ('post-primary') tuberculosis. Stead[23] has summarized the evidence that: (1) reactivation of dormant infection is the main cause of active disease in adults, in countries with a low incidence of tuberculosis; (2) primary infection with the tubercle bacillus confers enhanced, though partial, protection against re-infection. Factors contributing to reactivation are summarized in Table 7.2. Much less commonly the primary lesion progresses to produce clinical disease that is very similar to post-primary tuberculosis. The commonest site of reactivation is in the upper zone of the lung, and is thought to be due to relatively high pO_2 in these regions, relative to other pulmonary segments. (Tubercle bacilli grow better in the presence of a high oxygen tension.) Caseous necrosis of tuberculous lesions, softening or liquefaction of the caseous material due to hydrolytic enzymes derived from dying phagocytic cells and cavitation by discharge of caseous material into bronchi are characteristic features of post-primary tuberculosis. An explosive increase in the bacilliary content of tuberculous lesions follows cavitation. This is due to a combination of an increase in the oxygen tension and elimination by drainage via the bronchial tree, of caseous material which contains chemical constituents inhibiting mycobacterial growth[24]. While a closed caseous lesion contains 10^4 bacilli/g, up to 10^9 organisms may be contained within a single tuberculous cavity[25]. Cavitation also makes a tuberculous patient infectious to others ('sputum-positive').

Rupture of caseous lesions (tuberculous hilar lymph nodes or foci developing in the vasa vasorum of pulmonary veins) into pulmonary veins may result in dissemination of infection throughout the body with the formation of multiple granulomatous lesions in the lung, liver, spleen and meninges. This is called miliary tuberculosis and is often fatal due to meningeal involvement.

The timetable of tuberculosis

While human tuberculosis is protean in its manifestations, studies on the pattern of tuberculosis during the pre-chemotherapy era allowed the piecing together of a sequence of events following initial infection, called 'the timetable

Table 7.3 Natural history of untreated primary tuberculosis (modified after Wallgren [26] and Seaton *et al.* [8])

Time after infection	*Clinical features*
3–8 weeks	Conversion to tuberculin positivity. Minority develop illness and erythema nodosum. Large majority develop healed silent lesions
3–12 months	Miliary tuberculosis. Tuberculous meningitis (commonest in children under 1 year). Pleural effusion (rare in children, commonest in young adults)
1–5 years	Post-primary pulmonary lesion: apical lung lesion. Skeletal TB (spine, bone and joints)
5 – 15 years	Late manifestations: Genitourinary TB. Cutaneous TB (lupus vulgaris)

of tuberculosis'[26]. While tuberculosis does not behave with absolute uniformity, the timetable summarized in Table 7.3 illustrates, in general terms, the natural history of this disease. Observations of tuberculosis occurring after primary infection acquired during adolescence, based on 54 000 subjects studied during the British Medical Research Council BCG vaccine trial, spanning 1950–1970[27], are similar to Wallgren's original observations.

MECHANISMS OF ANTI-TUBERCULOUS IMMUNITY (see Table 7.4)

Introduction

Robert Koch showed that primary tuberculous infection in a naive guinea pig was accompanied by the formation of a progressive local granuloma with spread of infection to regional lymph nodes. Re-infection of an animal who already had a primary infection resulted in an accelerated local lesion becoming maximal at 72 h, followed by rapid healing, without lymphatic spread. Naturally infected hosts develop cutaneous delayed hypersensitivity to (antigens of) the tubercle bacillus, coincident with developing immunity. Chase[28] showed that delayed hypersensitivity was transferred by lymphocytes of immune animals but not by serum. Lymphocytes from immune animals were similarly shown to be capable of adoptively transferring immunity to tuberculosis in small rodents[29]. Lymphocytes important for mycobacterial immunity were further identified as T cells. Lurie[30], in a series of classical studies, demonstrated that macrophages from *M. tuberculosis*-infected rabbits showed an enhanced capacity to control the growth of tubercle bacilli introduced into anterior chambers of rabbit eyes, compared to macrophages from naive animals. Several studies by Mackaness[31] showed that specific immunity to intracellular bacteria depended on antigen-specific activation of lymphocytes which produce soluble factors (lymphokines) that activate macrophages and enhance their ability to control the growth of, or kill, intracellular bacteria. T-cell-derived lymphokines also contribute to granuloma formation by attracting and retaining mononuclear phagocytes to the site of T-cell activation (see ref. 32 for a review).

Table 7.4 Components of antimycobacterial immunity in humans as inferred from observations in patients with impaired immunity

	Result
(A) *T cell deficiency states*	
1. Renal transplant recipients. HIV-infected patients	1. Increased susceptibility to reactivation of tuberculosis 2. Infections with opportunistic mycobacteria (e.g. *M. avium intracellulare*)
2. Lepromatous leprosy; acquired specific T cell anergy to *M. leprae* (? due to suppressor T cells)	1. Multibacillary disease 2. Requires longer duration of drug therapy for cure than in patients with tuberculoid leprosy
(B) *Macrophage defects*	
1. Silicosis – inhalation of silica destroys pulmonary macrophages (i.e. local defences destroyed but systemic defences intact)	Severe cavitatory TB *localized* to lung[a]
2. Poorly characterized primary macrophage defect	1. Progressive, fatal BCG infection[b] 2. Fatal disseminated MAI infection[c]
3. Chronic gramulomatous disease (see text)	1. Several reports of disseminated BCG infection 2. No reports of MAI infection
4. Macrophage defects seen at late stage of HIV infection (see text)	1. Contributes to disseminated MAI infection which occurs in patients with AIDS 2. Contributes to disseminated BCG infection

[a] Snider, D. E. (1978) *Am. Rev. Resp. Dis.*, **118**, 455–60
[b] Fisher, A. *et al.* (1980) *Clin. Immunol. Immunopathol.*, **17**, 296–306
[c] Uchiama, N. *et al.* (1981) *J. Pediatr.*, **98**, 785–8

Genetic factors controlling the susceptibility to tuberculosis

Non-MHC-linked genes

The first clear evidence for genetic factors controlling susceptibility to tuberculosis was provided by studies in inbred rabbits by Lurie and co-workers[33]. Innate resistance, operating at the level of the macrophage, controls the initial growth of mycobacteria before T-cell-mediated immunity has developed. A single autosomal dominant gene, located on the centromeric portion of the first chromosome of mice, confers resistance to infection by intracellular pathogens including BCG, *M. avium*, *Leishmania* and *Salmonella typhimurium*[34,35]. This so-called Bcg gene exists in two allelic forms: Bcg.r (resistant) and Bcg.s (susceptible). All wild mice bear the Bcg.r gene, as do about half of inbred mouse strains (exemplified by C3H/He mice) and are resistant to intravenous challenge with BCG bacilli, with very little bacterial growth in organs such as the spleen, liver and lungs. Bcg.s bearing mice (e.g. BALB/c) show exponential growth of BCG within solid organs during the first few weeks following similar challenge. Analysis of restriction fragment linkage patterns, has allowed the identification of a linkage group containing several known genetic loci. A structurally homologous region has been identified on a conserved region of the human chromosome 2, probably in the segment q32–37, initiating speculation about the existence of a human equivalent of the Bcg gene.

Resistance conferred by the Bcg gene remains intact after total-body irradiation, but is sensitive to chronic injection of silica, which destroys macrophage function. The Bcg.r gene allows macrophage control of intracellular bacterial growth without participation of a T cell response or an inflammatory response, by a mechanism which is not yet elucidated. The effect of the gene is pleiotropic, however, and manifests as increased oxidative activity of macrophages and their ability to act as accessory cells supporting antigen- or mitogen-induced, T cell proliferation. Bcg.s bearing mice, in contrast, develop larger BCG or foreign-body-induced pulmonary granulomata which secreted increased amounts of IL-1. Genetically susceptible (Bcg.s) mice eventually control the bacterial challenge by developing T-cell-mediated responses. In contrast, the acquisition of specific T-cell-mediated immunity is delayed[36] in resistant (Bcg.r) mice, and is thought to be due to the poor replication of mycobacteria in these hosts[37].

Genetic susceptibility to tuberculosis in humans

The contribution of 'nature' and 'nurture' to susceptibility to tuberculosis are difficult to separate in outbred populations. They are, in particular, difficult to dissociate from external factors such as diet, overcrowding, occupation and exposure to environmental (non-pathogenic) mycobacteria (which might induce partial immunity due to antigens shared with pathogenic species). The largest fall in mortality and morbidity from tuberculosis in the UK coincided with rapid socioeconomic development during the first half of the twentieth century, well before chemotherapy was introduced in 1950 and without any specific anti-tuberculous measures being adopted[8]. The Lubeck disaster[38] provides evidence supporting inherited variation of susceptibility to tuberculosis. In 1926, well before anti-tuberculous drugs were available, 241 babies in the small German town of Lubeck were inoculated with virulent tubercle bacilli, instead of BCG vaccine, by mistake. Seventy-six children died of tuberculosis. The others developed minor lesions which resolved, and none of them developed tuberculosis during 12 subsequent years of observation. In 1926, Lubeck was a small town where most citizens were interrelated and hence provided a relatively homogeneous community. The infecting dose and strain (hence virulence) of the ingested tubercle bacilli was identical; yet the large majority of infants inoculated remained healthy, suggesting variability of innate resistance to tuberculosis. Kallman and Reisner[39], in a family study of patients with tuberculosis, including 308 twin pairs comprising 78 identical and 230 dizygotic pairs, showed that if one twin had tuberculosis the chances of the second twin developing the disease were 87% in the former and 26% in the latter; a striking difference. Racial differences to susceptibility and the clinical course of tuberculosis have been documented for many years (reviewed in ref. 40). Rich[41] found that tuberculosis in black populations ran a more rapid clinical course with an associated greater degree of caseous necrosis. The higher incidence of tuberculosis in blacks has been ascribed to poverty and overcrowding[42]. However, in a seminal contribution Stead *et al.*[40] showed that blacks living under similar social circumstances to whites, were twice as likely to be infected by *M. tuberculosis*, as evidenced by recent tuberculin conversion. Yet the incidence of clinical tuberculosis in these individuals, in the absence of chemotherapy, was no different in the two racial groups. At a cellular level this resistance to tuberculosis in humans appears to be a composite of innate resistance (presumably due to ingestion and destruction by unstimulated macrophages) and T-cell dependent acquired immunity. This is analogous to the situation in mice, summarized earlier. There is considerable evidence that macrophages from different subjects vary in their capacity to control the growth of intracellular *M. tuberculosis*[43,44]. Crowle and Elkins[45] have also shown that the rate of intracellular replication of virulent *M. tuberculosis* is higher in macrophages from black subjects than in cells from white donors.

The interaction of genetic, environmental (and cultural) factors on susceptibility to tuberculosis is well illustrated by the work of Davies[46] on the relationship between vitamin D deficiency and reactivation of tuberculosis in Asian immigrants to the UK. Immigrants to the UK from the Indian subcontinent have rates of tuberculosis 20–30 times that of the indigenous white population. The rate of extrapulmonary (lymph node) TB among Asian immigrants is even more strikingly elevated, compared to that of whites (relative risk of 140). This increase correlates with vitamin D deficiency occurring in dark-skinned Asians when they migrate to northern latitudes with poor sunlight. Asians, whose diet is deficient in cholecalciferol, depend primarily on sunlight-induced cutaneous synthesis of this vitamin. Dark skin reduces sunlight-induced synthesis of vitamin D; hence pigmented races living in northern latitudes are more susceptible to clinical vitamin D deficiency if dietary intake is inadequate. West Indians living in the UK, in contrast, have serum vitamin D concentrations matching those of indigenous whites due to adequate dietary intake of the vitamin and have only a 3–4-fold increased risk of tuberculosis, compared to whites. As discussed later, the biologically active form of vitamin D_3 (1,25 dihydroxy vitamin D_3) is locally synthesized by macrophages in granulomatous lesions and is capable of inducing tuberculostasis within human monocytes and (to a lesser extent) macrophages. Hence it is suggested that the depletion of the serum vitamin D_3 level is associated with a decline in cell-mediated immunity to *M. tuberculosis* resulting in reactivation of dormant lesions.

MHC-linked immune responses to tuberculosis

T cells recognize foreign antigens physically associated with self major histocompatibility complex (MHC) antigens. MHC class II antigens (found on antigen-presenting cells) vary in the efficiency with which they bind and present foreign antigens to CD4 (helper) T cells, to initiate an immune response. Hence it is not surprising that the immunogenicity of different mycobacterial antigenic determinants (epitopes) varies according to the MHC phenotype of the host. Weak associations between HLA class I alleles and tuberculosis have been reported in several studies[47–49] but the HLA alleles implicated vary in different populations, suggesting that the associations are due to linkage disequilibrium with putative susceptibility genes, rather than a direct effect. Singh *et al.*[50] reported a significant segregation of pulmonary tuberculosis with HLA-DR2 in Indian families with several affected individuals. In a recent study from Indonesia a positive association was also reported between sputum-positive tuberculosis and HLA-DR2, but the reported relative risk was modest[51]. High antibody responses to an epitope on a 38 kDa protein antigen of *M. tuberculosis* (which acts as a phosphate transport protein) were also associated with HLA-DR2 as shown in the same study. T-cell proliferative responses to PPD are higher in HLA-DR3 subjects[52] and strong cutaneous delayed hypersensitivity to tuberculin from *M. tuberculosis* is associated with HLA-DR4[53]. Using the 65 kDa heat shock protein of *M. tuberculosis* and *M. leprae*, which show 95% sequence homology, it has been shown that different MHC class II alleles govern the recognition of different epitopes on the same molecule, by $CD4^+$ T cells[54–56]. These observations have yet to be extended to a population level.

In conclusion, the evidence cited above for tuberculosis and that summarized elsewhere[52] for leprosy suggest the existence of MHC-linked immune response genes influencing T-cell responsiveness and susceptibility to mycobacterial diseases. However, as yet the picture is fragmentary and it is highly likely that: (a) susceptibility to tuberculosis in humans is multifactorial involving MHC and non-MHC linked genes and (b) antigenic determinants inducing protective (and/or tissue damaging) T-cell responses, vary with the HLA phenotype of the host.

T lymphocyte subsets and their activation by antigens (reviewed in ref. 57)

As highlighted by the HIV epidemic, T lymphocytes are essential for acquired immunity to intracellular bacteria. The antigen receptor of T cells comprises seven polypeptide chains forming the T cell receptor (TCR)-CD3 complex[57]. Most T cells bind antigen via a transmembrane protein made up of two glycosylated polypeptide chains called an α chain (45–55 kDa) and a β chain (37–45 kDa) joined together by disulphide bonds, forming the T cell receptor. Each α and β chain consists of extracellular N-terminal domains of variable amino-acid composition which make up their free terminal ends (and together forming an antigen-binding region that is unique to each T cell clone) and a constant region which is attached to the membrane; a structure analogous to that of immunoglobulin molecules. The variable portions of the α and β chains form the antigen binding site that confers unique antigen specificity to each individual T cell and its progeny. A small proportion (approximately 5% of peripheral blood T cells in humans) bear TCR formed not by α and β chains but by two different polypeptides called γ (35–43 kDa) and δ (40 kDa) chains. $\alpha\beta$ and $\gamma\delta$ T-cell receptors respectively, are associated with the CD3 protein complex which is made up of subunits called CD3-γ, CD3-δ, CD3-ε, CD3-ζ and CD3-η chains[58]. T cells recognize antigens in association with MHC glycoproteins (see below) via the $\alpha\beta$– or $\gamma\delta$–TCR, following which signals are transduced into the lymphocyte cytoplasm by the CD3 complex[57]. This results in the T cells being activated.

Unlike immunoglobulin receptors of B cells which can bind free antigen, TCR only recognize antigens which are physically associated with proteins encoded by autologous MHC genes and expressed on the surface of other cells. About two-thirds of peripheral T cells (in humans) have on their surface CD4 glycoproteins, and are called helper T cells, as this group of cells can help the function and differentiation of other types of immunologically competent cells. $CD4^+$ T cells only recognize antigen which has been taken up and processed by specialized antigen-presenting cells (which include macrophages) and expressed on the cell surface bound to MHC class II antigens (HLA, DR, DP and DQ molecules). About one-third of human peripheral T cells lack CD4 surface glycoprotein but express the CD8 molecule on their surface. TCRs of $CD8^+$ T cells only recognize foreign antigens which are bound to self MHC class I molecules, that are expressed on the surface of most nucleated cells. It is believed that MHC class I antigens within vesicles of the endoplasmic reticulum pick up processed antigen intracellularly, following which they reach the cell surface by reverse pinocytosis.

MHC genes, and hence the glycoproteins coded by them, are highly polymorphic. A given antigen may not be able to bind to all allelic forms of MHC proteins. Furthermore, T cells will only recognize antigen binding on to those allelic forms of MHC molecules shared with antigen-bearing cells. This genetic restriction hence governs the antigenic determinants that can be recognized by the T cells of any individual. Therefore, different antigens of complex organisms such as mycobacteria may vary in their immunogenicity for individual members of the human species, depending on the MHC haplotype of the host; a point of obvious relevance to the design of vaccines containing a few purified antigens of pathogenic organisms.

A number of adhesion molecules including CD4 (ligand: MHC class II molecules), CD8 (ligand: MHC class I molecules), CD2 (ligand: LFA 3–leucocyte functional antigen 3), CD18/CD11a (ligand: ICAM-1–intercellular adhesion molecule), enhance the efficiency of interactions between T cells and other cells such as antigen-presenting cells, endothelial cells and target cells for cytolysis.

A major function of $CD4^+$ cells is to enhance or help the function of other immunologically active cells by producing soluble factors or interleukins (IL) (see ref. 59) (*viz.* IL-2 which helps T cell growth; IL3 which acts on pluripotent precursor cells in bone marrow; B cell stimulating factors IL-4 and IL-5; interferon gamma (γIFN) which has antiviral properties and activates macrophages; and TNFα) (see later section for discussion of the role of cytokines in anti-mycobacterial immunity). In addition, $CD4^+$ cells can also directly lyse antigen-bearing target cells in a MHC class II restricted manner (see later). In mice, T helper cells are further subdivided into (1) TH1 cells which produce IL-2, γIFN and TNFα and are mainly involved in cell-mediated immunity, inflammation and delayed type hypersensitivity reactions (DTH); (2) TH2 cells, which produce IL-4 and IL-5 and primarily help B cells to produce antibodies[59]. Recent work in murine leishmaniasis has indicated that TH1 or TH2 subsets may be preferentially expanded and produce beneficial (protective immunity) or harmful (disease progression) effects in the host[60,61].

The main functional characteristic of $CD8^+$ T cells is the ability to lyse target cells expressing foreign (e.g. viral) antigens associated with self MHC class I molecules. However, CD8 T cell clones often secrete cytokines including γIFN and TNFα, and can activate macrophages. CD8 T cells capable of suppressing immune responses have been described, especially in lepromatous leprosy[62,63].

Role of T cell subsets in antimycobacterial immunity

The three subsets of T cells which are implicated in antimycobacterial immunity are $CD4^+$, $CD8^+$ and γδ-receptor bearing T cells. Depletion studies using monoclonal antibody treatment of thymectomized mice as well as adoptive transfer studies of T cells selectively depleted of $CD4^+$ or $CD8^+$ cells have shown that the major protective subset is $CD4^+$ (reviewed in refs 103 and 104). However, in these experiments $CD8^+$ cells were shown to have a protective effect, albeit of a lesser magnitude. $CD8^+$ cells were also shown to be particularly effective in protecting recipients against aerosol challenge with *M. tuberculosis* while $CD4^+$ cells were more effective in controlling infections following challenge via an intravenous route.

Murine $CD4^+$ T cell lines and clones specific for *M. tuberculosis* produce IL-2 and γIFN but not B cell stimulating factors (reviewed in 103 and 110) and are capable of adoptively transferring delayed type hypersensitivity. Hence they conform to the so-called TH1, T-cell phenotype.

Identification of antigens inducing T-cell responses (reviewed in ref. 64)

Since T-cell responses appear critical for protective immunity to tuberculosis three approaches have been applied to identify mycobacterial antigenic determinants capable of stimulating T cells of healthy contacts or patients with high levels of cell-mediated immunity to tuberculosis. The first is to affinity purify mycobacterial antigens recognized by murine monoclonal antibodies and to subsequently test proliferative responses of polyclonal T cells or T cell clones from mycobacteria-reactive individuals. Seven protein antigens of *M. tuberculosis* which are immunodominant in mice were initially identified by monoclonal antibodies from different laboratories[65]. These proteins had molecular weights of 71, 65, 38, 23, 19, 14 and 12 kDa. Recently, monoclonal antibodies have been produced which identify a fibronectin binding protein (55 kDa)[66] and the 23 kDa superoxide dismutase[67] of *M. tuberculosis.*

The second approach arose from difficulties caused by the inability to cultivate *M. leprae in vitro*. Young *et al.*[68] inserted genomic fragments of *M. leprae* and *M. tuberculosis* into *E. coli* using the λgt11 phage vector and produced a number of recombinant antigens. *E. coli* clones producing these antigens were identified by screening with a panel of monoclonal antibodies to mycobacterial antigens assembled by the WHO[69]. These methods allowed the generation of recombinant mycobacterial antigens which could be used to determine the specificity of T cells responding to whole bacterial lysates of *M. tuberculosis* or *M. leprae*. T cell clones with specificity for the r19 kDa and r65 kDa antigens of *M. tuberculosis* have been described using the above approach[70]. Munk *et al.*[71] showed that purified 71 kDa, 65 kDa, 19 kDa and 12 kDa proteins induce T cell responses in freshly isolated polyclonal T cells of healthy individuals. This approach was further extended by constructing sets of recombinant DNA clones containing overlapping fragments of mycobacterial DNA and examining the reactivity of panels of monoclonal antibodies[72] or proliferative responses of polyclonal or monoclonal T cell populations[73]. This approach has allowed the mapping of B and T cell epitopes within individual recombinant proteins like the 65 kDa antigen of mycobacteria. Furthermore, since T cell epitopes consist of short linear sequences of amino acids, synthetic peptides can be made and used in T cell proliferative assays, to obtain complementary data for identifying T cell epitopes. To avoid the labour of synthesizing large numbers of overlapping peptides, predictive theories have been developed to help identify amino acid motifs which are likely to comprise T cell epitopes. The application of such theories to identify T cell epitopes of the 65 kDa protein of *M. tuberculosis* is reviewed by Lamb *et al.*[64]. Such studies indicate that the T cell epitopes recognized by an individual depends on the MHC class II haplotype, reflecting the ability of the hypervariable domains of chains of MHC class II molecules to bind and present antigen to CD4 T cells.

An unexpected finding was that several mycobacterial proteins identified using the above approach had extensive amino acid sequence homologies with highly conserved 'heat shock' or stress proteins that are synthesized in large amounts by bacteria and eukaryotic cells, including human cells. For example, the 65 kDa heat shock protein of *M. tuberculosis* corresponds to the Gro EL protein of *E. coli* and shows 95% sequence homology with that of *M. leprae*[74,75] and shows about 50% amino acid identity with its human analogue. Stress proteins are synthesized in increasing amounts by mycobacteria when subjected to harmful stimuli which probably include the toxic free radicals produced by activated macrophages within tuberculous granulomata. Limiting dilution studies have shown that about a fifth of human peripheral blood T cells responding to *M. tuberculosis* recognize the 65 kDa HSP implying that this antigen may play a significant role in antimycobacterial immune responses. It has been argued that priming by highly conserved bacterial antigens like 'heat shock' proteins of intestinal or environmental bacteria may induce (partial) protective immune responses to pathogenic mycobacteria. Alternatively, since *M. tuberculosis* is highly virulent to humans, and BCG or environmental bacteria induce at best incomplete protection, it is likely that antigens which are critical for effective protective immunity are unique to the pathogenic mycobacterial species. The role of immune responses to bacterial stress proteins with homologies to human counterparts, in the pathogenesis of autoimmune diseases such as rheumatoid arthritis, is outside the scope of this review and the reader is referred elsewhere[76].

Recombinant antigens and affinity-purified antigens have one major disadvantage. Their selection depends on recognition by mouse B cells which are the precursors of hybridomas producing the relevant monoclonal antibodies. Since epitopes recognized by T and B cells often differ[77], and since immunogenicity for mice may not reflect relevance to human T cell responses, a third method was developed, to directly assess immunogenicity of the whole range of mycobacterial antigens without a bias introduced by preselection using serological methods. Mycobacterial lysates were separated by electrophoresis in SDS polysaccharide gels. The fractionated antigens were elctrophoretically transferred onto nitrocellulose sheets (Western blotted). The nitrocellulose sheet can be cut up into narrow bands, solubilized and used to assess T cell responses by *in vitro* proliferation assays[78]. Figure 7.1 shows the result of probing the response of (polyclonal) peripheral blood T cells with a sonicate of *M. tuberculosis* fractionated by SDS-PAGE and immunoblotted onto nitrocellulose. Clear peaks of T cell responses can be identified. By comparing proliferation profiles of patients with TB with their healthy contacts it may be possible to identify putative protective antigens. Here, too, variation of the immunodominance of antigenic fractions between individuals may reflect their MHC class II haplotype.

It has been known from the time of Robert Koch that killed mycobacteria elicit delayed hypersensitivity but do not in general induce protective immunity. In contrast, inoculation with viable mycobacteria is more efficient in inducing protective T cell responses[79,80]. Hence interest has focused on antigens secreted by live tubercle bacilli[66]. However, recently it has been demonstrated that protein–peptidoglycan complexes purified from cell walls of *M. tuberculosis* induce strong proliferative responses in peripheral blood T cells of patients with tuberculosis and their healthy tuberculin-positive contacts. T cell clones responsive to proteins of cell wall peptidoglycan complex were also shown to respond to the secreted antigens found in early log phase culture filtrates of tubercle bacilli grown *in vitro*[81]. One of these antigens is a 30 kDa fibronectin-binding protein which is present on the mycobacterial cell surface, is secreted into culture filtrate, and may play a role in mycobacterial adherence to human cells[66]. Similarly, in the case of *M. leprae* too, highly purified cell walls antigens are recognized by a high proportion of *M. leprae*-specific T cells in the blood and lesions of patients with tuberculoid leprosy. These observations imply that mycobacterial vaccines containing purified cell walls have the potential for being developed into successful vaccines of use in populations with a high incidence of HIV, in which live vaccines would be hazardous.

Role of cytokines in antimycobacterial immunity

From the classical work of Mackaness[82] grew the concept that T-cell-produced soluble factors (cytokines, interleukins) induced macrophage activation which resulted in a slowing of intracellular bacterial growth or killing of bacteria. These so-called macrophage-activating factors also caused inhibition of macrophage migration, resulting in their accumulation to form a granuloma[83,84]. When recombinant cytokines became available, γIFN was identified as capable of activating oxidative and non-oxidative microbiocidal potential of macrophages. Recombinant γIFN is capable of inducing striking

(a)

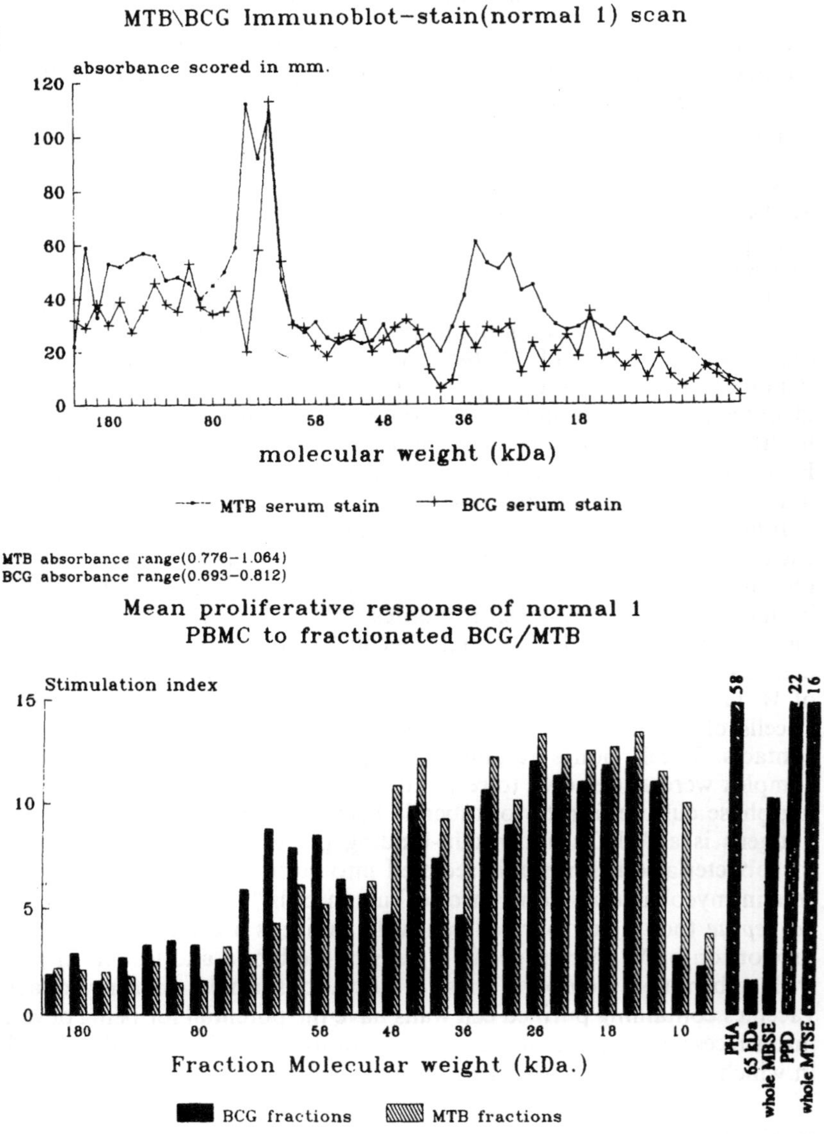

Figure 7.1 The pattern of T cell proliferative responses and serological responses to different molecular weight fractions of sonicated BCG or *M. tuberculosis* (MTB), produced by patients with tuberculosis: **(a)** and **(b)** show results for two individual patients. In each, the lower panel shows the degree of T cell proliferation to SDS-PAGE separated bacterial sonicates blotted to nitrocellulose membranes. Each molecular-weight band was solubilized and used to stimulate peripheral blood lymphocytes (see ref. 78 for detailed methods used). The five bars on the right of the panel show degree of proliferation to PHA, soluble 65 kDa HSP of *M. tuberculosis*, PPD, and soluble unfractionated sonicates of BCG (MBSE) and MTB (MTSE), respectively, for comparison. The upper panel shows scans of parallel nitrocellulose strips stained with the serum of each patient, using an immunoperoxidase method, to show the peak of antibody reactivity to the same molecular weight fractions

(b)

MTB\BCG Immunoblot-stain(patient 7)

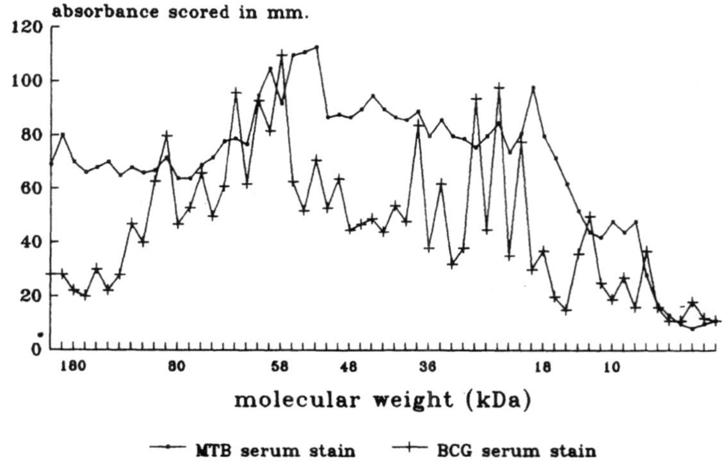

MTB absorbance range(0.480–0.603)
BCG absorbance range(0.686–0.827)

Mean proliferative response of patient 7
PBMC to fractionated BCG/MTB

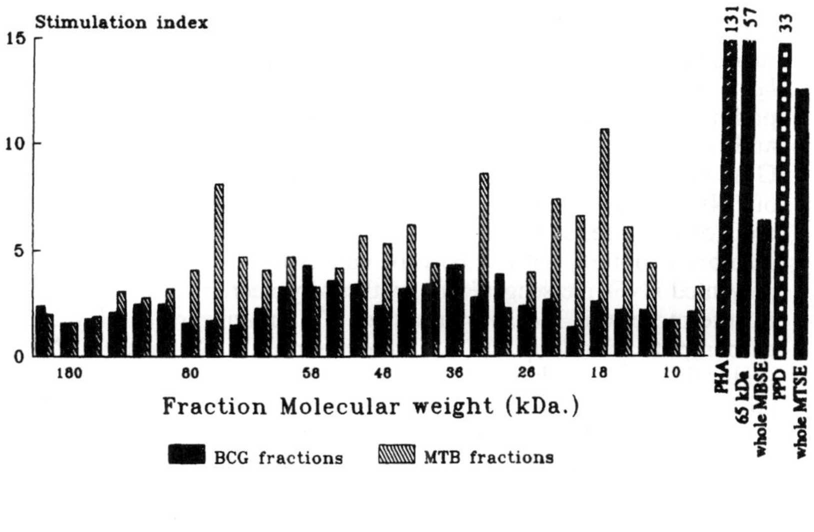

mycobacteriostasis within murine, bone-marrow-derived or peritoneal macrophages[85]. This effect is reduced in the presence of corticosteroids and appears to involve non-oxidative mechanisms as it is not blocked by scavengers of toxic oxygen radicles. However, γIFN has little bacteriostatic effect on *M. tuberculosis*-infected human macrophages, and may even enhance the growth of some virulent strains within human macrophages, in spite of activating these cells to be capable of killing other intracellular pathogens such as leishmania and inducing enhanced tumoricidal capacity of these cells[86]. γIFN is also incapable of controlling the growth of *M. avium* complex within human macrophages[87].

A growing list of cytokines have been shown to activate mononuclear phagocytes, increasing their microbicidal potential. A snapshot of current information is summarized in Table 7.5. Much of the data has been derived in animal experimental models, especially using murine macrophages. As is evident in the data summarized for γIFN, it is not possible to extrapolate from experimental results derived in mice to immune mechanisms within human macrophages. *M. tuberculosis* is not a natural pathogen for wild mice, presumably due to the greater efficiency of murine anti-mycobacterial immunity.

Two cytokines will be commented on in detail:

(a) Role of TNFα in anti-mycobacterial immunity

This multifunctional cytokine is synthesized by murine and human macrophages infected with mycobacteria. TNFα is synthesized as a 26 kDa transmembrane precursor which is subsequently cleaved into the 17 kDa secreted form. It is also released by $CD4^+$ T cells responsive to mycobacterial antigens. *In vivo* experiments have shown that TNFα plays a pivotal role in murine immunity to BCG and *M. avium* infection[16,88]. Treatment of mice infected with *M. bovis* BCG, with polyclonal rabbit anti-TNFα, causes the disappearance of preformed granulomata as well as prevents the formation of new granulomata and converts the infection from a paucibacillary to a multibacillary form. Granuloma formation of BCG-infected mice coincides with local synthesis of TNFα by the macrophages within granulomata, but serum levels of TNFα did not increase, suggesting that most of the TNFα remained localized (? membrane-bound) within the tuberculous lesions. The antibody treatment prevented TNFα messenger RNA synthesis by macrophages within granulomata. Furthermore, this locally synthesized TNFα appears to play a role in an autoamplification loop, as (1) TNFα enhances γIFN-induced TNFα mRNA synthesis by macrophages; (2) TNFα acts synergistically with IL-2 to induce γIFN production by T cells[89]; (3) macrophages exposed to 1,25-vitamin D3 (see later) or γIFN exhibit increased release of TNFα when stimulated within mycobacterial cell wall components (lipo-arabino mannans). Interestingly, exogenous TNFα, as a continuous perfusion of pharmacologically active doses delivered *in vivo* over 20 days or as an *in vitro* treatment for murine macrophages, fails to enhance mycobacterial growth inhibition. This suggests that mycobacteria-infected macrophages are maximally exposed to endogenous TNFα and are hence unresponsive to exogenous TNFα.

Recent work has shown that mRNA of TNFα and γIFN can be detected

Table 7.5 Role of cytokines in anti-mycobacterial immunity*

Cytokine	*In-vitro effect*		*In-vivo effect*	
	Mouse	*Man*	*Mouse*	*Man*
γIFN	Growth inhibition (better with prestimulated Mϕ)	Variable effects: Often growth of virulent strains of MTB increased. No effects on MAI	—	Intralesional injection in lepromatous leprosy induces bacterial killing
TNFα	No effect on its own but synergizes with γIFN and 1,25(OH)2-vitaminD_3	Growth inhibition of AIDS-associated strains of MAI. No effect on MTB	Exogenous TNFα. **Blocking of endogenous TNFα increases susceptibility to MAI and BCG**	
IL-2	No effect	Growth inhibition of AIDS associated strains of MAI. Synergizes with TNFα	Growth inhibition of BCG	Intralesional injection in lepromatous leprosy induces bacterial killing
CSF-GM	No effect	Growth inhibition of MTB at 100 u/ml and MAI at 10 u/ml	No data	No data
IL-4	Growth inhibition if added before infection to bone marrow derived Mϕ. (γIFN antagonizes effect). No effect on peritoneal Mϕ	Synergizes with TNFα or CSF-GM	No data	No data
IL-6	Growth inhibition if added before infection	No data	No data	No data
1,25$(OH)_2$ vitamin D_3	No effect at physiological concentrations	10^{-9} to 10^{-7} mol/l concentrations induce growth inhibition in blood monocytes. Less effect on macrophages. **Greatest effect of all cytokines tested on human cells**	—	Calcitriol treatment caused healing of cutaneous TB
α/β IFN	No effect	αIFN: no effect	No data	No data

* Effects refer to *M. tuberculosis* except where otherwise indicated

in pleural granulomata from patients with tuberculous pleurisy[90]. The locally synthesized γIFN and TNFα are both concentrated in the pleural compartment and do not spill over in significant amounts into the serum. Mycobacterial lipo-arabino mannan[91] and 46 kDa and 20 kDa protein fractions of *M. tuberculosis*[92] are potent stimulators of TNFα production from pleural mononuclear cells and monocyte-derived macrophages. Since pleural TB is well known to be paucibacillary, and since in the pre-chemotherapy era it was found that only 10% develop active tuberculosis within the first year and a third may remain healthy for a prolonged period[93], it is tempting to speculate that endogenously synthesized TNFα plays a pivotal role in the control of mycobacterial growth by human mononuclear phagocytes. It has been claimed that *in vitro* treatment of human monocytes or macrophages with exogenous TNFα fails to enhance their anti-mycobacterial potential[94]. However, it is probably impossible to have an *M. tuberculosis*-infected human macrophage that is not already maximally exposed to endogenously synthesized TNFα. Hence the above-described *in vitro* experiments are not physiologically sound. In our laboratory we are investigating the effect of abrogation of endogenous TNFα production on the mycobacteriostatic potential of human mononuclear phagocytes. Recent data indicate that TNFα may act synergistically with vitamin D_3 and γIFN in inducing anti-mycobacterial activity in human monocyte-derived macrophages[95].

In murine experimental systems depletion of endogenous TNFα by anti-TNF antibody treatment *in vivo* increases susceptibility to *M. avium*[88]. Against this less virulent organism, exogenous recombinant TNFα is also protective in mice[88]. Bermudez and Young[96], using a relatively avirulent strain of *M. avium* derived from AIDS patients, showed that TNFα and IL-2 were synergistic in inducing control of *M. avium* infection, in human macrophages. However, these strains are of low virulence and show poor replicating potential with macrophages of healthy donors. In contrast, strains of *M. avium* complex derived from non-HIV-infected patients are more virulent for normal human macrophages, and the significance of the observation of Bermudez and Young[96] for the large majority of MAI strains is disputed[97,98].

(b) Role of vitamin D_3(b) metabolites in anti-mycobacterial immunity[99]

Serum levels of vitamin D_3 are derived from dietary intake or cutaneous synthesis, on exposure to ultraviolet light. Cutaneous synthesis of vitamin D_3 is less efficient in dark-skinned races. Serum vitamin D_3 is hydroxylated into the physiologically active form by sequential hydroxylation of carbons at the 25 and 1 positions, occurring in the liver and kidney, respectively. In addition to this, macrophages within granulomatous lesions efficiently convert $25(OH)D_3$ to the $1,25(OH)_2$ derivative. Activation of macrophages by γIFN or endotoxin, and possibly even by mycobacterial lipo-arabinomannan, upregulates their 1-hydroxylase activity and increases synthesis of the active form of vitamin D_3. Cadranal *et al.*[100] have shown that pulmonary alveolar lavage cells from an anephric patient with pulmonary TB were capable of synthesizing $1,25(OH)_2D_3$.

In vitro, physiological concentrations of $1,25(OH)_2D_3$, reduces the growth of *M. tuberculosis* within human and murine macrophages. According to Rook, $1,25(OH)_2D_3$ is, to date, the most potent activator of anti-mycobacterial activity in human monocytes and (to a lesser extent) within macrophages. The effect is additive with that of γIFN and TNFα[95]. However, even using optimal concentrations of all three agents the effect appears to be modestly bacteriostatic and is incapable of fully explaining immunity from tuberculosis. The experimental data summarized above provide an explanation for (1) the association of low serum vitamins D_3 and increased susceptibility to reactivation of tuberculosis (see earlier); (2) reports of the cure of lupus vulgaris (cutaneous TB) being achieved with vitamin D therapy in the pre-chemotherapy era[101]; and (3) elevated serum Ca^{2+} levels seen in some patients with renal TB.

The possible role of activated vitamin D_3 synthesized with tuberculous granulomata in a complex autocrine activation pathway involving TNFα and γIFN have been discussed in the section dealing with TNF. The role of TNFα and vitamin D_3 in producing immunopathological lesions in tuberculosis has been reviewed by Rook[99].

Concluding remarks on the role of cytokines in TB

Despite the enormous and diverse efforts made to define the role of cytokines in anti-mycobacterial immunity, their precise significance is uncertain. The best degree of bacterial growth inhibition is in murine bone marrow-derived macrophages activated with rγIFN[102]. This is of the order of 1 log unit and appears to be bacteriostatic rather than sterilizing. The degree of growth inhibition demonstrated in human macrophages is much less striking and variable; at best it is modestly bacteriostatic. Much effort is being expended in chasing the holy grail of the right balance of known and unknown cytokines acting in a precise sequence to enable human mononuclear phagocytes to kill tubercle bacilli. The reality as presently evident is as follows:

1. Technical factors make it difficult to design *in vitro* experiments to assess anti-mycobacterial efficacy of human mononuclear phagocytes. First, it is not possible to have human mononuclear phagocytes infected with tubercle bacilli that are not substantially, if not maximally, activated by autocrine pathways as discussed earlier. Hence the critical experiments may require blocking of these pathways rather than attempting to study the effects of exogenous cytokines. Secondly, a granuloma *in vivo*, is a 'miniature organ' that is continually exposed to fresh migrant monocytes, T cells and other effector cells: a situation difficult to mimic in a test tube. It is quite clear that monocytes have greater bactericidal potential than mature macrophages or inactive 'epithelioid' macrophages.

2. Epidemiological evidence summarized earlier provides strong evidence that human anti-tuberculous immunity is not sterilizing but is bacteriostatic in nature. Bacteriostasis is a key feature of murine anti-tuberculous immunity where many bacteria may persist for long periods in a dormant form[19–21]. In practice, if the net bacterial growth *in vivo* is less than the numbers converted to dormancy, effective immunity would be achieved. Bacteria dormant for long periods may die of starvation or inanition.

Indeed, it is well known that the likelihood of reactivation of primary TB in humans declines with age. Presumably this is due to the above process.

Role of cytolytic cells (CTL) in anti-mycobacterial immunity

The failure, *in vitro*, to achieve effective mycobacterial growth inhibition or killing with lymphokine-activated human macrophages, as described above, has led to the speculation of the role of cytolytic T cells in anti-mycobacterial immunity.

A considerable body of experimental evidence indicates that CD8 (cytolytic) T cells are required in addition to CD4 T lymphocytes for effective immunity against a variety of intracellular parasites[103]. It is also now well established that CD4-positive T cell clones and polyclonal lines are capable of lysing antigen-presenting cells (including macrophages) that bear the relevant antigen on their surface. Recently we have shown that T cell lines induced by several days of *in-vitro* stimulation with PPD or a sonicate of *M. tuberculosis* can lyse autologous macrophages[104]. Mycobactrerial antigen-bearing target macrophages are lysed to a greater extent than those untreated with antigen or bearing an irrelevant antigen such as streptokinase. The main cytolytic cells in this system are CD4 T cells and the mycobacterial antigen-specific component of macrophage lysis is MHC class II restricted[104,105]. When antigen-activated CD4 cells are added to antigen-pulsed macrophages *in vitro* such killing seems to be the rule, and the cytolysis starts by 4 h and is complete by 12–16 h[106].

The ability of patients with tuberculosis to generate mycobacterial antigen-induced cytolotyic cells was related to their clinical state[104]. Those with tissue-damaging tuberculosis (i.e. cavitatory pulmonary TB or caseous extrathoracic disease) generated T lymphoblasts with high levels of cytolytic capacity, but patients with non-cavitating pulmonary infiltrates or disseminated (miliary) tuberculosis showed poor antigen-specific cytolysis. We have also observed two patients with recurrent mycobacterial infection refractory to treatment, caused in one case by *M. tuberculosis* and the other by *M. avium-intracelluare* and not associated with a recognized impairment of cell-mediated immunity, who were unable to generate cytolytic T cells capable of killing autologous macrophages pulsed with mycobacterial antigens. Both patients had strong T cell proliferative responses and cutaneous delayed hypersensitivity responses to mycobacterial antigen[104]; (also R. A. Thompson, D. J. Lipscombe and D. S. Kumararatne, unpublished data).

Patients with HIV have impaired proliferative responses to mycobacterial antigens during later stages of HIV disease (CDC III–IV). Mycobacterial antigen-specific cytolytic capacity generated *in vitro* from peripheral blood mononuclear cells in healthy controls was significantly higher than in asymptomatic HIV-infected individuals (CDC groups II and III) and was still further reduced in symptomatic (CDC group IV) patients (M. Forte, J. Passi, D. S. Kumararatne and J. S. H. Gaston, manuscript in preparation).

Our data are consistent with the view that antigen-non-specific cytolytic cells generated in response to mycobacterial antigens contribute to tissue damage within tuberculous lesions, while mycobacterial antigen-specific cytolytic cells may contribute to protective immunity. This is comparable to the distinction made by Rook and associates between tissue damaging, non-protective, 'Koch-type' hypersensitivity and 'listeria type' hypersensitivity, which is protective[107].

How may cytolytic T cells contribute to antimycobacterial immunity? Tissue macrophages and non-professional phagocytes which may become infected with intracellular bacteria have lower antibacterial potential than freshly emigrated blood monocytes. Therefore it is suggested that lysis of effete infected phagocytes liberates bacteria contained within them, which are then available for uptake and killing by young immunocompetent macrophages. Secondly, exposure of extracellular bacteria to toxic products of necrotic tissue within caseous lesions may inhibit their growth[108]. It is well recognized that closed caseous lesions have lower numbers of viable tubercle bacilli than in open cavities or within infected macrophages seen in disseminated tuberculosis of patients with impaired T cell function (e.g. in AIDS patients). *M. leprae*, which is an obligate intracellular parasite, would of course be unable to survive extracellularly. Thirdly, activation of intracellular processes leading to cell death within target monocytes (e.g. endonuclease which induces cleavage of target-cell DNA and apoptotic cell death) might concomitantly damage intracellular bacteria and cause their demise. Finally, repeated cycles of phagocytosis, and liberation by cytolysis, may result in reduced mycobacterial replication and induce dormancy.

Recent work in lepromatous leprosy[109] provides data supporting a role for cytolytic T cells *in vivo*. Induction of a cutaneous cell-mediated immune response in patients with lepromatous leprosy by intradermal injection of PPD, γIFN, or recombinant IL-2, leads to the infiltration of lesions with CD4 and CD8 T cells. Over 1–4 days macrophages containing numerous leprosy bacilli appear to die, and this is associated with a striking reduction of viable leprosy bacilli. The bacilli remaining within such lesions show fragmentation by electron microscopy. Systemic administration of recombinant IL-2 produces a similar reduction in bacillary load. This is, however, not accompanied by a correction of anergy to antigens of *M. leprae*, hence suggesting a protective role for antigen-non-specific (natural killer type or lymphokine-activated killer type) cytolytic cells, in producing the antibacterial effect.

One of the mycobacterial antigens inducing CTL responses has been identified as the 65 kDa heat shock protein (HSP) of *M. tuberculosis* and target epitopes recognized by CTL of HLA-DR3 positive donors has been localized to the N-terminal 65 amino acid residues of this molecule[105]. Of greater importance is our preliminary observation that *M. bovis* (BCG) bacilli, capable of intracellular survival within macrophages, are inhibited or killed when these cells were lysed by CD4-positive effector cells and that the 65 kDa HSP was more effective than PPD in inducing this response[110]. Kaufmann's group has shown that $CD8^+$ murine T cell lines are capable of inhibiting mycobacterial growth, when added to infected macrophages, by a mechanism independent of γIFN[111].

Theoretically, lysis of infected macrophages by CTL could also contribute to bacterial dissemination. However, bacillaemia and disseminated disease appears to occur most readily in HIV-infected subjects who have poor CTL responses.

Role of $\gamma\delta$ receptor-bearing T cells in mycobacterial immunity

The large majority of T cells recognize foreign antigens bound to autologous MHC antigens (class I or class II) via T cell receptors comprising disulphide-bond linked α and β chains. Approximately 5% of peripheral T cells express an alternative T cell receptor composed of disulphide-linked γ and δ chains[57]. In the mouse $\gamma\delta$ T cells are found mainly in the skin, intestinal epithelium and lung, and form a minority subset (1–3%) in the circulation. In humans $\gamma\delta$ T cells are more uniformly distributed and comprise about 1–5% of the peripheral lymphocyte pool. In humans, as in the mouse, genes coding for the variable regions of γ and δ chains are limited, compared to the number available for α and β TCR chains. By implication the number of antigens recognized by $\gamma\delta$ T cells is likely to be limited. Relatively little is known about the antigens recognized by $\gamma\delta$ T cells. Furthermore $\gamma\delta$ T cells antigen recognition seems to be, in the main, MHC unrestricted[111].

Activated $\gamma\delta$ T cells are enriched in murine lymph nodes draining sites injected with antigens from *M. tuberculosis* and lungs of animals infected with aerosols containing this organism[113]. $\gamma\delta$ T cells are also enriched in granulomatous lesions of leprosy[114] and leishmaniasis, as well as among mycobacterial-antigen-reactive lymphocytic infiltrates from the synovial tissue of patients with rheumatoid arthritis[115]. $\gamma\delta$ T cells are also a common resident of caseous tuberculous lymph nodes[116]. A high proportion of murine $\gamma\delta$ T-cell hybridomas derived from foetal thymocytes recognize the 65 kDa HSP of *M. tuberculosis*[117]. However, only a small proportion of human $\gamma\delta$ T cells recognize this heat shock protein, though a high proportion recognize as yet undefined antigens of *M. tuberculosis* which are protease-resistant and hence are possibly carbohydrate in nature[118].

Gram-positive and Gram-negative bacteria, including *S. aureus*, group A streptococci and *Listeria monocytogenes*, induce the expansion of human $\gamma\delta$ cells[119]. Recent data[120] indicate that monocytes infected with live *M. tuberculosis* or *Salmonella typhimurium* are more efficient than dead bacteria at inducing human $\gamma\delta$ T-cell expansion. In contrast, heat-killed organisms preferentially induced $CD4^+$, $\alpha\beta$ T-cell expansion. The nature of the stimulating antigen is unknown and may be produced during intracellular bacterial growth. Alternatively, it has been suggested that bacterial superantigens analogous to staphylococcal enterotoxin may polyclonally activate $\gamma\delta$-bearing T cells. $\gamma\delta$ T-cell expansion is supported by IL2; there is little other information on the cytokine-dependence of $\gamma\delta$ T-cell growth and differentiation.

These cells can secrete cytokines [IL-2, γIFN, lymphotoxin (TNFβ)][119] and can lyse macrophage targets in an antigen-specific as well as non-specific manner. We and others have shown that mycobacterial antigen-stimulated polyclonal T cell lines show 'NK-like' killing of antigen-unpulsed targets[104,105] and 'NK' activity has been demonstrated to be high, in mononuclear cells of tuberculous pleural exudates[121]. Such activity may be due to $\gamma\delta$ T cells.

Thus $\gamma\delta$ T cells may be an ontogenically early form of immune response to intracellular bacterial pathogens, and may produce their effects via cytolysis of infected phagocytic cells or by cytokine production.

Mechanisms of mycobacterial growth inhibition

Despite much research these mechanisms are poorly understood.

Case for and against reactive oxygen species

Monocytes, and to a lesser extent macrophages, can be activated by bacterial ingestion to produce reactive oxygen species such as superoxide and hydrogen peroxide. In the presence of myeloperoxidase found within granules of monocytes, activated halide and 'OH' radicals capable of killing a variety of microbial pathogens are also generated. γIFN and other cytokines can activate these pathways of monocytes and to a lesser extent of tissue macrophages. Classical data indicate that virulent M. tuberculosis strains can be killed *in vitro* by hydrogen peroxide[122], but a recent study[123] showed that *M. tuberculosis* H37Rv, *M. avium*, *M. kansasii* and *M. cheloni* are completely resistant to activated oxygen species, hydroxyl radicals and halide ions generated *in vitro* by an Fe-dependent xanthine-oxidase system. Mycobacteria possess a superoxide dismutase capable of inactivating O_2^-. Recent work has indicated that the phenolic cell-wall glycolipid of *M. leprae* acts as a scavenger of lethal oxygen radicals[124]. Furthermore, attenuation of virulent strains of *M. tuberculosis* coincides with a change in their cell wall lipid, which makes this ineffective at scavenging active oxygen radicals ('the attenuation indicator lipid' of Goren)[125]. Scavengers of oxygen radicals, including superoxide dismutase, catalase, histidine, etc., do not reverse mycobacterial growth inhibition within γIFN-activated murine macrophages. The interaction of mycobacteria with chronic granulomatous disease (CGD) provides an interesting paradox. As described earlier, neutrophils of CGD patients which are unable to generate toxic O_2 radicals have a modest bactericidal capacity against virulent tubercle bacilli, and the similar property of healthy neutrophils cannot be reversed by scavengers of free radicals. We have also recently observed a patient with CGD who was immunized at birth with BCG and developed a healed BCG lesion and skin test converted. His blood monocytes and macrophages can control the growth of intracellular BCG growth equivalent to macrophages from normal donors (R. A. Thompson , D. S. Kumararatne and G. Rylance, unpublished observations). Hence a considerable body of data suggests that non-oxidative mechanisms within macrophages may be responsible for mycobacterial growth inhibition (or killing). Nevertheless, several cases of fatal disseminated BCG infection have been reported in patients with CGD[126]. In contrast there have been no reported instances to date of MAI infection in patients with CGD[127]. Although CGD is a rare disorder, MAI is widely distributed in the environment and is capable of commonly causing nosocomial disease in patients with HIV infection. Hence on epidemiological grounds it is likely that children with CGD are exposed to MAI infection but are resistant. A possible explanation to the above paradox may lie in the genetic heterogeneity of CGD. It may be that some patients with CGD have an impairment of non-oxidative as well as oxidative defence mechanisms. Alternatively, patients with CGD who developed disseminated BCG infection may have an additional genetic phenotype analogous to that of Bcg.s mice. Investigating the mycobacterial growth inhibitory capacity of the monocytes of CGD patients *in vitro* may provide a useful way of dissecting antimycobacterial immune mechanisms in humans.

There is little information on the non-oxidative mechanisms of mycobacterial growth inhibition. Recently, generation of nitric oxide by oxidation of L-arginine has been shown to be microbicidal, in murine macrophages[128]. γIFN and TNF α or β synergistically increase reactive nitrogen intermediates (RNI) within murine macrophages. Muramyl dipeptide of mycobacteria does the same, acting in synergy with γIFN. Unpublished evidence for the role of RNI in the inhibition of intracellular *M. tuberculosis* and intracellular *M. leprae* has been cited in a recent review[128].

According to a recent report murine T cell clones which are non-cytolytic can activate leishmaniacidal activity in macrophages by direct contact without the apparent participation of secreted products (cytokines)[129], highlighting yet another possible mechanism of antibacterial activity against intracellular bacteria.

As described below, *M. tuberculosis* infection is seen at an early stage of HIV infection while MAI infection occurs only in severely immunocompromised patients with AIDS. It is tempting to speculate that MAI infection requires impaired macrophage function *in addition* to T cell deficiency, while the latter effect is sufficient to reactivate infection by the more virulent *M. tuberculosis.*

Concluding synthesis of current views on human anti-tuberculous immunity

Human tuberculosis usually follows the inhalation of very small numbers of bacteria (one to three bacteria) in droplet nuclei which are small enough to reach the alveoli. In those individuals with 'innate' macrophage-based resistance to tuberculosis these bacteria are rapidly destroyed before sufficient antigen is generated to sensitize T cells. Local generation of TNFα and other cytokines by infected macrophages may be a crucial part of this process. If bacterial multiplication overcomes this initial inhibitory process macrophages die, and the disgorged bacilli are ingested by freshly emigrated monocytes. As this process continues, a silent bacillaemia results in the dissemination of mycobacteria to other permissive sites. Experimental evidence indicates that this bacillaemia occurs about 20 days after the primary aerosol infection, and its magnitude is small (10^2–10^3 bacilli)[130]. When sufficient bacterial antigen is produced to result in T cell activation, cell-mediated immunity is enhanced at each of the metastatic foci. This probably includes granuloma formation, action of cytokines, activity of cytolytic CD4, CD8 and γδ T cells and NK/LAK-type effector cells. The combined effect of all these processes contributes to tissue damage and bacterial growth inhibition. The immune

Table 7.6 Mycobacteria causing disease in HIV-infected individuals

Mycobacterium tuberculosis	*M. fortuitum*
M. avium complex	*M. gordonae*
M. leprae	*M. asiaticum*
M. kansasii	*M. malmoense*
M. scrofulaceum	*M. xenopi*
M. szulgai	*M. bovis* (bacille Calmette-Guérin)
M. flavescens	

response probably induces a small proportion of tubercle bacilli to revert to a dormant state, presumably at the centre of granulomatous foci. Exogenous reinfection by inhalation of a large number(?) of virulent tubercle bacilli, or reactivation of endogenous foci by waning immunity (e.g. old age or HIV infection), results in progressive disease. Epidemiological and experimental evidence suggests that enhancement of T cell immunity by BCG immunization, natural primary TB infection or exposure to environmental mycobacteria does not prevent reinfection but reduces the risk of haematogenous spread of bacteria[130].

MYCOBACTERIAL DISEASE IN PATIENTS WITH HUMAN IMMUNODEFICIENCY VIRUS (HIV) INFECTION

Introduction

The course of HIV infection is frequently complicated by mycobacterial infection. *Mycobacterium tuberculosis* and *Mycobacterium avium* complex (MAC) are the most frequently identified pathogens. The former is not strictly an opportunistic infection, being a common infection in patients with apparently intact immunity, but is able to take advantage of even modest immune impairment. Alternatively, disseminated MAC occurs only with severe impairment of immunity, and has been closely associated with end-stage HIV infection. The incidence of both infections shows considerable variation according to geographical location and socioeconomic group. Other mycobacterial infections, some due to organisms previously not associated with human disease and generally considered non-pathogenic, have also been described in HIV-infected individuals (Table 7.6).

Epidemiology of tuberculosis in HIV-infected patients

Tuberculosis was seen infrequently in AIDS patients during the initial phase of the HIV epidemic in the USA. The annual incidence of new tuberculosis cases had fallen steadily from 1945 onwards, and was largely confined to certain high-risk groups. However, the expected annual decline in numbers of new cases halted in 1984 and has increased modestly since then[131]. Significant clumping of new cases occurred in areas with a high incidence of HIV infection. In New York, for instance, the annual incidence of tuberculosis doubled from 1979 to 1985, at which time 46% of cases occurred in individuals with AIDS or ARC[132]. The majority of these patients were i.v. drug abusers, a group already known to have a high past exposure to *M. tuberculosis* (as measured by delayed-type hypersensitivity to PPD). Skin test surveys also indicate that Haitians have a high prevalence of prior tuberculous infection, and a study of Haitian patients with AIDS in South Florida showed that 60% developed tuberculosis[133]. In comparison, only 2.7% of white homosexual males from the same area, which was a group with low prior exposure to tuberculosis, had the disease. Conversely, a study of 71 newly diagnosed cases of tuberculosis in Florida found that 31% of patients were HIV positive[134]; the majority of these individuals were Haitian. Similarly in San Fracisco, where a doubling in the incidence of tuberculosis occurred from 1982 to 1987, 29% of tuberculous patients were found to be HIV seropositive[135].

These population-based studies suggest that co-infection with HIV leads to the reactivation of latent tuberculous foci. This has been most clearly demonstrated in a study of tuberculin skin test positive drug addicts, in New York City[136]. Seven of 62 HIV seropositive addicts developed tuberculosis during the study period, compared to none of 49 HIV negative addicts. The risk of tuberculosis was 7.9% per year, 10-fold the yearly age-specific and race-specific rates reported for New York City for 1980–1986.

There is no evidence that HIV infection increases the risk of acquiring primary or secondary exogenous tuberculous infection. However, once exposed such individuals might reasonably be expected to be at high risk of progressive disease. Progressive primary and secondary exogenously acquired tuberculosis has been clearly demonstrated in patients with other cellular immunodeficiency conditions, although as yet is not well documented with HIV infection.

Experience in several African countries suggests that tuberculosis in HIV-infected individuals has become a major health problem. HIV seropositivity rates of 17–55% in newly diagnosed tuberculosis cases have been reported from several African countries[137–139]. A recent study from Zambia found that 49% of all newly diagnosed tuberculosis patients were HIV-1 seropositive, compared to 10% seropositivity for blood donors from the same area[140]. In Nairobi, 18% of HIV positive individuals requiring emergency admission to hospital were found to have active tuberculosis, and this accounted for 40% of all tuberculous cases requiring admission during the period of the study[141]. In comparison only 9% of tuberculosis patients attending the outpatient clinic were found to be HIV positive, emphasizing that tuberculous infection in HIV positive individuals tends to be more severe. In the Ivory Coast a high incidence of tuberculosis has been noted in HIV-1- and HIV-2-induced individuals[142]. Several African countries have now reported increased annual incidence rates for tuberculosis. The magnitude of the problem has become immense. In Uganda for instance, where the tuberculosis incidence doubled from 1984 to 1987, it is now estimated that 40000–50000 new cases of HIV-related tuberculosis may occur each year[143].

Clinical features

As discussed earlier, cellular-immune responses to tuberculous infection are responsible for both immunological defence and for tissue-damaging hypersensitivity, which contributes significantly to the clinical picture. Therefore, the clinical presentation of tuberculosis in HIV-infected individuals may be considerably modified by the degree of cellular immunodeficiency.

The association of tuberculosis with HIV infection was initially described in patients with severe immunodeficiency; most either had AIDS at the time tuberculosis was diagnosed or progressed to AIDS within a few months[133,144–146]. In these patients the clinical features of tuberculosis were frequently atypical; extrapulmonary sites are affected in approximately 60–70% of patients, pulmonary involvement occurred in 70% of patients and both pulmonary and extrapulmonary sites were affected in 30%. The chest radiographic appearances are frequently considered atypical; apical cavitation is unusual, while a diffuse or miliary picture is seen in 60% of patients (Figure 7.2)[147]. Hilar lymphadenopathy is often prominent, and as this feature is unusual in persistent generalized lymphadenopathy (PGL) or *Pneumocystis carinii* pneumonia it is a helpful clinical pointer to a diagnosis of tuberculosis. Patients with normal chest radiographs, yet proven pulmonary tuberculosis, have been described.

In 1987 the CDC added extrathoracic tuberculosis to its list of AIDS-defining opportunistic infections[148].

Subsequently studies have shown that, at the time tuberculosis is diagnosed, up to 75% of patients with HIV infection show no sign of AIDS or ARC[134,149]. These patients are more likely to present with characteristic pulmonary tuberculosis. However, in comparison to HIV seronegative tuberculosis patients, these otherwise asymptomatic HIV positive individuals still demonstrate atypical featues such as a tendency to produce diffuse pulmonary disease, extrathoracic involvement and a higher incidence of negative tuberculin skin tests.

Several studies in Africa have assessed the clinical presentation of tuberculosis there, and also found that extrapulmonary disease is more common in HIV-infected individuals. In a study of 206 HIV seropositive tuberculosis patients from Zambia, 123 patients had pulmonary disease, 67 had pleural and 16 had pericardial involvement[140]. Forty-nine per cent of all patients with tuberculosis were HIV seropositive while seropositivity rates in those with pleural and pericardial disease were 81% and 84% respectively. Where diagnostic facilities, including HIV serodiagnosis, are scarce tuberculosis may readily be mistaken for advanced HIV infection with the danger that effective treatment may not be offered[141].

Diagnosis

As the clinical features are frequently atypical, tuberculosis should be considered in the differential diagnosis of most clinical conditions, including pneumonitis, lymphadenitis, hepatosplenomegaly, meningitis and brain abscess. Nevertheless, over 70% of patients will still have pulmonary involvement. Pulmonary tuberculosis may be confused with *Pneumocystis carinii* pneumonia, but in the latter mediastinal lymphadenopathy does not occur.

As with non-HIV-infected tuberculosis patients the tuberculin skin test is of doubtful value. In countries where BCG is not routinely offered a positive

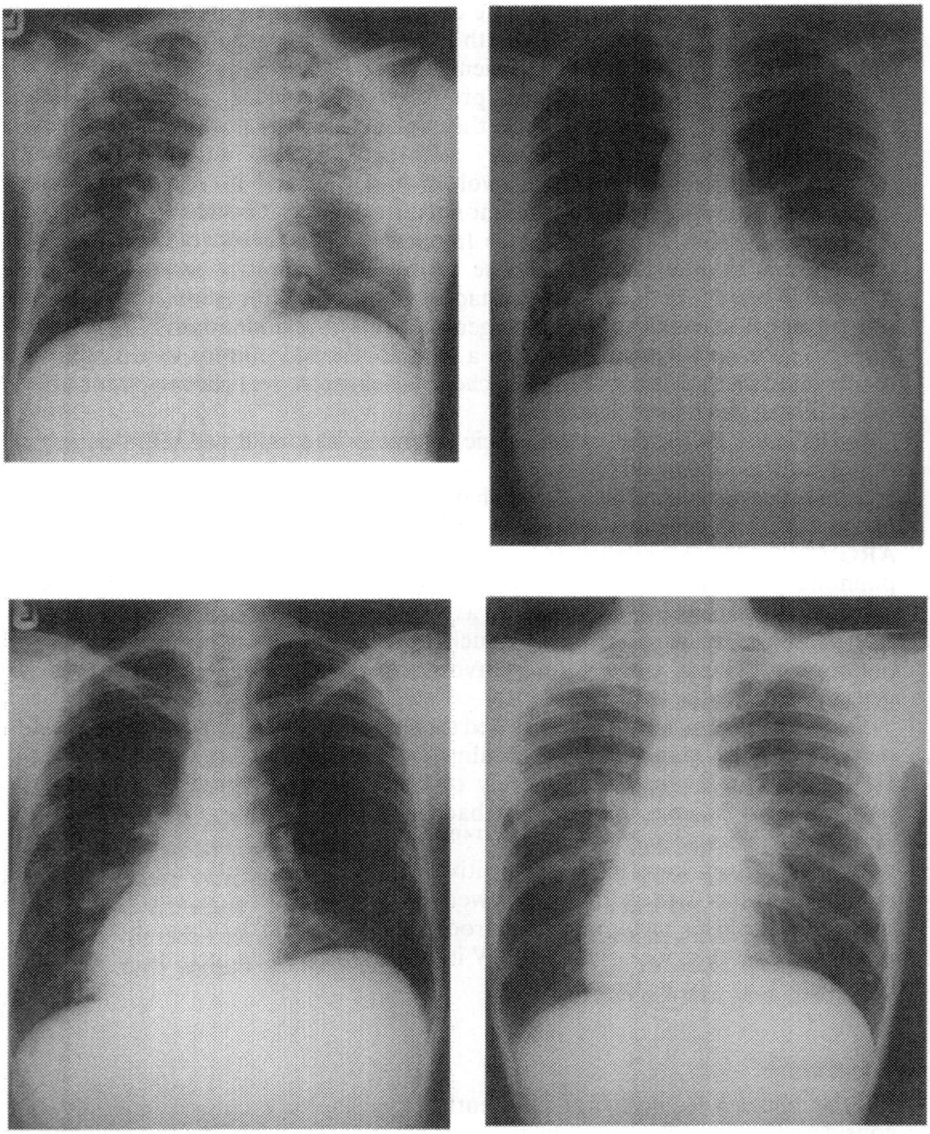

Figure 7.2 The atypical radiological appearances of pulmonary tuberculosis in patients with HIV infection

tuberculin test may be taken as evidence of tuberculous infection, and in asymptomatic patients prophylactic isoniazid be offered[150,151] (see below). However, a negative tuberculin test does not exclude tuberculosis, and HIV-infected individuals with tuberculosis – particularly those with advanced disease – are more likely to have negative tests than non-HIV-infected individuals[146].

Diagnosis rests on microbiological methods. Some studies have suggested that sputum smear and culture from patients with pulmonary disease is less sensitive than in non-HIV-infected individuals[134]. This has been attributed to the poor pulmonary cavitation which is found, denying extracellular growth, which can result in an explosive increase in mycobacterial numbers. Theuer *et al.*[149] in a study of newly diagnosed tuberculosis patients, found smear-positive rates of 47% and 51%, and culture-positive rates of 88% and 95%, in HIV positive and HIV negative patients respectively. In this study there was no significant difference in clinical and radiographic appearances between the patient groups.

M. tuberculosis can be readily demonstrated from liver biopsy, bone marrow, broncho-alveolar lavage fluid (BAL) and other infected tissues. *M. tuberculosis* bacteraemia is more frequently seen in HIV-infected individuals than other tuberculous patients[152]. The organism remains intracellular within macrophages; consequently a detection system which utilizes lysis/centrifugation is most effective.

A number of antibody and antigen detection serodiagnostic tests are being developed for tuberculosis, but currently there are no data evaluating their effectiveness in HIV-infected individuals.

Management

Current experience suggests that tuberculosis in HIV-infected individuals responds satisfactorily to standard antituberculous regimes containing three or four drugs given for 6–9 months (rifampicin plus isoniazid for 6–9 months, including either or both pyrazinamide and ethambutol of the first 2 months)[150,151]. Concern has been expressed about the duration of antituberculous therapy and the need for long-term chemoprophylaxis, as is required for *P. carinii* pneumonia. However, with such regimes rapid sterilization of sputum and radiological improvement has occurred in patients with advanced HIV infection[149,153]. Furthermore relapse has only been rarely reported. In one recent study this occurred in only three of 66 patients with advanced HIV infection and tuberculosis followed up for 82.3 patient years[153]. Poor compliance was considered important in each of these cases. These results suggest that continued chemoprophylaxis with isoniazed after completion of chemotherapy may not be necessary, at least in developed countries with low rates of tuberculosis transmission. However, in developing countries re-infection rates are likely to be much greater, and further long-term studies of isoniazid chemoprophylaxis are required in such settings.

Drug failure is extremely rare provided a three-drug regime is used from the outset. In the above study only one case occurred, in a patient with an isoniazid-resistant organism who was intolerant of rifampicin. There is a single report[154] of a patient who was commenced on isoniazid and rifampicin for what was shown to be a fully sensitive isolate. Compliance was considered good, yet he later relapsed with a rifampicin-resistant isolate. Both isolates had an identical phage type.

Although tuberculosis most frequently occurs before a diagnosis of AIDS is established, and despite effective chemotherapy, the median survival of such patients is only 16 months[153]. This is little better than the 14.4 month median survival of patients after a first episode of *P. carinii* pneumonia[155]. The majority of such patients die of non-tuberculous opportunistic infections and other HIV-related conditions. As previously described, *M. tuberculosis* is a potent inducer of TNFα production and release from mononuclear phagocytes[156]. In turn TNFα can effectively induce HIV-1 transcription in monocytes and T cells, increasing HIV production and theoretically increasing the immunodeficiency (reviewed in ref. 157).

Chemoprophylaxis should be considered in any HIV-infected individual with evidence of tuberculous infection in the absence of clinical disease[150]. There is considerable evidence supporting the use of isoniazid chemoprophylaxis in non-HIV positive individuals and experience to date supports a 1-year course of isoniazid in HIV positive individuals. However, tuberculous disease has been recorded following isoniazid chemoprophylaxis[158]. Moreover, the high risk of progressive disease from exogenous reinfection may require lifelong chemoprophylaxis. A further complication to a policy of chemoprophylaxis for individuals with positive tuberculin skin tests occurs in countries where BCG vaccination is offered to children.

Mycobacterium avium complex (MAC)

Epidemiology

The *Mycobacterium avium* complex includes *Mycobacterium avium* and *Mycobacterium intracellulare*, which are morphologically and biochemically indistinguishable. They are environmental organisms recognized to cause disease in birds, and are not infrequently found as commensals in the human gastrointestinal tract[159]. Until recently, MAC was mainly recognized as a cause of cervical adenitis in children and pulmonary infection in individuals with pre-existing lung disease[160]. Less than 50 cases of disseminated disease had been described in the world literature before 1980[161]. The past 10 years has seen an explosive increase in the incidence of disseminated MAC infection occurring in AIDS patients. Studies in the USA have recognized MAC infection in up to one-third of AIDS patients at some time during the course of their illness[162–164]. Postmortem studies show that up to 53% of AIDS patients have disseminated MAC infection, indicating that a large proportion of such infections are not recognized clinically[163,165]. There is, however, considerable geographical variation in the incidence of MAC infection. A careful study in Uganda was unable to identify any case of MAC infection and very few cases have been identified in other parts of Africa[166]. Similarly the incidence of MAC infection varies considerably throughout the UK, being frequently recognized in London but much less so in other areas with moderate numbers of patients.

The MAC may be divided into a large number of serotypes[167]. Remarkably, disseminated MAC infections in AIDS patients are almost invariably caused by a small number of serotypes, most frequently serotypes 1, 4 and 8[168]. These serotypes are less frequently represented in non-AIDS MAC infection, and do not reflect the pattern of environmental serotypes[169,170].

The MAC may also be distinguished at the molecular level. A recent study, using species-specific gene probes, demonstrated that 98% of 45 patients with AIDS were infected with *M. avium*, while 40% of isolates from non-HIV-infected individuals were *M. intracellulare*[171]. DNA probes which distinguish restriction fragment length polymorphisms (RFLP) allow accurate genetic identification of specific MAC strains. Using such probes, 73% of MAC strains from 45 AIDS patients were indistinguishable by RFLP analysis[172]. Furthermore, the banding pattern of these isolates was quite distinguishable from that of MAC derived from the stool of healthy individuals and from 60% of non-AIDS-derived MAC isolates. RFLP analysis and serotyping of MAC isolates frequently show poor correlation, as demonstrated by the finding of different serotypes giving identical banding patterns. Nevertheless, it is likely that the commonly identified serotypes represent a few common strains.

The mode of MAC transmission has not yet been defined. It is generally believed that MAC infection occurs through colonization of the gastrointestinal (GI) tract. This view is supported by finding extensive involvement of the GI tract in many patients with disseminated MAI, and the observation that GI colonization may precede disseminated disease by some weeks[173]. However, RFLP analysis of MAC isolates, as discussed above, suggests that the normal commensal strains are not responsible for invasive disease[172]. Therefore it appears most likely that newly acquired infection is responsible for disseminated MAC, and this is likely to occur through contaminated food or drink. The respiratory tract is another established route of infection, and isolated pulmonary disease can progress to disseminated disease[174].

Clinical features

In contrast to tuberculosis, MAC infection usually occurs in patients with advanced HIV infection, often following previous AIDS-defining opportunistic infection. However, with improved prophylaxis against *Pneumocystis carinii* and other pathogens, disseminated MAC is increasingly seen in some patients as the first significant opportunistic infection. These patients are likely to have very low circulating CD4 T cells and defective mononuclear cell function which readily allows MAC to grow intracellularly within the latter. The clinical picture most often attributed to MAI infection is one of persisting, or recurrent, fever for weeks to months, weight loss, sweats, rigors and often diarrhoea[175]. Malabsorption may occur, and a Whipple's disease-like state has been identified. Generalized lymphadenopathy and hepatosplenomegaly are often present.

Liver function abnormalities and pancytopenia are common, and total and CD4 T lymphocyte counts are usually extremely low. In this setting MAI can be readily demonstrated from blood, faeces, duodenal aspirates, sputum, bone marrow and liver biopsy. Sustained bacteraemia, with large numbers of organisms (colony counts often greater than 10^4/ml) is frequently seen[176]. Blood culture, therefore, is an effective means of establishing the diagnosis. Using modern methods of lysis/centrifugation, to release the organism from circulating monocytes (which may increase the colony counts up to 5-fold), and radiorespirometric detection the sensitivity of blood culture approaches 100%.

Survival for untreated patients with disseminated MAC infection rarely exceeds 11 months. However, because these patients usually have other opportunistic infections or HIV-related complications the contribution of MAC to their demise has been uncertain. For instance, a postmortem study of 12 patients with disseminated MAC found that death could be directly attributed to MAC in only one individual, the remaining 11 patients died of other opportunistic infections or HIV-related disease[177].

Management

With the currently available drugs treatment of MAC is difficult and often unsatisfactory. Unlike *M. tuberculosis* MAC isolates show highly variable *in vitro* drug sensitivities which do not correlate with clinical efficacy[175]. This is clearly influenced by considerable species and strain variation. For instance, *M. avium* isolates from AIDS patients, as identified by gene probe, were less sensitive to rifampicin, ethambutol and streptomycin than *M. intracellulare* isolated frrom non-AIDS cases[171]. Further complications arise from the tendency of MAC isolates to change morphologically, e.g. from yellow pigment-producing to unpigmented variants or opaque to transparent colonial variants, during *in vitro* culture[178,179] A corresponding change in drug susceptibility occurs with these morphological changes. Overall most AIDS-associated MAC isolates are resistant to conventional first-line anti-tuberculous drugs (rifampicin, isoniazid and ethambutol) used as single agents, but are sensitive to clofazimine, amikacin and rifabutin, and less so to ethionamide[175]. Some *in vitro* activity has also been demonstrated for ciprofloxacin and the new macrolides such as azithromycin[180,181].

Early experiences with three or more drugs regimes, including rifabutin and clofazamine, were disappointing. Treatment had little or no clinical effect and failed to control bacteraemia in the majority of patients[163]. However, rifabutin was given in a dosage of only 150 mg/day and the mean duration of therapy was only 6 weeks. In a subsequent study rifabutin and clofazamine, in combination with ethambutol and isoniazid, were given for longer periods and effectively controlled bacteraemia in five of seven patients and significantly improved symptoms in six of seven patients[174]. In a further study, using rifabutin in a higher dosage of 300–600 mg/day plus clofazamine, isoniazid and ethambutol, clearing of mycobacteraemia was demonstrated in 22 of 25 patients, and 18 patients had an excellent symptomatic response[182]. Others have found that the combination of amikacin, ethambutol and rifampicin is clinically effective[183].

Despite clinical improvement with antimycobacterial therapy the survival of these patients is not improved beyond that expected in untreated patients.

All are severely immunocompromised and develop other HIV-related complications.

The poor clinical response found with antituberculous drugs has encouraged the possible use of immunological treatment with cytokines. As discussed before, considerable uncertainty surrounds the effectiveness of various cytokines against MAC infection both *in vitro* and in animal models (Table 7.4). Of the available cytokines, TNFα shows most consistent antimycobacterial activity against MAC[88,96]. However, elevated TNFα levels are found in the serum of AIDS patients and from HIV-infected monocytes in culture[184,185]. Furthermore TNFα induces HIV replication within cultured monocytes and T cells, and therefore is an unlikely candidate for cytokine therapy[197]. Interferon-gamma, which shows variable antimycobacterial ability *in vitro*, has been given to two patients with disseminated MAC infection[186]. In one patient there was a temporary fall in MAC bacillaemia with a rapid rise on discontinuation; in the other there was no fall during therapy, but a sustained rise afterwards. Experience to date is therefore not very encouraging.

Other mycobacteria

Several other mycobacteria have been isolated from HIV-infected individuals and implicated as causing disease. *M. kansasii* has caused disseminated disease in a number of patients[187,188], as has infection with organisms generally considered non-pathogenic such as *M. gordonae* and *M. xenopi*[189,190]. Hirschel *et al.* described a fatal infection with a novel, unidentified mycobacterium[191]. Such organisms would previously have been considered as contaminants when isolated from clinical specimens, but in the context of HIV infection any mycobacterial isolate should be considered seriously.

BCG has been given to many HIV-infected individuals, largely without any deleterious effect. However, several cases of disseminated BCG have been described[192,193]. Most interesting was a 36-year-old homosexual man with AIDS who developed BCG adenitis 30 years after vaccination[194]. This suggested that, like virulent *M. tuberculosis*, BCG can remain dormant for many years.

The clinical spectrum of leprosy reflects underlying cellular immune responsiveness to *M. leprae*. It might therefore be expected that concurrent HIV infection would have a significant impact on the clinical picture, particularly in areas where the tuberculoid form of the disease is predominant. However, although HIV infection has been described in lepropsy patients in Zambia[195] there is currently insufficient information to predict the impact HIV will have on the clinical presentation.

Influence of HIV infection on macrophage function

Mononuclear cells bear CD4 receptors and act as an important reservoir for infection[196]. In so doing the HIV virus may alter the function of a cell which is the cornerstone of defence against many pathogens.

There is now considerable evidence that cytokines may influence HIV expression[197]. In particular TNFα, which is produced by mononuclear cells under the influence of endotoxins, viruses and certain bacteria, can upgrade HIV expression through the pleitrophic cellular transcription factor NF-kB, which binds to the core enhancer region of HIV long terminal repeat (LTR). Other cytokines which enhance HIV expression include IL6 and GM CSF[197,198].

HIV-infected monocytes appear to have impaired function. They show abnormal cytokine secretion, defective chemotaxis[199], reduced phagocytosis[200] and reduced ability to generate reactive oxygen species[201]. Crowle *et al.*[202,203] have demonstrated that macrophages from HIV-infected individuals are more permissive to the intracellular growth of *M. avium*, which is only partially explained by a lack of the serum inhibitory factor found in normal individuals, which can prevent intracellular MAC growth.

References

1. Snider, D. E. (1989). Introduction. Research towards global control and prevention of tuberculosis with an emphasis towards vaccine development. *Rev. Infect. Dis.*, **11**, S336–8
2. Wells, W. F. (1934). On airborne infection. II. Droplets and droplet nuclei. *Am. J. Hyg.*, **20**, 611
3. Ratcliffe, J. L. and Palladino, V. S. (1953). Tuberculosis induced by droplet nuclei infection. *J. Exp. Med.*, **97**, 61–8
4. Riley, R. L. (1961). Airborne pulmonary tuberculosis. *Bact. Rev.*, **25**, 243–8
5. Hoak, V. N., Baker, J. H., Sorenson, K. and Kent, M. C. (1968). The epidemiology of tuberculosis infections in a closed environment. *Arch Environ Health*, **16**, 26
6. Lurie, M. B. (1964). *Resistance to tuberculosis: experimental studies in native and acquired defensive mechanisms* (Cambridge, Mass: Harvard University Press)
7. Dickinson, J. M., Lefford, M. J., Lloyd, J. and Mitchison, D. A. (1963). The virulence in the guinea pig of tubercle bacilli from patients with tuberculosis in Hong Kong. *Tubercle*, **44**, 446–51
8. Seaton, A., Seaton, D. and Leitch, G. A. (1984). In *Crofton and Douglas Respiratory Diseases*, 4th edn (Oxford: Blackwell Scientific Publications), chapter 13, pp. 367–94
9. Mitchison, D. A. (1990). Infectivity of patients with pulmonary tuberculosis during chemotherapy. *Eur. Resp. J.*, **3**, 385–6
10. Bloch, H. (1948). The relation between phagocytic cells and human tubercle bacilli. *Am. Rev. Tuberc.*, **58**, 667–70
11. Montgomery, L. G. and Lemon, W. (1933). The cellular reaction of the pleura to infection with *M. tuberculosis. J. Thorac. Cardiovasc. Surgery*, **2**, 429–38
12. Jones, G. S., Amirault, H. J. and Anderson, B. R. (1990). Killing of *M. tuberculosis* by neutrophils: a nonoxidative process *J. Infect. Dis.*, **162**, 700–4
13. Schlesinger, L. S. and Horwitz, M. A. (1990). Phagocytosis of leprosy bacilli is mediated by complement receptors CR1 and CR3 on human monocytes and complement component C3 in serum. *J. Clin. Invest.*, **85**, 1304–14
14. Schlesinger, L. S., Bellinger-Kawahara, C. G., Payne, N. R. and Horwitz, M. A. (1990). Phagocytosis of *Mycobacterium tuberculosis* is mediated by human monocyte complement receptors and complement component C3. *J. Immunol.*, **144**(7), 2771–80
15. Schwartz, R. P., Naai, D., Vogel, C. W. and Yeager, H. Jr (1988). Differences in uptake of mycobacteria by human monocytes: a role for complement. *Infect. Immun.*, **56**, 2223–7
16. Kindler, V., Sappino, A. P., Cran, G. E., Piguet, P. F. and Vassalli, P. (1989). The inducing role of TNFα in the development of bactericidal granulomas during BCG infection. *Cell*, **56**, 731–40
17. Kovacs, C. J. (1991). Fibrogenic cytokines: the role of immune nucleators in the development of scar tissue. *Immunol. Today*, **12**, 17
18. Strom, L. (1955). A study of cutaneous absorption of BCG vaccine labelled with phosphate in subjects with or without immunity. *Acta Tuberc. Scand.*, **31**, 141
19. McCune, R. M. and Tompsett, R. (1956). Fate of *M. tuberculosis* in mouse tissue as determined by the microbial enumeration technique. 1. The persistence of drug susceptible tubercle bacilli in the tissues despite prolonged antimicrobial therapy. *J. Exp. Med.*, **104**, 737–62

20. Grosset, J. (1978). Experimental data on short course chemotherapy for tuberculosis. *Bull. Int. Union Tuberc.*, **53**, 265–7
21. Toman, K. (1981). Bacterial persistence in leprosy. *In. J. Leprosy*, **49**, 205
22. Mitchison, D. A. (1979). Basic mechanisms of chemotherapy for tuberculosis, *Chest*, **76** (Suppl.), 771–81
23. Stead, W. W. (1989). Pathogenesis of tuberculosis: clinical and epidemiological perspective. *Rev. Infect. Dis.*, **11**, S366–8
24. Dannenberg, A. M. (1989). Immune mechanisms in the pathogenesis of pulmonary tuberculosis. *Rev. Infect. Dis.*, **11**, S369–78
25. Cannetti, G. (1965). Present aspects of bacterial resistance in tuberculosis. *Am. Rev. Respir. Dis.*, **92**, 687
26. Wallgren, A. (1948). The timetable of tuberculosis, *Tubercle*, **29**, 245
27. Sutherland, I. (1968). The ten year incidence of clinical tuberculosis following 'conversion' in 2550 individuals aged 14–19 years. TSRU progress report (KNCV, POB 146, The Hague)
28. Chase, M. W. (1945). The cellular troughs of cutaneous hypersensitivity to tuberculin. *Proc. Soc. Exp. Biol. Med.*, **59**, 134
29. Lefford, M. J. (1975). Transfer of adoption immunity to tuberculosis in mice. *Infect. Immun.*, **11**, 1174
30. Lurie, M. B. (1942). Studies on the mechanism of immunity to tuberculosis. *J. Exp. Med.*, **75**, 247
31. Mackaness, G. B. (1968). The immunology of anti-tuberculous immunity. *Am. Rev. Resp. Dis.*, **97**, 337
32. Unanne, E. R. (1980). Co-operation between mononuclear phagocytes and lymphocytes in immunity. *N. Engl. J. Med.*, **303**, 977
33. Lurie, M. B., Zappazodi, P., Dannenberg, A. M. and Weiss, G. H. (1952). On the mechanism of genetic resistance to tuberculosis and its mode of inheritance. *Am. J. Hum. Genet.*, **4**, 302–14
34. Schurr, E., Bushman, E., Malo, D., Gros, P. and Skamene, E. (1990). Immunogenetics of mycobacterial infections: mouse–human homologies. *J. Infect. Dis.*, **161**, 634–9
35. Plant, J. E., Blackwell, J. M., O'Brien, A. D., Bradley, D. J. and Glynn, A. A. (1982). Are the Lsh, Ity disease resistance genes at one locus on mouse chromosome 1? *Nature*, **297**, 510–11
36. Grove, I. M., Stokes, R. W. and Collins, F. M. (1985). Only two out of fifteen strains of BCG follow the Bcg pattern. In: Skamene, E. (ed.), *Progress on Leukocyte Biology*, Vol. 3: *Genetic Control of Host Resistance to Infection and Malignancy* (New York: Liss), p. 285
37. Stokes, R. W. and Collins, F. M. (1990). Passive transfer of immunity to Mycobacterium avium in susceptible and resistant strains of mice. *Clin. Exp. Immunol.*, **81**, 109–15
38. Mims, C. A. (1987). *The Pathogenesis of Infectious Diseases*, 3rd edn. (London: Academic Press), pp. 71–87
39. Kallman, F. J. and Reisner, D. (1943). Twin studies on the significance of genetic factors in tuberculosis. *Am. Rev. Tuberc.*, **47**, 549
40. Stead, W. W., Senner, J. W., Reddich, W. J. and Lofgren, J. P. (1990). Racial differences in susceptibility to infection by *M. tuberculosis. N. Engl. J. Med.*, **322**, 422
41. Rich, A. R. (1951). *The Pathogenesis of Tuberculosis*, 2nd edn. (Springfield, IL: Charles C. Thomas), pp. 131–48
42. Bates, J. H. (1982). Tuberculosis susceptibility and resistance. *Am. Rev. Respir. Dis.*, **125**, 20
43. Rook, G. A. W., Steele, J., Ainsworth, M. and Champion, B. R. (1986). Activation of macrophages to inhibit proliferation of *M. tuberculosis. Clin. Exp. Immunol.*, **59**, 333–8
44. Crowle, A. J. (1988). The tubercle bacillus – human macrophage relationship, studies *in vitro*. In Bendinelli, ? and Friedman, ? (eds), *M. tuberculosis. Interactions with the Immune System.* (New York: Plenum Press), pp. 99–131
45. Crowle, A. J. and Elkins, N. (1990). Relative permissiveness of macrophages from black and white people for virulent tubercle bacilli. *Infect. Immun.*, **58**, 632–8
46. Davies, P. D. (1985). A possible link between vitamin D deficiency and impaired host defense to *M. tuberculosis. Tubercle*, **66**, 301–6
47. Selby, R., Barnard, J. M., Buehler, S. K., Crumley, J., Larsen, B. and Marshall, W. H. (1978). Tuberculosis associated with HLA B8 Bfs in a Newfoundland community study. *Tissue Antigens*, **11**, 403–8
48. Al-arif, L. I., Goldstein, K. A., Affronti, L. F. and Janicki, B. W. (1978). HLA BW15 and tuberculosis in a North American black population. *Am. Rev. Respir. Dis.*, **120**, 1275–8
49. Hafez, M., El-Salab, S., El-Shennawy, F. and Bassiony, M. R. (1985). HLA antigens and

tuberculosis in the Egyptian population. *Tubercle*, **66**, 35–40

50. Singh, S. P. N., Mehra, N. K., Dingley, H. B., Pandi, J. N. and Vaidya, M. C. (1983). HLA-linked control of susceptibility to pulmonary tuberculosis and association with HLA DR types. *J. Infect. Dis.*, **148**, 676–81
51. Bothamley, G. H., Swanson Beck, J., Schreuder, G. M. T., D'Amaro, J., de Vries, L. R. P., Kardjito, T. and Ivanyi, J. (1989). Association of tuberculosis and *M. tuberculosis* specific antibody levels with HLA. *J. Infect. Dis.*, **159**, 549
52. de Vries, R. R. P. (1989). Regulation of T cell responsiveness against mycobacterial antigens by HLA Class 2 immune response genes. *Rev. Infect. Dis.*, **11**, S400
53. Ottenhoff, T. H. M., Torres, P., de las Agves, J. T., Fernandez, R., van Embden, W., de Vries, R. R. and Stanford, J. L. (1986). Evidence for an HLA Dr4 associated immune response gene for *M. tuberculosis*. A clue to the pathogenesis of rheumatoid arthritis? *Lancet*, **2**, 310–13
54. Thole, J. E. R., van Schooten, W. C. A., Reuben, W. J., Hermans, P. W. M., Jansen, A. A. M., de Vries, R. R. P., Kolk, A. H. J. and van Embden, J. D. A. (1988). Use of recombinant antigens expressed in *E. coli* K12 to napB-cell and T-cell epitopes on the immunodominant 65 kD protein of *M. bovis* BCG. *Infect. Immun.*, **56**, 1633–40
55. Lamb, J. R., Ivanyi, J., Rees, A. D. M., Rothbardi, J. B., Howland, K., Young, R. A. and Young, D. B. (1987). Mapping of T cell epitopes using recombinant antigens and synthetic peptides. *EMBO J.*, **6**, 1245–9
56. Gaston, J. S. H., Life, P., Jenner, P. J., Coleston, M. J. and Bacon, P. A. (1990). Recognition of a mycobacteria specific epitope in the 65 kD heat shock protein by synovial fluid derived T cell clones. *J. Exp. Med.*, **171**, 831–41
57. Danska, J. S. (1989). The T cell receptor: structure, molecular diversity and somatic localisation. *Curr. Opinion Immunol.*, **2**, 81–6
58. Koyasu, S., D'adanio, L. Clayton, L. K. and Reinberg, E. L. (1991). T cell receptor isoforms and signal transduction. *Curr. Opinion Immunol.*, **3**, 32–9
59. Mosmann, T. R. and Coffman, K. L. (1987). Two types of mouse helper T-cell clones: implications for immune regulation. *Immunol. Today*, **8**, 223–7
60. Scott, P., Natoritz Coffmann, R. L., Pearce, E. and Sher, A. (1988). Immunoregulation in cutaneous leishmaniasis T cell lines that transfer protective immunity or exacerbation belong to different T helper subsets and respond to distinct parasite antigens. *J. Exp. Med.*, **168**, 1675
61. Heinzel, F. P., Sadik, M. D., Holaday, B. J., Coffmann, R. L. and Locksley, R. M. (1989). Reciprocal expression of interferon γ or interleukin 4 during resolution or progression of murine leishmaniasis. Evidence for the expansion of distinct helper T cell subsets. *J. Exp. Med.*, **169**, 59–72
62. Ottenhoff, T. H. M., Elferink, D. G., Klatser, P. R. and de Vries, R. R. P. (1986). Cloned suppressor T cells from a lepromatous leprosy patient suppress *M. leprae* reactive helper T cells. *Nature*, **322**, 462–4
63. Modlin, R. L., Kato, H., Mehra, V., Nelson, E. E., Xue-dong, F., Rea, T. H., Pattengale, P. K. and Bloom, B. R. (1986). Genetically restricted suppressor T cell clones derived from lepromatous leprosy lesions. *Nature*, **322**, 459
64. Lamb, J. R., Lathigra, R. and Rothbard, J. B. (1989). Identification of mycobacterial antigens recognised by T lymphocytes. *Rev. Infect. Dis.*, **II**, S443–7
65. Engers, H. D. and Workshop participants (1985). Results of a WHO workshop to characterise antigens recognised by mycobacterium specific monoclonal antibodies. *Infect. Immun.*, **48**, 603
66. Abou Zeid, C., Ratcliffe, T. L., Wilker, H. G., Harboe, M., Bennendsen, J. and Rook, G. A. W. (1988). Characterisation of fibronectin-binding antigens released by *M. tuberculosis* and *M. bovis* BCG. *Infect. Immun.*, **56**, 3046–51
67. Zhang, Y., Lathigra, R., Garbe, T., Catty, D. and Young, D. (1991). Cloning and characterisation of the superoxide dismutase gene from *M. tuberculosis. Mol. Microbiol.* (In press)
68. Young, R. A., Mehra, V., Swater, D., Buchanan, T., Clark Curtess, J., Davis, R. W. and Bloom, B. R. (1985). Genes for the major protein antigens of the Leprosy parasite *M. leprae. Nature*, **316**, 450–2
69. Engers, H. D. (1986). Results of a WHO sponsored workshop to characterise antigens

recognised by *Mycobacterium* specific monoclonal antibodies. *Infect. Immun.*, **52**, 718
70. Oftung, F., Mustafa, A. S., Husson, R., Young, R. A. and Godal, T. (1987). Human T cell clones recognise two abundant *M. tuberculosis* protein antigens expressed by *E. coli*, *J. Immunol.*, **138**, 297
71. Munk, M. G., Schoel, B. and Kaufmann, S. H. E. (1988). T cell responses of normal individuals towards recombinant protein antigens of *M. tuberculosis*, *Eur. J. Immunol.*, **18**, 1835
72. Mehra, V., Swatson, D. and Young, R. A. (1986). Efficient mapping of protein antigenic determinants. *Proc. Natl. Acad. Sci. USA*, **83**, 7013–17
73. Lamb, J. R., Ivanyi, J., Rees, A. D. M., Rothbard, J. B., Howland, K., Young, R. A. and Young, D. B. (1987). Mapping of T cell epitopes using recombinant antigens and synthetic peptides. *EMBO J.*, **6**, 1245–9
74. Young, D. B., Lathigra, R. B., Hendrix, R., Sweetser, D. and Young, R. A. (1988). Stress proteins are immune targets in leprosy and tuberculosis. *Proc. Natl. Acad. Sci. USA*, **85**, 4267–70
75. Shinnick, T. (1987). The 65-kilodalton antigen of *M. tuberculosis*. *J. Bacteriol.*, **169**, 1080–8
76. Morimoto, R. I., Tissieres, A. and Georgopulos, C. (eds) (1990). *Stress Proteins in Biology and Medicine.* (Cold Spring Harbor, New York: Cold Spring Harbor Press)
77. Berzofsky, J. A., Reichman, L. K. and Killion, D. J. (1979). Distinct Hr2 linked Ir genes control both antibody and T cell responses to different determinants on the same antigen myoglobin. *Proc. Natl. Acad. Sci. USA*, **76**, 4046–50
78. Abou-Zeid, C. E., Filley, C. and Rook, G. A. W. (1987). A simple new method for using antigens separated by polyserylamide gel electrophoresis to stimulate lymphocyte in vitro after converting bands cut from Western-blots into antigen bearing particles. *J. Immunol Methods*, **98**, 5
79. Blandon, R. V., Lifford, M. J. and Mackaness, G. B. (1969). Host response to Calmette-Guerin bacillus infection in mice. *J. Exp. Med.*, **129**, 1079–107
80. Rook, G. A. W., Steele, J., Barnass, S., Mace, J. and Stanford, J. L. (1986). Responsiveness to live *M. tuberculosis* and common antigens of sonicate-stimulated T cell lines from normal donors. *Clin. Exp. Immunol.*, **63**, 105
81. Barnes, P. F., Mehra, V., Hirshfield, G. R., Fong, S. T., Abou Zeid, C., Rook, G. A. W., Hunter, S. W., Brennan, P. J. and Modlin, R. L. (1989). Characterisation of T cell antigens associated with the cell-wall protein–peptido-glycan complex of *M. tuberculosis*. *J. Immunol.*, **143**, 2656–62
82. Mackaness, G. B. (1969). The influence of immunologically committed lymphoid cells on macrophage activity *in vivo*. *J. Exp. Med.*, **129**, 973–92
83. Ando, M., Dannenberg, A. M. and Shina, K. (1972). Macrophage accumulation, division, maturation and digestive and microbicidal capacities in tuberculous lesions. Rates at which mononuclear cells enter and divide in primary BCG lesions. *J. Immunol.*, **109**, 8–19
84. David, J. R. and David, R. R. (1972). Cellular hypersensitivity and immunity: inhibition of macrophage migration and the lymphocyte mediators. *Prog. Allergy*, **16**, 300–449
85. Flesch, I. and Kaufmann, S. H. E. (1987). Mycobacterial growth inhibition by gamma interferon activated bone marrow macrophages and differential susceptibility among strains of *M. tuberculosis*. *J. Immunol.*, **138**, 4408
86. Douvas, G. S., Hooper, D. L., Valter, A. E. and Crowle, A. J. (1985). Gamma interferon activates human macrophages to become tumoricidal and leishmanicidal but enhances replication of macrophage associated mycobacteria. *Infect. Immun.*, **50**, 1–8
87. Toba, H., Crawford, J. T. and Ellner, J. J. (1989). Pathogenicity of mycobacterium avium for human monocytes: absence of macrophage-activating factor activity of gamma interferon. *Infect. Immun.*, **57**, 329
88. Dennis, M. (1991). Modulation of *Mycobacterium avium* growth *in vivo* by cytokines: involvement of tumour necrosis factor in resistance to atypical mycobacteria. *Clin. Exp. Immunol.*, **83**, 466–71
89. Scheurich, P., Thoma, B., Ucer, U. and Pfizenmaier, J. (1987). Immunoregulatory activity of recombinant human TNF alpha, induction of TNF alpha receptors of human T cells and TNF alpha mediated enhancement of T cell responses. *J. Immunol.*, **138**, 1786
90. Barnes, P. F., Fong, S. J., Brennan, P. J., Twomey, P. E., Mazumder, A. and Modlin, R. C. (1990). Local production of tumor necrosis factor and IFN-γ in tuberculosis pleuritis. *J. Immunol.*, **145**, 149–54
91. Moreno, C., Taverne, J., Mehlert, A. J., Bate, C. A. W., Brearly, A., Meager, A., Rook, G.

A. W. and Playfair, J. H. L. (1989). Lipoarabinomannan from *M. tuberculosis* induces the production of TNFα from human and murine macrophages. *Clin. Exp. Immunol.*, **76**, 240
92. Wallis, R. S., Amit, T., Ahmasseb, M. and Ellner, J. J. (1991). Induction of interleukin 1 and tumor necrosis factor by mycobacterial proteins: the monocyte western blot. *Proc. Natl. Acad. Sci. USA*, **87**, 3348–52
93. Roper, W. H. and Waring, J. J. (1955). Primary serofibrinous pleural effusion in military personnel. *Am. Rev. Tuberc.*, **71**, 616
94. Rook, G. A. N. (1990). The role of activated macrophages in protection and immunopathology of tuberculosis. *Res. Microbiol.*, **141**, 253–6
95. Dennis, M. (1991). Killing of *M. tuberculosis* within human monocytes: activation by cytokines and calcitriol. *Clin. Exp. Immunol.*, **84**, 200–6
96. Bermudez, L. E. and Young, L. S. (1988). Recombinant tumour necrosis factor alone or in combination with interleukin-2 but not gamma-interferon is associated with killing of *M. avium* complex from AIDS patients. *J. Immunol.*, **140**, 3006
97. Crowle, A. J. (1990). Intracellular killing of mycobacteria. *Res. Microbiol.*, **141**, 231–6
98. Ellner, J. J. (1990). Source of variability in assays of microbiology with mononuclear phagocytes: of mice and men. *Res. Microbiol.*, **141**, 237–40
99. Rook, G. A. W. (1988). The role of vitamin D in tuberculosis. *Am. Rev. Resp. Dis.*, **138**, 768–70
100. Cadranel, J., Hance, A. J., Milleron, B., Paillrd, F., Akoun, G. M. and Garabodian, M. (1988). Vitamin D metabolism in tuberculosis: production of 1,25(OH)2 D3 by cells recovered by bronchoalveolar lavage and the role of this metabolite in calcium homeostasis. *Am. Rev. Respir. Dis.*, **138**, 984–9
101. MacRae, D. (1947). Calciferol treatment of lupus vulgaris. *Br. J. Dermatol.*, **59**, 333
102. Rees, R. J. W. and D'Arcy Hart, P. (1961). Analysis of the host parasite equilibrium in chronic murine tuberculosis by total and viable bacillary counts. *Br. J. Exp. Pathol.*, **42**, 83
103. Kaufmann, S. H. E. (1988). $CD8^+$ T lymphocytes in intracellular microbial infection. *Immunol Today*, **9**, 168–74
104. Kumararatne, D. S., Pithie, A. D., Drysdale, P., Gaston, J. S. H., Kiessling, R., Iles, P. B., Ellis, C. J., Innes, J. A. and Wise, R. (1990). Specific lysis of mycobacterial antigen-bearing macrophages by Class II MHC-restricted polyclonal cell lines in healthy donors or patients with tuberculosis. *Clin. Exp. Immunol.*, **80**, 314–23
105. Ottenhoff, T. H. M., Kale-Ab, B., Van Embden, J. A., Thole, J. E. R. and Kiessling, R. (1988). The recombinant 65 kD heat shock protein of *M. bovis* (BCG)/*M. tuberculosis* is a target molecule for $CD4^+$ cytotoxic T lymphocytes that lyse human monocytes. *J. Exp. Med.*, **168**, 1947–52
106. Rahelu, M. (1991). Cytolytic T cell responses to mycobacterial antigens. MSc thesis, University of Birmingham, UK
107. Rook, G. A. W. and Stanford, J. L. (1981). The heterogeneity of the immune response to mycobacteria and the relevance of the common antigens to their pathogenicity. *Ann. Immunol.*, **132D**, 155–64
108. Dubos, R. J. (1955). Properties and structures of tubercle bacilli concerned in their pathogenicity. *Symp. Soc. Gen. Microbiol.*, **5**, 103
109. Kaplan, G. and Cohn, Z. A. (1991). Leprosy and cell mediated immunity. *Curr. Opin. Immunol.*, **3**, 91–6
110. Kale, ab B., Kiessling, R., Van Embden, J. D. A., Thole, J. E. R., Kumararatne, D.S., Wondimu, A. and Ottenhoff, T. H. M. (1990). Induction of antigen specific CD4 HLA-DR restricted cytotoxic T lymphocytes as well as non specific nonrestricted killer cells by the recombinant mycobacterial 65 kD heat shock protein. *Eur. J. Immunol.*, **20**, 369
111. De Libero, G., Flesch, I. and Kaufmann, S. H. E. (1988). *Mycobacteria* reactive Lyt 2^+ T cell lines. *Eur. J. Immunol.*, **18**, 59
112. Raulet, D. H. (1989). The structure, function and molecular genetics of the $\gamma\delta$ T cell receptor. *Annu. Rev. Immunol.*, **7**, 175
113. Janis, E. M., Kaufmann, S. H. E., Schwartz, R. H. and Pardoll, D. M. (1989). Activation of $\gamma\delta$ T cells in the primary immune response to *M. tuberculosis*. *Science*, **244**, 713
114. Modlin, R. L., Primez, C., Hofman, F. M., Torigiani, K., Uyemura, K., Rea, T. H., Bloom, B. R. and Brenner, M. B. (1989). $\gamma\delta$ lymphocytes bearing antigen-specific receptors accumulate in human infectious disease lesions. *Nature*, **339**, 544
115. Holoshitz, J., Koning, F., Coligan, J. E., De Bruyn, J. and Strober, S. (1989). Isolation of

CD4⁻, CD8⁻ mycobacteria-reactive T lymphocyte clones from rheumatoid arthritis synovial fluid. *Nature*, **339**, 226

116. Falini, B., Flenghi, L., Pileri, P., Pelicci, P., Fagiolo, M., Martelli, M. F., Moretta, L. and Ciccone, E. (1989). Distribution of T cells bearing different forms of the T cell receptor $\gamma\delta$ in normal and pathological human tissues. *J. Immunol.*, **143**, 2480
117. O'Brian, R. L., Pat Happ, M., Dallas, A., Palmer, E., Kubo, R. and Born, W. K. (1989). Stimulation of a major subset of lymphocytes expressing T cell receptor $\gamma\delta$ by an antigen derived from *M. tuberculosis. Cell*, **57**, 667–74
118. Pfeffer, K., Schock, B., Gulle, H., Kaufmann, S. H. E. and Wagner, H. (1990). Primary responses of human T cells to mycobacteria: a frequent set of $\gamma\delta$ T cells are stimulated by protease-resistant ligands. *Eur. J. Immunol.*, **20**, 1175–9
119. Munk, E. M., Gatrill, A. J. and Kaufmann, S. H. E. (1990). Target cell lysis and IL2 secretion by $\gamma\delta$ T lymphocytes after activation by bacteria. *J. Immunol.*, **145**, 2434–9
120. Havler, D. V., Ellner, J. J., Chervenak, K. A. and Boone, W. H. (1991). Selective expansion of human T cells by monocytes infected with live *M. tuberculosis. J. Clin. Invest.*, **87**, 729–33
121. Ota, T., Okubo, Y. and Sekiguchi, M. (1990). Analysis of immunologic mechanisms of high natural killer cell activity in tuberculous pleural effusions. *Am. Rev. Resp. Dis.*, **142**, 29–33
122. Jackett, P. S., Abez, V. R. and Lowrie, D. B. (1980). The susceptibility of strains of *M. tuberculosis* to catalase-mediated peroxidative killing. *J. Gen. Microbiol.*, **121**, 381–6
123. Yamada, Y., Saito, H., Tomioka, H. and Jidoi, J. (1987). Susceptibility of micro-organisms to active oxygen species: sensitivity to the xanthine oxidase mediated antimicrobial system. *J. Gen. Microbiol.*, **133**, 2007–14
124. Chan, J., Fujiwara, T., Brennan, P., McNeil, M., Turco, S. T., Sibille, J., Snapper, M., Aisin, P. and Bloom, B. R. (1989). Microbial glycolipids: possible virulence factors that scavenge oxygen radicals. *Proc. Natl. Acad. Sci. USA*, **86**, 2453–7
125. Goren, M. B., Brokl, O. and Schaefer, W. B. (1974). Lipids of putative relevance to virulence of *M. tuberculosis*: phthiocerol dimycocersate and attenuation indicator lipid. *Infect. Immun.*, **9**, 150–8
126. Kolayashi, Y., Komazawa, Y., Kobayashi, M., Matsumoto, T., Sakura, N., Ishikawa, K. and Usui, T. (1984). Presumed BCG infection in a boy with chronic granulomatous disease. *Clin. Paediatr.*, **23**, 586
127. MEDLINE (*Index Medicus* database) search 1975–1991
128. Nathan, C. F. and Hibbs, J. B. (1991). Role of nitric acid synthesis in macrophage antimicrobial activity. *Curr. Opin. Immun.*, **3**, 65–70
129. Sypek, J. P. and Wyler, D. J. (1990). T cell hybridomas reveal two distinct mechanisms of anti-leishmanial immunity. *Infect. Immun.*, **58**, 1146–52
130. Wiegeshaus, E., Balasubramaniam, V. and Smith, D. W. (1989). Immunity to tuberculosis from the perspective of pathogenesis. *Infect. Immun.*, **57**, 3671–6
131. Centres for Disease Control (1988). Tuberculosis, final data – United States, 1986. *Morbid. Mortal. Weekly Rep.*, **36**, 817–20
132. Handwerger, S., Mildvan, D., Senie, R. and McKinley, F. W. (1987). Tuberculosis and the acquired immunodeficiency syndrome at a New York City Hospital: 1978–1985. *Chest*, **92**(2), 176–80
133. Pitchenik, A. E., Cole, C., Russell, B. W., Fischl, M. A., Spira, T. J. and Snider, D. E. (1984). Tuberculosis, atypical mycobacteriosis and the acquired immunodeficiency syndrome among Haitian and non-Haitian patients in South Florida. *Ann. Intern. Med.*, **101**, 641–5
134. Pitchenik, A. E., Burr, J., Suarez, M., Fertel, D., Gonzalez, G. and Moas, C. (1987). Human T-cell lymphotrophic virus-III (HTLV-III) seropositivity and related disease amongst 71 consecutive patients in whom tuberculosis was diagnosed. *Am. Rev. Respir. Dis.*, **135**, 875–9
135. Theuer, C. P., Chaisson, R. E., Schecter, G. F. and Hopewell, P. C. (1988). Human immunodeficiency virus infection in tuberculosis patients in San Francisco. *Am. Rev. Respir. Dis.*, **137**, 121a
136. Selwyn, P. A., Hartel, D., Lewis, V. A., Schoenbaum, E. E., Vermund, S. H., Klein, R. S., Walker, A. T. and Friedland, G. H. (1989). A prospective study of the risk of tuberculosis amongst intravenous drug users with human immunodeficiency virus infection. *N. Engl. J. Med.*, **320**, 545–50
137. Mann, J., Snider, D., Francis, H. *et al.* (1986). Association between HTLVII/LAV infection and tuberculosis in Zaire. *J. Am. Med. Assoc.*, **256**, 346

138. Mbolidi, C. D., Cathebras, P. and Vohito, M. D. (1988). Parallel increase in the prevalence of pulmonary tuberculosis and infection with HIV in Bangui. *Presse Med.*, **17**, 872–3
139. Van de Perre, P., Rouvroy, D., Lepage, P. *et al.* (1984). Acquired Immunodeficiency syndrome in Rwanda. *Lancet*, **2**, 62–5
140. Elliot, A. M., Luo, N., Tembo, G., Halwindi, B., Steenbergen, G., Machiels, L., Pobee, J., Nunn, P., Hayes, R. J. and MacAdam, P. W. J. (1990). Impact of HIV on tuberculosis in Zambia – a cross sectional study. *Br. Med. J.*, **301**, 412–15
141. Gilks, C. F., Brindle, R. J., Otieno, L. S., Bhatt, S. M., Newnham, R. S., Simani, P. M., Lule, G. N., Okelo, G. B. A., Watkins, W. M., Waiyaki, P. G., Were, J. O. B. and Warrell, D. A. (1990). Extrapulmonary and disseminated tuberculosis in HIV-1-seropositive patients presenting to the acute medical services in Nairobi. *AIDS*, **4**, 981–5
142. De Cock, K. M., Gnoare, E., Adjorlobi, G., Brann, M. M., Lafontaine, M. F., Yesso, G., Bretton, G., Coulibaly, I. M., Gershy-Damet, G. M., Bretton, R. and Heyward, W. L. (1991). Risk of tuberculosis in patients with HIV-1 and HIV-2 infections in Abidjan, Ivory Coast. *Br. Med. J.*, **302**, 496–498
143. Goodgame, R. W. (1990). AIDS in Uganda – clinical and social features. *N. Engl. J. Med.*, **323**, 383–9
144. Chaisson, R. E., Schecter, G. F., Theuer, C. P., Rutherford, G. W., Echenberg, D. F. and Hopewell, P. G. (1987). Tuberculosis in patients with the acquired immunodeficiency syndrome. *Am. Rev. Respir. Dis.*, **136**, 570–4
145. Sunderam, G., McDonald, R. J., Maniatis, T., Oleske, J., Kapila, R. and Reichman, L. B. (1986). Tuberculosis as a manifestation of the acquired immunodeficiency syndrome (AIDS). *J. Am. Med. Assoc.*, **256**, 362–6
146. Duncanson, F. P., Hewlett, D., Maayan, S., Estepan, H., Perla, E. N., McLean, T., Rodriguez, A., Miller, S. N., Lenox, T. and Wormser, G. P. (1986). Mycobacterium tuberculosis infection in the acquired immunodeficiency syndrome. A review of 14 patients. *Tubercle*, **67**, 295–302
147. Pitchenik, A. E. and Rubinson, H. A. (1985). The radiographic appearance of tuberculosis in patients with the acquired immune deficiency syndrome (AIDS) and pre-AIDs. *Am. Rev. Resp. Dis.*, **131**, 393–6
148. Centers for Disease Control (1987). Revision of the CDC Surveillance Case Definition for Acquired Immunodeficiency. *Morbid. Mortal. Weekly Rep.*, **136**, 3s–9s
149. Theuer, C. P., Hopewell, P. C., Elias, D., Schecter, G. F., Rutherford, G. W. and Chaisson, R. E. (1990). Human immunodeficiency virus infection in tuberculous patients. *J. Infect. Dis.*, **162**, 8–12
150. American Thoracic Society (1987). Mycobacterioses and the acquired immunodeficiency syndrome. *Am. Rev. Resp. Dis.*, **136**, 492–6
151. Centre for Disease Control (1989). Tuberculosis and human immunodeficiency virus infection: recommendations of the advisory committee for the elimination of tuberculosis. (ACET) *Morbid. Mortal. Weekly Rep.*. **38**, 236–8, 243–50
152. Barker, T. W. and McCabe, W. R. (1990). Bacteraemia due to *Mycobacterium tuberculosis* in patients with HIV infection. *Medicine*, **69**, 375–83
153. Small, P. M., Schecher, G. F., Goodman, P. C., Sande, M. A., Chaisson, R. E., and Hopewell, P. C. (1991). Treatment of tuberculosis in patients with advanced HIV infection. *N. Engl. J. Med.*, **324**, 289–94
154. Dylewski, J. and Thibert, L. (1990). Failure of tuberculous chemotherapy in an HIV infected patient. *J. Infect. Dis.*, **162**, 778–79
155. Lemp, G. F., Payne, S. F., Neal, D., Temelso, T. and Rutherford, G. W. (1990). Survival trends for patients with AIDS. *J. Am. Med. Assoc.*, **263**, 402–6
156. Rook, G. A. W., Taverne, J., Leveton, C. and Steele, J. (1987). The role of gamma interferon, vitamin D3 metabolites and tumour necrosis factor in the pathogenesis of tuberculosis. *Immunology*, **62**, 229–34
157. Rosenberg, Z. F. and Fauci, A. S. (1990). Immunopathogenic mechanisms of HIV infection: cytokine induction of HIV expression. *Immunol. Today*, **11**, 176–80
158. Johnston, S. C., Stamm, C. P. and Hicks, C. B. (1990). Tuberculous psoas muscle abscess following chemoprophylaxis with isoniazid in a patient with HIV infection. *Rev. Infect. Dis.*, **12**, 754–6
159. Portaels, F. (1988). Isolation of mycobacteria from healthy persons' stools. *Int. J. Leprosy*, **56**, 468–71

160. Wolinsky, E. (1979). Nontuberculous mycobacteria and associated diseases. *Am. Rev. Resp. Dis.*, **119**, 107–9
161. Horsburgh, C. R. Jr, Mason, U. G. III, Farhi, D. C. and Iseman, M. D. (1985). Disseminated infection with *Mycobacterium avium intracellulare*: a report of 13 cases and a review of the literature. *Medicine*, **64**, 36–48
162. Macher, A. M., Kovacs, J. A., Gill, V., Roberts, G. D., Ames, J., Park, C. H., Straus, S., Lane, H. C., Parillo, J. E., Fauci, A. S. and Masur, H. (1983). Bacteraemia due to *Mycobacterium avium intracellulare* in the acquired immunodeficiency syndrome. *Ann. Intern. Med.*, **99**, 782–78
163. Hawkins, C. C., Gold, J. W. M., Whimbey, E., Kiehn, T. E., Brannon, P., Camarata, R., Brown, A. E. and Armstrong, D. (1986). *Mycobacterium avium* complex infections in patients with the acquired immunodeficiency syndrome. *Ann. Intern. Med.*, **105**, 184–8
164. Lerner, C. W. and Tapper, M. L. (1984). Opportunistic infection complicating acquired immunodeficiency syndrome. *Medicine*, **63**, 155–64
165. Wallace, J. M. and Hannah, J. B. (1988). *Mycobacterium avium* complex infection in patients with the acquired immunodeficiency syndrome. A clinicopathological study. *Chest*, **93**, 926–32
166. Okello, D. O., Sewankambo, N., Goodgame, R., Aisu, To, Kwezi, M., Morrissey, A. and Ellner, J. J. (1990). Absence of bacteraemia with *Mycobacterium avium intracellulare* in Ugandan patients with AIDS. *J. Infect. Dis.*, **162**, 208–210
167. Wolinsky, E. and Schaefer, W. B. (1973). Proposed numbering scheme for mycobacterial serotypes by agglutination. *Int. J. System Bacteriol.*, **23**, 182–3
168. Kiehn, T. E., Edward, F. F., Brannon, P., Tsang, A. Y., Maio, M., Gold, J. W. M., Wimbey, E., Wong, B., McClatchy Jk and Armstrong, D. (1985). Infections caused by Mycobacterium avium complex in immunocompromised patients: diagnosed by blood culture and faecal examination, antimicrobial susceptibility tests, and morphological and seroagglutination characteristics. *J. Clin. Microbiol.*, **21**, 168–173
169. Wolinsky, E. and Rynearson, T. K. (1967). Mycobacteria in soil and their relationship to disease associated strains. *Am. Rev. Resp. Dis.*, **97**, 1032–7
170. Horsbergh, C. R., Cohn, D. L. and Roberts, R. B. (1986). *Mycobacterium avium–Mycobacterium intracellulare* isolates from patients with or without acquired immunodeficiency syndrome. *Antimicrob. Ag. Chemother.*, **30**, 955–7
171. Guthertz, L. S., Damsker, B., Bottone, E. J., Ford, E. G., Midura, T. F. and Janda, J. M. (1989). *Mycobacterium avium* and *Mycobacterium intracellulare* infections in patients with and without AIDS. *J. Infect. Dis.*, **160**, 1037–41
172. Hampson, S. J., Portaels, F., Thompson, J., Green, E. P., Moss, M. T., Hermon-Taylor, J. and McFadden, J. J. (1989). DNA probes demonstrate a single highly conserved strain of *Mycobacterium avium* infecting AIDS patients. *Lancet*, **1**, 65–8
173. Young, L. S., Inderlied, C. B., Berlin, O. G. and Gottlieb, M. S. (1986). Mycobacterial infections in AIDS patients, with an emphasis on the *Mycobacterium avium* complex. *Rev. Infect. Dis.*, **8**, 1024–33
174. Agins, B. D., Berman, D. S., Spicehandler, D., El Sadr, W., Simberkoff, M. S. and Rahal, J. J. (1989). Effect of combined therapy with ansamycin, clofazamine, ethambutol and isoniazid for *Mycobacterium avium* infection in patients with AIDS. *J. Infect. Dis.*, **159**, 784–7
175. Young, L. S. (1988). *Mycobacterium avium* complex infection. *J. Infect. Dis.*, **157**, 863–7
176. Wong, B., Edwards, F. F., Kiehn, T. E., Whimbey, E., Donnelly, H., Bernard, E. M., Gold, J. W. W. and Armstrong, D. (1985). Continuous high-grade *Mycobacterium avium–intracellulare* bacteraemia in patients with the acquired immunodeficiency syndrome. *Am. J. Med.*, **78**, 35–40
177. Klatt, E. C., Jensen, D. F. and Meyer, P. R. (1987). Pathology of *Mycobacterium avium–intracellulare infection* in acquired immunodeficiency syndrome. *Hum. Pathol.*, **18**, 709–14
178. Kuze, F. and Uchihira, F. (1984). Various colony-formers of *Mycobacterium avium–intracellulare. Eur. J. Respir. Dis.*, **65**, 402–10
179. Stormer, R. S. and Falkinham, J. O. III (1989). Differences in antimicrobial susceptibility of pigmented and unpigmented colonial variants of *Mycobacterium avium. J. Clin. Microsc.*, **27**, 2459–65
180. Khardori, N., Rolston, K., Rosenbaum, B., Hayat, S. and Bodey, G. P. (1989). Comparative *in-vitro* activity of twenty antimicrobial agents against clinical isolates of *Mycobacterium avium* complex. *J. Antimicrob. Chemother.*, **24**, 667–73

181. Inderlied, C. B., Kolonoski, P. T., Wu, M. and Young, L. S. (1989). *In vitro* and *in vivo* activity of azithromycin [CP 62993] against the *Mycobacterium avium* complex. *J. Infect. Dis.*, **159**, 994–97
182. Hoy, J., Mijch, A., Sandland, M., Grayson, L., Lucas, R. and Dwyer, B. (1990). Quadruple-drug therapy for *Mycobacterium avium–intracellulare* bacteraemia in AIDS patients. *J. Infect. Dis.*, **161**, 801–5
183. Baron, E. J. and Young, L. S. (1986). Amikacin, ethambutol, and rifampicin for treatment of disseminated *Mycobacterium avium–intracellulare* infections in patients with AIDS. *Diagn. Microbiol. Infect. Dis.*, **5**, 215–20
184. Wright, S. C., Jewett, A., Mitsuyasu, R. and Bonavida, B. (1988). Spontaneous cytotoxicity and tumour necrosis factor production by peripheral blood monocytes from AIDS patients. *J. Immunol.*, **141**, 9–104
185. Lahdevirta, J., Maury, C. P. J., Teppo, A.-M. and Repo, H. (1988). Elevated levels of circulating cachectin/tumour necrosis factor in patients with acquired immunodeficiency syndrome. *Am. J. Med.*, **85**, 289–91
186. Squires, K. E., Murphy, W. F., Madoff, L. C. and Murray, H. F. (1989). Interferon-gamma and *Mycobacterium avium-intracellulare* infection. *J. Infect. Dis.*, **159**, 599–600
187. Sherer, R., Sable, R., Sonnenberg, M. *et al.* (1986). Disseminated infection with *Mycobacterium kansasii* in the acquired immunodeficiency syndrome. *Ann. Intern. Med.*, **105**, 710–2
188. Hirasuna, J. D. (1987). Disseminated *Mycobacterium kansasii* infection in the acquired immunodeficiency syndrome. *Ann. Intern. Med.*, **107**, 784
189. Tecson-Tumang, F. T. and Bright, J. L. (1984). *Mycobacterium xenopi* and the acquired immunodeficiency syndrome. *Ann. Intern. Med.*, **100**, 461–2
190. Chan, J., McKitrick, J. C. and Klein, R. S. (1984). *Mycobacterium gordonae* in the acquired immunodeficiency syndrome. *Ann. Intern. Med.*, **101**, 400
191. Herschel, B., Chang, H. R., Mach, N. *et al.* (1990). Fatal infection with a novel, unidentified mycobacterium in a man with the acquired immunodeficiency syndrome. *N. Engl. J. Med.*, **323**, 109–12
192. Centre for Disease Control (1986). Disseminated *Mycobacterium bovis* infection from BCG vaccination of a patient with acquired immunodeficiency syndrome. *Morbid. Mortal. Weekly Rep.*, **34**, 227–8
193. Von Reyn, C. F., Clements, C. J. and Mann, J. M. (1987). Human Immunodeficiency virus infection and routine childhood immunisation. *Lancet*, **2**, 669–72
194. Reyes, J., Perez, C., Lamaury, I., Janbon, F. and Bertrand, A. (1989). Bacille Calmette-Guerin adenitis 30 years after immunization in a patient with AIDS. *J. Infect. Dis.*, **160**, 727
195. Meeran, K. (1989). Prevalence of HIV infection among patients with leprosy and tuberculosis in rural Zambia. *Br. Med. J.*, **298**, 364–5
196. Meltzer, M. S., Skillman, D. R., Hoover, D. L., Hanson, B. D., Turpin, J. A., Kalter, D. C. and Gendelman, H. E. (1990). Macrophages and the human immunodeficiency virus. *Immunol. Today*, **1**, 217–23
197. Poli, G., Bressler, P., Kinter, A., Duh, E., Timmer, W. C., Rabson, A., Justement, J. S., Stanley, S. and Fauci, A. S. (1990). Interleukin 6 induces human immunodeficiency virus expression in infected monocytic cells alone and in synergy with tumour necrosis factor-alpha by transcriptional and post-transcriptional mechanisms. *J. Exp. MED.*, **172**, 151–8
198. Folks, T. M., Justement, J., Kinter, A., Dinarello, A. and Fauci, A. S. (1987). Cytokine-induced expression of HIV-1 in a chronically infected promyelocyte cell line. *Science (Wash. DC)*, **238**, 800
199. Smith, P. D., Ohura, K., Masur, H., Lane, F. C., Fauci, A. S. and Wahl, S. M. (1984). Monocyte function in the acquired immunodeficiency syndrome. *J. Clin. Invest.*, **74**, 2121
200. Bender, B. S., Davidson, B. L., Kline, R., Brown, C. and Quinn, T. C. (1988). Role of the mononuclear phagocyte system in the immunopathogenesis of human immunodeficiency virus infection and the acquired immunodeficiency syndrome. *Rev. Infect. Dis.*, **10**, 1142
201. Spear, G. T., Kiessler, H. A., Rothenberg, L., Phair, J. and Landay, A. L. (1990). Decreased oxidative burst activity of monocytes from asymptomatic HIV-infected individuals. *Clin. Immunol. Immunopathol.*, **54**, 184
202. Crowle, A. J. and Poche, P. (1989). Inhibition by normal human serum of *Mycobacterium avium* multiplication in cultured human macrophages. *Infect. Immun.*, **57**, 1332–5
203. Crowle, A. J., Cohn, D. L. and Poche, P. (1989). Defects in sera from acquired immunodeficiency syndrome (AIDS) patients with and from non-AIDS patients with *Mycobacterium avium* infection which decrease macrophage resistance to *M. avium*. *Infect. Immun.*, **57**, 1445–51

8
Prospects for vaccination against HIV infection

K. H. G. MILLS

INTRODUCTION

Control of the escalating AIDS epidemic is most likely to be achieved by the development of successful vaccination strategies aimed at the prevention of primary HIV infection in seronegative individuals. In other viral diseases of humans, notably polio, hepatitis B, measles, mumps and smallpox, inactivated or attenuated whole virus or subunit vaccines are highly effective and have greatly reduced the incidence of these diseases[1]. However, there are a number of characteristics of the infection with HIV which may permit the virus to escape or down-regulate a potentially protective immune response and thereby complicate vaccine development. (1) HIV can infect individuals as free or cell-associated virus by intravenous or mucosal routes, and once in the body can be transmitted as free virus and between cells[2,3]. (2) Interaction of the HIV surface envelope (*env*) protein with the CD4 receptor on T-helper (Th) cells[4-6] enables the virus preferentially to infect the cell responsible for the induction and maintenance of immune responses, and upon which successful vaccination depends. (3) Like other retroviruses, HIV integrates its genetic information into the genome of its host cell[7]; these cells can become latently infected[8,9] and in the absence of synthesis of new viral proteins may not stimulate an anti-HIV immune response. (4) The induction of HIV-enhancing antibodies enables the virus to infect monocytes via complement or Fc receptor-mediated uptake of antigen–antibody complexes[10-12]. Furthermore, replication of the virus within monocyte/macrophage vacuoles and infection of central nervous system tissue may permit the virus to escape immune control[2,13,14]. (5) Antigenic variation, in particular in the putative protective surface *env* protein, also enables the virus to escape immunity. An examination of geographically distinct HIV-1 strains and sequential isolates from persistently infected individuals has revealed evidence of point mutations, deletions and insertions in the HIV genome which result in a large number of antigenically distinct variants[15–18]. These unique features of the infection with HIV are likely to seriously compromise the possibility of controlling the infection by post-exposure vaccination of HIV positive individuals. However, considerable progress has been made in the development and testing of vaccines aimed at preventing primary HIV infection.

Candidate HIV vaccines include inactivated whole virus preparations, purified native glycoproteins and recombinant proteins expressed in a variety of vectors and antigen-presenting systems. Since the nature of the protective immune response to HIV remains to be defined, each vaccine must be tested for its ability to induce a variety of humoral and cell-mediated immune responses. These immunogenicity studies can be readily performed in small animals. In contrast, the testing of HIV vaccine efficacy has necessitated the development of non-human primate lentivirus infection models. Outside of humans only the chimpanzee[19] and gibbon ape[20] can be infected with HIV-1 and the infection in these non-human primates does not lead to an AIDS-like disease. However, a closely related lentivirus of monkeys, the simian immunodeficiency virus (SIV), induces disease in macaques and provides an acceptable alternative model[21–23].

NATURE OF A PROTECTIVE IMMUNE RESPONSE

The body responds to an invading microorganism such as a virus by the generation of humoral (B cell) and cell-mediated (T cell) immune responses directed against a variety of epitopes on the foreign antigens[24]. Humoral responses include the production of antibodies capable of binding to the virus and where the epitope is a functionally important region such as the receptor binding or membrane fusion domain of a viral surface protein, the antibody will be capable of neutralizing or preventing infectivity of the virus. Alternatively virally infected cells can be eliminated by mechanisms involving antibody-dependent cellular cytotoxicity (ADCC) natural killer (NK) cells or MHC-restricted cytotoxic T lymphocytes (CTL) (see Chapter 4). Finally, the induction and regulation of these effector functions are dependent on lymphokines released by antigen-specific Th cells. Following encounter with foreign antigen, memory T and B cells are generated which enable the immune system to respond quickly to the microorganism bearing the foreign antigen and thereby eliminate it. This is the theoretical basis of successful anti-viral vaccination strategies[25].

Unlike antibodies which bind antigen directly, T cells recognize linear determinants on denatured antigen, in association with MHC proteins, following processing in an antigen-presenting cell (APC). In general, Th cells are $CD4^+$ MHC class II-restricted and recognize exogenous antigen, processed in endosomes and readily provided by immunization with soluble antigen or shed from virally infected cells[26]. In contrast $CD8^+$ CTL are MHC class I-restricted and recognize antigen processed by the endogenous route following infection of the target cell with a replicating virus[27] or in exceptional circumstances by immunization with synthetic peptides[28]/lipopeptides[29] or soluble proteins presented as immune stimulating complexes (ISCOMs)[30]. Therefore both the qualitative and the quantitative nature of an immune response generated by vaccination is dependent on the nature of the immunogen. Live vectors, lipid-based or particulate antigen-presenting systems each have their merits for stimulating different arms of the immune response.

In most viral systems where a protective immune response has been demonstrated, antibodies against virus surface proteins are considered to play a key role[31]. Although CTL have also been implicated in protection, their role is more likely to be in the control of disease progression through the clearance of virally infected cells[32,33]. Furthermore, in certain viral diseases virus-specific CTL can contribute to disease pathology by the destruction of tissues expressing viral antigens[34].

PROTECTIVE IMMUNITY TO HIV

The possible mechanisms of protective immunity to HIV remain to be defined. Following HIV infection in humans a wide range of humoral and cellular immune responses are generated; antibodies mediating *in vitro* virus neutralization, inhibition of CD4–gp120 interaction or cellular cytotoxicity and cells mediating MHC-restricted and non-restricted lytic activity as well as helper function have all been documented[33,35]. Although there is some indication that certain of these responses decline with disease progression, it is not clear which, if any, of these anti-HIV immune responses influence the course of infection. The ability of the virus to latently infect certain cells[2,8,9,13], to rapidly mutate its envelope protein in infected individuals[15–17] and to induce antibodies which enhance infection[10–12] may help it to escape a potentially protective immune response. Alternatively its tropism for the $CD4^+$ T cell[4–6], which up-regulates almost all immune responses, may be a critical factor in the evasion of immunity. Indeed abnormal Th function has been documented in HIV-infected individuals long before a reduction in the number of $CD4^+$ T cells is evident[36] (see Chapter 5). This may be one of the major obstacles in attempts to control HIV infection by post-exposure immunotherapy. However, studies in animal models indicate that it should be possible to induce a protective immune response to at least a limited range of virus variants, by vaccination of seronegative individuals.

In addition to studies of anti-HIV immunity in infected humans, extensive investigations have been reported on the immune responses to HIV proteins in experimental animals. An important component of a protective immune response to HIV is considered to be the neutralizing antibody response against the surface *env* glycoprotein. A large number of studies have centred on a hypervariable region, called the V3 or GPGR loop, which appears to be the immunodominant neutralizing antibody epitope in HIV-infected individuals[35,37,38]. However, antibodies to alternative functionally important and more conserved regions of *env*, such as the CD4 binding domain of gp120 or the region of gp41 implicated in fusion activity or antibodies mediating ADCC, may be required for a broadly protective immune response.

Poor reproducibility of the *in vitro* HIV neutralization assay and an overemphasis on the use of synthetic peptides to map antibody epitopes has seriously compromised the search for the protective immune responses.

In contrast to the humoral responses where the protective antibody epitopes are usually on the exposed regions of viral surface proteins, T cells can recognize conserved internal proteins as well as variable surface viral glycoproteins[27,33]. MHC class I or class II-restricted T cell epitopes have been identified on HIV *env*, *gag*, *pol* and *nef* proteins[33]. HIV *gag*-specific class I-restricted $CD8^+$ CTL have been detected at high frequency in a large proportionof HIV-infected individuals, and there is some evidence that the activity declines with disease progression[39–41] (see Chapter 4). Furthermore there is evidence from *in vitro* experiments that $CD8^+$ CTL can control HIV replication in $CD4^+$ T cells[42]. Although antibody responses to *env* are considered to be the main protective mechanism against HIV infection, it is possible that CTL, directed against early-expressed HIV regulatory proteins[43], may be able to eliminate the infected cell before release of new viral particles. In other viral infections, such as influenza, CTL have been shown to play a role in viral clearance and disease control[32]. However, proposals to boost cellular responses to HIV in seropositive individuals by vaccination are complicated by the possible accelerated destruction of host cells with viral antigens absorbed to their surface[33,44]. Furthermore, the requirements for a live vector, such as vaccinia virus recombinants[45], to generate $CD8^+$ class I-restricted CTL[27], also carry the risk of Th cell activation which is known to increase their susceptibility to HIV[9].

The role of HIV-specific MHC class II-restricted T cells in protective immunity to HIV is likely to be indirect, through the generation of anti-HIV antibodies by B cells and in the recall memory responses, where individuals are exposed to the virus at a time when the circulating antibody levels are low or undetectable. Although Th cell responses to HIV *env*, *gag* and *pol* have been demonstrated in HIV seropositive individuals, these responses are often weak and become undetectable as the infection progresses[46,47]. In contrast, consistent HIV-specific Th cell activity has been demonstrated in HIV human volunteers[48,49] and experimental animals[50–52] following immunization with recombinant or native HIV proteins or live recombinant HIV vaccines.

The fine specificity of Th cells that may be required for the generation of a protective immune response remains to be defined. Th cells specific for epitopes on any viral protein, including conserved regions of internal proteins, could theoretically regulate effector functions directed against putative protective epitopes on the more variable domains of the surface *env* glycoprotein. Studies in influenza[53,54] and hepatitis B[55] have shown that this type of intermolecular intrastructural antibody–T cell help can operate. However, a recent study has suggested that vaccination with recombinant HIV or SIV *gag* proteins, although capable of inducing *gag*-specific Th cells, did not result in the generation of an enhanced anti-*env* antibody response following a boost with inactivated HIV or challenge with live SIV[129]. This may suggest that the Th cells and antibody epitopes critical for protection may be confined to the *env* glycoprotein. If correct, this will considerably complicate the efforts to generate protective immunity to a wide range of HIV variants.

EXPRESSION SYSTEMS AND ADJUVANTS FOR RECOMBINANT HIV PROTEINS

The possible risks associated with an inactivated whole virus or live attenuated vaccine are likely to preclude their widespread use for immunization of HIV seronegative individuals. Furthermore the technical difficulties of producing highly purified native viral proteins has resulted in an emphasis being placed on the development of vaccines produced by recombinant DNA technology. A variety of genetic engineering approaches have been applied to the production of HIV synthetic vaccines[56]. Insertion of portions of the HIV genome in bacteria, yeast, insect or mammalian cells by a number of different expression systems[57] can result in the synthesis of high levels of the HIV protein, which is either secreted or can be purified from the disrupted cells. Once the purification methods have been carefully established it is relatively easy to produce large amounts of these recombinant proteins.

Alternatively, live recombinant HIV vaccines have been created by genetic recombination of portions of the HIV genome with that of attenuated viruses[45] or of intracellular bacteria[57]. The use of live vectors for delivery of HIV antigens has the advantage of prolonged exposure to the immune system, presentation of the antigen in a more native state and the possibility of inducing $CD8^+$ CTL. However, the disadvantages include poor 'takes' of the vaccine due to pre-existing immunity to the carrier virus or bacterium, and the possible risks associated with the use of a live vaccine. The vaccinia virus HIV recombinants have been most studied[45]; although capable of inducing HIV-specific CTL responses[27,33], their limited ability to boost primary responses and to generate neutralizing antibodies may account for their failure in vaccine trials in non-human primates (see below).

A major disadvantage of the purified native or recombinant subunit vaccines, and well illustrated by animal immunization studies with gp120, is their poor immunogenicity in alum, the only universally accepted adjuvant for human use[58-60]. A number of alternative adjuvants and antigen-presenting systems currently being examined are aimed at one or more of the following: (1) to maintain the antigen at the site of injection for a prolonged period by creating a depot; (2) to augment the immune response through the stimulation of macrophages and T cells and (3) to facilitate antigen uptake by antigen-presenting cells (APC).

Alum precipitation or the incorporation of the antigen into water in oil emulsions (e.g. Freund's adjuvant) or the less toxic oil in water emulsions (e.g. Syntex[61,62] or Ribi[63,64] adjuvant systems) facilitates depot formation. Muramyl dipeptide (MDP), the active but non-toxic component of *Mycobacteria* in complete Freund's or monophosphoryl lipid A (MPL), a detoxified derivative of lipid A, the active constituent of bacterial endotoxin, boost immune responses to the injected antigen mainly through the stimulation of IL-1 production by macrophages[61,63,65]. These compounds also stimulate the production of γ-IFN and other lymphokines by T cells[61,63,65,66]. The overall effect is to up-regulate antigen presentation and Th cell function.

The incorporation of soluble antigens into liposomes[67], immune stimulating complexes[30,68] (ISCOMS) or binding to the surface of squalene–pluronic emulsion microspheres[61] facilitate their uptake by APC. Furthermore there is some evidence that certain of these systems can help exogenous antigen to gain access to the MHC class I presentation pathway for the stimulation of CD8$^+$ CTL[30]. The introduction of HIV sequences into yeast Ty:virus-like-particles (VLPs)[51,69] or poliovirus chimeras[70], or fusion to hepatitis core particles[71], have also been used to deliver HIV antigens in a multivalent particulate form. Although HIV-specific immune responses have been demonstrated using these systems, constraints on the length and/or conformation of the HIV insert may limit their broad application.

ANIMAL MODELS

The development of successful vaccination strategies for the prevention or control of HIV infection in humans is critically dependent on the availability of a relevant animal model. The ideal model would be one where an AIDS-like disease is reproducibly induced following HIV inoculation by intravenous (i.v.) or mucosal routes; unfortunately such a model is not available. Although chimpanzees can be infected with HIV, the absence of disease in this model[19,72], not only prevents the testing of strategies aimed at modifying disease, but may also undermine its relevance for assessing the ability of a vaccine to prevent primary infection. Furthermore, the limited availability of this endangered species questions their continued use for testing candidate vaccines which have not shown efficiency in other primate models. Apart from gibbon apes[20], HIV-1 does not infect other non-human primates, and HIV-2, although capable of infection in macaques[73], does not induce disease in non-human primates. However, infection of monkeys with SIV can lead to an AIDS-like disease which is now considered to be the most suitable animal model of HIV infection in humans[21–23]. A number of different but closely related viruses have been isolated from macaques, African green monkeys, sooty mangabeys and mandrills[22]. The biological and genetic characteristics of these SIVs are closely related to HIV, and there is considerable sequence homology in the major structural and regulatory proteins[74,75]. Like HIV, SIV binds to the CD4 receptor on a subpopulation of T cells and on other cells such as monocytes. The virus is tropic for these cells[75] and can eventually lead to immunodeficiency disease following long-term persistent infection[22].

Non-primate models for AIDS have also been examined; these include lentivirus infection of sheep, cows, horses and cats (reviewed by Letvin[23]). Of these, the feline immunodeficiency virus (FIV) model is probably the most promising; FIV-infected cats develop AIDS-like disease symptoms, especially when co-infected with feline leukaemia virus[76]. A number of vaccine trials are under way in this model.

A murine model for AIDS would have considerable advantages both for large-scale preliminary vaccine testing and for the possibility of manipulating the immune system. Severe combined immunodeficient (SCID) mice reconstituted with fetal liver/bone marrow and thymus[77,78] or with human peripheral blood lymphocytes (PBL)[79,80] can be infected with HIV-1. Although the SCID mice have considerable potential for rapid screening of anti-HIV drugs, and may be useful for dissecting the nature of the protective immune response to HIV, the failure to completely reconstitute a functional human immune system, especially with the PBL approach, may be a major limitation of this model for vaccine testing.

VACCINE TRIALS IN CHIMPANZEES

Chimpanzees have been used to test the efficacy of a number of candidate HIV vaccines, including purified native or recombinant *env* or *gag* proteins and vaccinia virus recombinants expressing HIV *env* or *env* and *gag* genes; until recently all vaccines tested were unsuccessful at preventing HIV infection (Table 8.1). However, in a recent report, Berman and colleagues[81] demonstrate that immunization with recombinant gp120, but not gp160, in alum could protect chimpanzees against HIV-1 challenge. At the time of challenge the two protected animals had higher neutralizing antibody titres (1/320–1/640) than the two unprotected animals (1/60). Previous failures with native[72] or recombinant[82] gp120 or vaccinia virus HIV recombinants[83] may have been related to the higher virus challenge doses or poorer quality of the immunogen. Although HIV-specific cell-mediated immunity and binding antibodies were documented in the unsuccessful trials, neutralizing antibody levels were weak or undetectable[50,60,72,82–84]. The lack of protection with recombinant gp160 has also been attributed to possible induction of enhancing antibodies directed against the transmembrane region of the glycoprotein, or the failure to generate antibodies to the V3 loop[81]. Antibodies to a synthetic peptide corresponding to this region were detected in the two gp120-immunized and protected animals on the day of challenge[81]. Further circumstantial evidence for role of antibodies to the V3 loop has recently been provided by Girard and colleagues, who have shown that from a group of animals immunized with various combinations of inactivated virus, HIV *env* recombinants and synthetic peptides, two animals that received a V3 peptide–KLH conjugate and gp160 were protected[85]. This finding awaits confirmation in more carefully controlled experiments.

The recent report[86] of a study with a recombinant HIV-1 core precursor p55 protein, demonstrated anti-*gag* antibody responses in two immunized chimpanzees. However, virus-neutralizing antibodies were not detected, and the results of live HIV challenge of one of the immunized animals demonstrated that the immune response generated with the *gag* protein did not protect against HIV infection.

Table 8.1 Summary of HIV vaccine studies in chimpanzees

Vaccine	*Adjuvant*	*Schedule (weeks)*	*Neutrolizing antibody*[a]	*Cell-mediated immunity*[b]	*Challenge dose ($TCID_{50}$)*[c]	*Number challenged*	*Number protected*	*Reference*
Recombinant gp120	Alum	0, 4, 10, 14, 28	+	+	100	2	0	82
Vaccinia-**env**	—	0, 8	–	+	3.2×10^5	3	0	83
Native gp120	Alum	0, 1, 9, 21, 35	+	+	40	1	0	72
Recombinant gp120	Alum	0, 4, 32	+++	+	40	2	2	81
Recombinant gp160	Alum	0, 4, 32	++	+	40 ($10\ CID_{50}$)	2	0	81
Recombinant P55	Alum	0, 4, 24	–	NR	10–30 CID_{50}	1	0	86

[a] – = Not detected, + → +++ = weak to strong response.
[b] Cytotoxic and/or proliferative T cell response; NR = not reported.
[c] $TCID_{50}$ = 50% tissue culture infectious dose, CID_{50} = 50% chimpanzee infectious dose.

VACCINE TRIALS IN MACAQUES

Following initial vaccine failures in the SIV macaque model, largely due to poor immunogens and high-dose virus challenge, five centres, three in the United States and two in the UK, have now reported at least partial protection against SIV infection in macaques (Tables 8.2 and 8.3). Partial protection against infection in two animals, and delayed disease in a further four, was first reported in 1989 by Desrosiers and colleagues[87] at the New England Regional Primate Center following immunization of six macaques with detergent-treated virus with tMDP in syntex vehicle as adjuvant. At the Delta Regional Primate Center Murphey-Corb and colleagues[88] reported protection in eight of nine animals immunized with formalin-treated whole SIV plus tMDP with or without alum. In contrast, studies at the California Primate Center showed that psoralen and UV light-inactivated SIV with tMDP failed to prevent infection but did appear to delay viraemia and disease[89]. A study at the National Institute for Biological Standards and Control (NIBSC) in the UK has demonstrated 100% protection against infection in eight animals immunized with a glutaraldehyde-fixed SIV-infected cell vaccine administered with quil A[90]. This has recently been followed up in a collaborative study between NIBSC and the Centre for Applied Microbiology Research (CAMR) at Porton, where protection against SIV challenge has been achieved in eight of eight animals using formalin-inactivated SIV incorporated in the syntex adjuvant formulation with tMDP (SAF-1) (Cranage *et al.*, in preparation).

The varying degree of protection seen with the different whole SIV vaccine trials probably reflects differences in the virus inactivation methods, the immunization schedules and the challenge dose. More successful protection was achieved using aldehyde-inactivated vaccines and a low-dose challenge (10 monkey infectious doses (MID_{50}))[88,90]. In contrast to detergent treatment, which will disrupt the virus and may denature conformational antibody epitopes, aldehyde fixation may serve to retain the *env* antigen on the viral surface. It has also been suggested[88] that a long rest period of up to a year before the final immunization may be critical for the generation of a protective immune response with inactivated SIV. However, experiments at NIBSC have shown that this can be reduced to as little as 8 weeks, at least in short-term protection against low-dose homologous challenge[90]. This is not to say that a broader and more sustained immune response may be achieved using a long rest interval; antibody diversity and affinity are known to increase following hyperimmunization and maturation of the memory B cells response[91,92].

Although not directly applicable to vaccination against HIV, two protection experiments have been reported with non-pathogenic or attenuated live retroviruses. A study of the National Bacteriological Laboratory in Stockholm has shown that infection of macaques with HIV-2, which resulted in transient viraemia, protected against the pathogenic effects of a subsequent SIV infection[73]. Similarly a transient infection with a non-pathogenic molecular clone (1A11) of SIV_{mac}, although not generating a protective immune response, did appear to delay disease symptoms[93].

Table 8.2 Summary of inactivated SIV vaccine studies in macaques

Vaccine	*Adjuvant*[a]	*Immunization schedule (weeks)*	*Neutralizing antibody*[b]	*Cell-mediated immunity*[c]	*Challenge*			*Number protected*	*Reference*
					Route[d]	*Dose (MID_{50})*[e]	*Number*		
Formalin–SIV_{mac}	SAF	0, 3, 6	+	NR	i.v.	10^5–10^6	4	0	87
Triton–SIV_{mac}	SAF	0, 3, 6, 23, 25	+	NR	i.m.	10^5–10^6	2	1	87
		0, 3, 6, 45, 47, 50	+	NR	i.m.	200	4	1	
Formalin–SIV_{delta}	tMDP ± alum	0, 3, 9, 58	+	NR	i.v.	10	9	8	88
Psoralen UV–SIV_{mac}	tMDP	0, 12, 32, 65	+	NR	i.v.	10^2–10^3	4	0	94
		0, 12, 32, 65	+	NR	mucosal	?	4	0	
β-Propiolactone–SIV_{mac}	—	0, 4, 12, 16, 36	+	NR	i.v.	10	3	1	95
	IFA	0, 4, 12, 16, 36	+	NR	i.v.	10	2	1	
	tMDP	0, 4, 12, 16, 36	+	NR	i.v.	10	3	3	
Glutaraldehyde fixed	quil A	0, 4, 8, 36	+	+	i.v.	10	4	4	90
SIV_{mac} infected cells		0, 4, 8, 16	+	+	i.v.	10	4	4	
Formalin–SIV_{mac}	SAF	0, 4, 8, 16	+	NR	i.v.	10 (SIV_{mac})	4	4	[f]
		0, 4, 8, 26	+	NR	i.v.	10 (SIV_{delta})	4	4	
		0, 4, 8, 32	+	+	i.v.	10 (SIV_{mac})	4	4	
		0, 4, 8, 32	+	+	i.v.	10 (HIV-2)	4	0	

[a] tMDP = threonyl muramyl dipeptide, IFA = incomplete Freund's adjuvant, SAF = syntex adjuvant formulation with tMDP.
[b] + = Detected.
[c] Cytotoxic and/or proliferative T cell responses; NR = not reported.
[d] i.v. = Intravenous, i.m. = intramuscular.
[e] MID_{50} = 50% monkey infectious dose (of homologous virus unless stated otherwise).
[f] Cranage *et al.*, in preparation.

Table 8.3 Summary of live/attenuated, recombinant and SIV subunit vaccine studies in macaques

Vaccine	*Adjuvant*	*Immunization schedule (weeks)*	*Neutralizing antibody*	*Cell-mediated immunity*	*Challenge*			*Number protected*	*Reference*
					Route	*Dose (MID_{50})*	*Number*		
Live/attentuated virus									
IAII SIV_{mac} genomic clone	—		—	NR	i.v.	10^3	4	0	93
Live recombinant									
Vaccinia SIV_{mac} *env*	—		+	NR	i.m.	200	3	0	89
Vaccinia SIV_{mac} *gag-env*	—		+	NR	i.m.	200	3	0	
Subunit									
env-enriched SIV_{delta}	tMDP + alum	0, 5, 58	NR	NR	i.v.	10	4	2	96
gag-enriched SIV_{delta}	tMDP + alum	0, 4, 57	NR	NR	i.v.	10	4	0	
SIV_{mac} *gag* p27: Ty-VLPs	Alum	0, 6, 12, 36	—	+	i.v.	10	4	0	[a]

Abbreviations as in Table 8.2.

[a] Mills *et al.*, in preparation.

Having demonstrated that it is possible to generate a protective immune response to SIV, a number of groups are now beginning to examine different parameters, such as the route of challenge, choice of adjuvant, nature of the protective antigen and mechanism of protective immunity. At the California Primate Centre attempts were made to compare i.v. and mucosal challenge[94]. Although the vaccine used for this study, psoralen and UV-inactivated SIV with tMDP, was not protective, the observation of earlier disease symptoms in the mucosally challenged animals suggests that it may be more difficult to protect against this route of infection[94]. In the majority of the vaccine trials discussed above, virus homologous to the immunogen has been used for challenge. However, a recent collaborative study carried out in the UK has demonstrated protection against challenge with a heterologous SIV strain, SIV_{delta}, but not against HIV-2, following immunization with formalin-inactivated SIV_{mac} in SAF-1 (Cranage *et al.*, in preparation).

Workers at the California Primate Centre have compared the effect of different adjuvants and have shown that immunization with β-propriolactone-inactivated SIV protected three of three animals when given with tMDP but only one of two with incomplete Freund's adjuvant (IFA) and one of three when given as aqueous antigen[95]. The question of SIV vaccine efficacy in different adjuvant formulations is also being addressed in a large collaborative study, coordinated by the EC programme for a vaccine against AIDS (project EVA) and involving eight centres and five countries.

In an attempt to identify the protective antigen in the whole SIV vaccine, Murphey-Corb and colleagues have shown that an *env*-depleted virus preparation failed to protect four macaques against infection, whereas the *env*-enriched fraction protected two of four animals[96]. A collaborative study between NIBSC and British Biotechnology demonstrated that a recombinant *gag* protein p27, expressed in yeast as SIV p27 Ty-VLPs, failed to protect against SIV challenge[129]. Finally vaccinia virus *env* or *env* and *gag* recombinants have also failed to protect against SIV infection[89]. Therefore, while it appears that *env* is the key component of a successful vaccine, it may not be straightforward to generate protective immunity using recombinant vaccines. It is possible that the heterogeneous and particulate nature of the whole SIV vaccines, with multiple copies of the *env* protein in their native conformation, may be difficult to duplicate with the recombinant approach.

In each of the successful vaccine trials in the SIV model, antibodies capable of neutralizing the virus *in vitro* have been demonstrated. However, neutralizing antibodies have also been found in the serum of unprotected animals at the time of challenge. Apart from one or two studies, cell-mediated responses have not been tested or reported[90]. Clearly the role of T cells and of antibodies that inhibit the function of the virus in ways other than that detected by *in vitro* neutralization assays, require more careful consideration in attempts to define the nature of the protective immune response to SIV.

CLINICAL TRIALS

Ideally a candidate vaccine should enter phase I clinical trials, for testing its immunogenicity and safety in healthy volunteers, only following demonstration of efficacy in a suitable animal model. It then enters a phase II trial where larger numbers of volunteers are used to determine the optimum immunization schedule and finally a phase III trial examines the efficacy in humans. However, because of the mounting pressure to tackle the AIDS epidemic several HIV candidate vaccines have entered phase 1 clinical trials in seronegative individuals or phase I/phase III trials in HIV positive patients with AIDS-related complex, before testing in primate models[97]. Indeed a number of retrospective trials in chimpanzees or macaques with certain of these vaccines, or their SIV equivalent, have resulted in failure to protect against homologous challenge.

The first trial of a HIV candidate vaccine in humans began in 1986, when Zagury and colleagues immunized seronegative volunteers with vaccinia virus recombinants expressing HIV *env*[98]. This vaccine produced only low levels of neutralizing antibodies and cell-mediated immunity; however, these responses could be considerably boosted using fixed autologous vaccinia-*env*-infected cells or soluble gp160[48,49]. In the United States phase I clinical trials are currently under way with recombinant baculovirus-expressed HIV gp160 (microGeneSys Corporation[99,100]) and live vaccinia virus recombinant expressing the *env* protein (Bristol Myers Inc. and Oncogen Corporation[101]). Recombinant gp120 expressed in yeast (Ciba-Geigy and Chiron and Biocine Co.) is also being tested in Switzerland[102]. In the UK trials are under way with two HIV core preparations; a synthetic peptide of p17 called HGP-30 (Virol Technology[103]) and a HIV *gag* p24 protein expressed in yeast as HIV p24: Ty-VLPs (British Biotechnology). Toxic side-effects and possible risks of generating autoantibodies or immunosuppression with *env* proteins have not yet been reported from any of the clinical trials. However, low levels of enhancing antibodies were detected in serum from individuals immunized with recombinant gp160[99]. In addition a proportion of HIV *env*-specific $CD4^+$ CTL clones generated from gp160 vaccines displayed cytolytic activity for autologous $CD4^+$ cells pulsed with gp120[104]. It is not known if these T cells could mediate lysis of normal $CD4^+$ T cells with gp120 absorbed to this surface *in vivo*.

Although consistent HIV-specific $CD4^+$ T cell responses have been generated with many of the candidate vaccines, the levels of humoral immunity reported have often been disappointing. Recombinant gp160 with alum induced proliferation and cytotoxic T cells, but antibody levels detected by ELISA were low, and neutralizing antibody activity was documented only in a minority of volunteers[99,100,104,105]. The vaccinia virus HIV *env* recombinant failed to induce neutralizing antibodies and only generated strong proliferative T cell responses in vaccinia naive individuals[101]. However, boosting with soluble gp160 generated anamnestic anti-*env* antibody levels, with neutralizing activity in a proportion of individuals, and strong T cell responses, irrespective of their pre-immunization vaccinia immune status[106]. Although the results from this study look promising, further phase I clinical trials should await further development and testing of the optimum expression systems, adjuvants and immunization protocol for recombinant *env* proteins in the non-human primate models.

Attempts at post-exposure immunotherapy by vaccination of HIV positive individuals have also begun. Salk[107] has proposed that it may be possible to reduce the virus load in HIV positive individuals by boosting the antiviral immune response during the asymptomatic phase of the infection. The vaccine being tested in HIV-infected individuals is inactivated *env*-depleted HIV emulsified in incomplete Freund's adjuvant[108]; this combination was reported to be capable of inducing resistance to reinfection in HIV positive chimpanzees[109]. However, attempts to modify the course of infection in macaques by post-exposure vaccination with inactivated SIV, known to be capable of inducing protection against SIV infection in naive animals, were unsuccessful[90,110].

FUTURE DIRECTIONS

The recent results with the inactivated whole virus vaccines in the SIV model are very encouraging, and demonstrate that it is possible to generate a protective immune response against a lentivirus infection in primates. However, the ability to protect against an i.v. challenge with a relatively low dose of SIV at the peak of the antibody response, 2 weeks after the last of four immunizations with an inactivated virus, requires considerable refinement. The emphasis in the animal model must now focus on the subunit recombinant vaccines, as well as methods of potentiating the protective immune response and circumventing the problem of antigenic variation. Protection against free and cell associated virus by i.v. and mucosal routes must also be considered when designing the optimum vaccination protocols. The generation of circulating antibodies capable of inhibiting virus binding to its receptor or its fusion with the cell membrane are likely to be central to the mechanism of protection against free virus by the i.v. route. However, *in vitro* neutralization antibody responses in the SIV vaccine trials have not always correlated with protection. Alternative assays aimed at detecting other functionally significant antibody- or cell-mediated immune responses need to be more fully explored. Secretory antibodies may be important in protection against mucosal challenge. Furthermore following exposure to cell-associated virus, complement- or antibody-dependent cytoxicity or NK activity may function to destroy the allogeneic virus-infected cells.

Although it remains to be confirmed, it seems likely that the *env* protein is the protective antigen; the optimum recombinant expression system and the most suitable adjuvant formulation must be defined using the non-human primate models. It has been suggested that a synthetic HIV vaccine should include only selective regions of the envelope protein that contain the key B and T cell epitopes, and that regions that generate undesirable responses should be excluded[35]. In particular, antigen-presenting systems containing the V3 loop, or other neutralizing antibody site on the *env* protein, are being considered as candidate vaccines[37,38,70,71,111,112]. However, despite the possible risks of induction of autoimmunity or immunosuppression[113] with *env* sequences, the attention must focus on the use of all or most of the gp120 protein, with the exclusion of the transmembrane portion gp41 on the basis of enhancing antibody production[12]. It may be important to include several functionally important and possibly conserved or conformationally dependent antibody epitopes and a wide range of T cell epitopes for recognition in association with different MHC haplotypes.

Studies with other viruses, such as influenza[114,115] and lymphocytic choriomeningitis virus[116], have shown the immune pressure from antibody and T cells can result in antigenic variation which allows the virus to escape immunity. Analysis of the immune response to HIV proteins indicates that this may also be a major stumbling block in effective HIV vaccine development[35,37,38,44,52]. Nevertheless, early results from the SIV model suggest that there is a certain degree of cross-reactivity in the protective immune responses. Vaccines with multiple or consensus sequences may be required for protection against diverse HIV-1 isolates, with a separate vaccine for HIV-2. Alternative strategies aimed at inhibiting the interaction between gp120 and CD4 with soluble CD4[23], or by the administration of anti-CD4 monoclonal antibodies[117], may in theory be capable of circumventing the problem of antigen variation, but are not without their own limitations and complications.

The immunogenicity trials with recombinant *env* proteins in humans and experimental animals have shown that the antibody levels, in particular those that neutralize HIV infectivity *in vitro*, are quite poor when alum is used as the adjuvant[58–60,105]. Although live vectors such as vaccinia virus[45,83], adenovirus[118], poliovirus[70] or *Salmonella*[119] may be useful for generating primary responses in naive individuals, boosting this response may require the use of recombinant protein incorporated into potent adjuvant formulations. Synthetic polymers[120], metabolizable oil-in-water emulsions[121], microparticles[122], ISCOMS[30,68] or liposomes in combination with encapsulated immune potentiating agents[123,124] are being tested in animals, and a number are undergoing toxicity testing in humans[125]. Finally, it may be possible to focus the HIV preparation onto B cells or other cells capable of presenting antigen *in vivo*, through surface immunoglobulin[126], class II MHC antigens[127] or complement receptors[128].

While the prospects for preventing primary HIV infection in seronegative individuals look increasingly promising, the possibility of clearing the virus from seropositive individuals by post-infection immunization seems more unlikely. Once inside the host cell, immunological mechanisms may function to control the virus for a prolonged period, but may be incapable of completely eliminating it.

References

1. Hilleman, M. R. (1985). Newer directions in vaccine development and utilization. *J. Infect. Dis.*, **151**, 407–19
2. Haase, A. T. (1986). Pathogenesis of lentivirus infections. *Nature*, **322**, 130–6
3. Bloom, B. R. (1987). Aids vaccine strategies. *Nature*, **327**, 193
4. Dagleish, A. G., Beverley, P. C. L., Clapham, P. R., Crawford, D. H., Greaves, M. F. and Weiss, R. A. (1984). The CD4 (T4) antigen is an essential component of the receptor for the AIDS retrovirus. *Nature*, **312**, 763–7

5. Klatzmann, D., Barre-Sinoussi, F., Nugeyre, M. T., Dauguet, C., Vilmer, E., Griscelli, C., Brun-Vezinet, F. B., Rouzious, C., Gluckman, J. C., Chermann, J-C. and Montagnier, L. (1984). Selective tropism of lymphadenopathy associated virus (LAV) for helper–inducer T lymphocytes. *Science*, **225**, 59–63
6. Fenyo, E. M., Albert, J. and Asjo, B. (1989). Replicative capacity, cytopathic effect and cell tropism of HIV. *AIDS*, **3** (Suppl. 1), S5–12
7. Cann, A. J. and Karn, J. (1989). Molecular biology of HIV: new insights into virus life-cycle. *AIDS*, **3**, (Suppl. 1), S19–34
8. Hoxie, J. A., Haggarty, B. S., Rackowsky, J. L., Pilsbury, N. and Levy, J. A. (1985). Persistent non-cytopathic infection of human lymphocytes with AIDS-associated retrovirus (ARV). *Science*, **229**, 1400–2
9. Rosenberg, Z. F. and Fauci, A. S. (1989). Induction of expression of HIV in latently or chronically infected cells. *AIDS Res. Hum. Retrovir.*, **5**, 1–4
10. Robinson, W. E., Monterfiori, D. C. and Mitchell, W. M. (1988). Antibody-dependent enhancement of human immunodeficiency virus type 1 infection. *Lancet*, **1**, 790–4
11. Homsy, J., Megar, M., Tateno, M., Clarkson, S. and Levy, J. A. (1989). The Fc and not CD4 receptor mediates antibody enhancement of HIV infection in human cells. *Science*, **244**, 1357–60
12. Robinson, W. E., Kawamura, T., Lake, D., Masuko, Y., Mitchell, W. M. and Hersh, E. M. (1990). Antibodies to the primary immunodominant domain of human immunodeficiency virus type 1 (HIV-1) glycoprotein gp41 enhance HIV-1 infection *in vitro*. *J. Virol.*, **64**, 5301–5
13. Orsenstein, J. M., Meltzer, M. S., Phipps, T. and Gendelman, H. E. (1988). Cytoplasmic assembly and accumulation of human immunodeficiency virus types 1 and 2 in recombinant human colony-stimulating factor-1-treated human monocytes: an ultrastructural study. *J. Virol.*, **62**, 2578–86
14. Price, R. W., Brew, B., Sidtis, J., Rosenblum, M., Scheck, A. C. and Cleary, P. (1988). The brain in AIDS: central nervous system HIV-1 infection and AIDS dementia complex. *Science*, **239**, 586–92
15. Hahn, B. H., Shaw, G. W., Taylor, M. E., Redfield, R. R., Markham, P. D., Salahuddin, S. Z., Wong-Staal, F., Gallo, R. C., Parks, E. S. and Parks, W. P. (1986). Genetic variation in HTLV-III/LAV over time in patients with AIDS or at risk for AIDS. *Science*, **232**, 1548–53
16. Saag, M. S., Hahn, B. H., Gibbons, J., Li, Y., Parks, E. S., Parks, W. P. and Shaw, G. M. (1988). Extensive diversity of human immunodeficiency virus type-1 *in vivo*. *Nature*, **334**, 440–4
17. Wain-Hobson, S. (1989). HIV genome variability *in vivo*. *AIDS*, **3** (Suppl. 1), S13–8
18. Myers, G., Rabson, A. B., Joseph, S. F., Smith, T. F. and Wong-Staal, F. (1990). *Human Retroviruses and AIDS 1990: A Compilation and Analysis of Nucleic Acid and Amino Acid Sequences* (Los Alamos, MN: Los Alamos National Laboratory)
19. Alter, H. J., Eichberg, J. W., Masur, H., Saxinger, W. C., Gallo, R., Macher, A. M., Lane, H. C. and Fauci, A. S. (1984). Transmission of HTLV-III infection from human plasma to chimpanzees: an animal model for AIDS. *Science*, **226**, 549–52
20. Lusso, P., Markham, P. D., Ranki, A., Earl, P., Moss, B., Dorner, F., Gallo, R. C. and Krohn, K. J. E. (1988). Cell-mediated immune response toward viral envelope and core antigens in gibbon apes (*Hylobates lar*) chronically infected with human immunodeficiency virus-1. *J. Immunol.*, **141**, 2467–73
21. Letvin, N. L., David, M. D., Sehgal, P. K., Desrosiers, R. C., Hunt, R. D., Waldron, L. M., MacKey, J. J., Schmidt, D. K., Chalifoux, L. V. and King, N. W. (1985). Induction of AIDS like diseases in macaque monkeys with T-cell tropic retrovirus STLV-III. *Science*, **230**, 71–3
22. Desrosiers, R. C. (1988). Simian immunodeficiency viruses. *Ann. Rev. Microbiol.*, **42**, 607–25
23. Letvin, N. L. (1990). Animal models for Aids. *Immunol. Today*, **11**, 322–6
24. Mills, K. H. G. (1989). Recognition of foreign antigen by T cells and their role in immune protection. *Curr. Opin. Infect. Dis.*, **3**, 804–14
25. Ada, G. L. (1988). What to expect of a good vaccine and how to achieve it. *Vaccine*, **6**, 77–9
26. Mills, K. H. G. (1986). Processing of viral antigens and presentation to class II-restricted T cells. *Immunol. Today*, **7**, 260–3
27. Rouse, B. T., Norley, S. and Martin, S. (1988). Antiviral cytotoxic T lymphocyte induction and vaccination. *Rev. Infect. Dis.*, **10**, 16–33
28. Aichele, P., Hengartner, H., Zinkernagel, R. M. and Schulz, M. (1990). Antiviral cytotoxic T cell response induced by *in vivo* priming with a free synthetic peptide. *J. Exp. Med.*, **171**,

1815–20

29. Deres, K., Schild, H., Wiesmuller, K-H., Jung, G. and Rammensee, H. G. (1989). *In vivo* priming of virus-specific cytotoxic T lymphocytes with synthetic lipopeptide vaccine. *Nature*, **342**, 561–4
30. Takahashi, H., Takeshita, T., Morein, B., Putney, S., Germain, R. N. and Berzofsky, J. A. (1990). Induction of CD8$^+$ cytotoxic T cells by immunization with purified HIV-I envelope protein in ISCOMs. *Nature*, **344**, 873–5
31. Dimmock, N. J. (1984). Mechanisms of neutralization of animal viruses. *J. Gen. Virol.*, **65**, 1015–22
32. Lukacher, A. E., Braciale, V. L. and Braciale, T. J. (1984). *In vivo* effector function of influenza virus-specific cytotoxic T lymphocyte clones is highly specific. *J. Exp. Med.*, **160**, 814–26
33. Mills, K. H. G., Nixon, D. F. and McMichael, A. J. (1989). T cell strategies in AIDS vaccines: MHC-restricted T cell responses to HIV proteins. *AIDS*, **3** (Suppl. 1), S101–10
34. Oehen, S., Hengartner, H. and Zinkernagel, R. M. (1991). Vaccination for disease. *Science*, **251**, 195–8
35. Bolognesi, D. P. (1989). HIV antibodies and vaccine design. *AIDS*, **3** (Suppl. 1), S111–18
36. Gurley, R. J., Ikeuchi, K., Byrn, R. A., Anderson, K. and Groopman, J. E. (1989). CD4$^+$ lymphocyte function with early immunodeficiency virus infection. *Proc. Natl. Acad. Sci., USA*, **86**, 1993–7
37. Goudsmit, J. (1988). Immunodominant B-cell epitopes of the HIV-I envelope recognized by infected and immunized hosts. *AIDS*, **2** (Suppl. 1), S41–5
38. Javaherian, K., Langlois, A. J., McDanal, C., Ross, K. L., Eckler, L. I., Jellis, C. L., Profy, A., Rusche, J. R., Bolognesi, D. P., Putney, S. D. and Matthews, T. J. (1989). Principal neutralizing domains of the human immunodeficiency virus type 1 envelope protein. *Proc. Natl. Acad. Sci., USA*, **86**, 6768–72
39. Nixon, D. F., Townsend, A. R. M., Elvin, J. G., Rizza, C. R., Gallwey, J. and McMichael, A. J. (1988). HIV-I gag-specific cytotoxic T lymphocytes defined with recombinant vaccinia virus and synthetic peptides. *Nature*, **336**, 484–7
40. Hoffenbach, A., Langlade-Demoyen, P., Dadaglio, G., Vilmer, E., Michel, F., Mayaud, C., Autran, B. and Plata, F. (1989). Unusually high frequencies of HIV-specific cytotoxic T lymphocytes in humans. *J. Immunol.*, **142**, 452–62
41. Koup, R. A., Sullivan, J. L., Levine, P. H., Brettler, D., Mahr, A., Mazzara, G., McKenzie, S. and Panicali, D. (1989). Detection of major histocompatibility complex class I-restricted HIV-specific cytotoxic T lymphocytes in the blood of infected hemophiliacs. *Blood*, **73**, 1909–14
42. Tsubota, H., Lord, C. I., Watkins, D. I., Morimoto, C. and Letvin, N. L. (1989). A cytotoxic T lymphocyte inhibits acquired immunodeficiency syndrome virus replication in peripheral blood lymphocytes. *J. Exp. Med.*, **169**, 1421–34
43. Culmann, B., Gomard, E., Kieny, M-P., Guy, B., Dreyfus, F., Saimot, A-G., Sereni, D., Sicard, D. and Levy, J-P. (1991). Six epitopes reacting with human cytotoxic CD8$^+$ T cells in the central region of the HIV-I Nef protein. *J. Immunol.*, **146**, 1560–5
44. Siliciano, R. F., Lawton, T., Knall, C., Karr, R. W., Berman, P., Gregory, T. and Reinherz, E. L. (1988). Analysis of host-virus interactions in AIDS with anti-gp120 T cell clones: effect of HIV sequence variation and a mechanism of CD4$^+$ cell depletion. *Cell*, **54**, 561–75
45. Charkrabarti, S., Robert-Guroff, M., Wong-Staal, F., Gallo, R. C. and Moss, B. (1986). Expression of the HTLV-III envelope gene by a recombinant vaccine virus. *Nature*, **320**, 535–7
46. Clerici, M., Stocks, N. I., Zajac, R. A., Boswell, R. N., Bernstein, D. C., Mann, D. L., Shearer, G. M. and Berzofsky, J. (1989). Interleukin-2 production used to detect antigenic peptide recognition by T-helper lymphocytes from asymptomatic HIV-seropositive individuals. *Nature*, **339**, 383–5
47. Schrier, R. D., Gnann, J. W., Landes, R., Lockshin, C., Richmann, D., Mccutchan, A., Kennedy, C., Oldstone, M. B. A. and Nelson, J. A. (1989). T cell recognition of HIV synthetic peptides in a natural infection. *J. Immunol.*, **142**, 1166–76
48. Berzofsky, J. A., Bensussan, A., Cease, K. B., Bourge, J. F., Cheynier, R., Zirimwabagabo, L., Salaun, J. J., Gallo, R. C., Shearer, G. M. and Zagury, D. (1988). Antigenic peptides recognized by T lymphocytes from AIDS viral envelope-immune humans. *Nature*, **334**, 706–8
49. Zagury, D., Bernard, J., Cheynier, R., Desportes, I., Leonard, R., Fouchard, M., Reveii, B., Ittele, D., Zirimwabagabo, L., Mbayo, K., Wane, J., Salaun, J-J., Goussard, B., Dechazai,

L., Burny, A., Nara, P. and Gallo, R. C. (1988). A group specific anamnestic immune reaction against HIV-1 induced by a candidate vaccine against AIDS. *Nature*, **332**, 728–31
50. Zarling, J. M., Morton, W., Moran, P. A., McClure, J., Kosowski, S. G. and Hu, S-L. (1986). T-cell responses to human AIDS virus in macaques immunized with recombinant vaccinia viruses. *Nature*, **223**, 344–6
51. Cease, K. B., Margalit, H., Cornette, J. L., Putney, S. D., Robey, W. G., Ouyang, C., Streicher, H. Z., Fischinger, P. J., Gallo, R. C., DeLisi, C. and Berzofsky, J. A. (1987). Helper T cell site identification in the AIDS virus gp120 envelope protein and induction of immunity in mice to the native protein using a 16-residue synthetic peptide. *Proc. Natl. Acad. Sci., USA*, **84**, 4249–53
52. Mills, K. H. G., Kitchin, P. A., Mahon, B. P., Barnard, A. L., Adams, S. E., Kingsman, S. M. and Kingsman, A. J. (1990). HIV p24-specific helper T cell clones from immunized primates recognize highly conserved regions of HIV-1. *J. Immunol.*, **44**, 1677–83
53. Russell, S. M. and Liew, F. Y. (1980). Cell cooperation in antibody responses to influenza virus. 1. Priming of helper T cells by internal components of the virion. *Eur. J. Immunol.*, **10**, 791–6
54. Scherle, P. A. and Gerhard, W. (1986). Functional analysis of influenza-specific helper T cell clones *in vivo*. T cells specific for internal viral proteins provide cognate help for B cell responses to haemagglutinin. *J. Exp. Med.*, **166**, 1114–28
55. Milich, D. R., McLachlan, A., Thornton, G. B. and Hughes, J. L. (1987). Antibody production to the nucleocapsid and envelope of the hepatitis B virus primed by a single synthetic T cell site. *Nature*, **329**, 547–9
56. Fields, B. N. and Chanock, R. M. (1989). What biotechnology has to offer vaccine development. *Rev. Infect. Dis.*, **11** (Suppl. 3), S519–23
57. Langley, D. and Spier, R. F. (1988). Is a vaccine against AIDS possible? *Vaccine*, **6**, 3–5
58. Page, M., Mills, K. H. G., Schild, G. C., Ling, C., Patel, V., McKnight, A., Barnard, A. L., Dilger, P. and Thorpe, R. (1991). Studies on the immunogenicity of Chinese hamsters ovary cell-derived recombinant gp120 (HIV-1_{IIIB}). *Vaccine*, **9**, 47–52
59. Anderson, K. P., Lucas, C., Hanson, C. V., Londe, H., Izu, A., Gregory, T., Ammann, A., Berman, P. W. and Eichberg, J. W. (1989). Effect of dose and immunization schedule on immune response of baboons to recombinant glycoprotein 120 of HIV-1. *J. Infect. Dis.*, **160**, 960–9
60. Arthur, L. O., Pyle, S. W., Nara, P. L., Bess, J. W., Gonda, J. C., Kelliher, J. C., Gilden, R. V., Robey, W. G., Bolognesi, D. P., Gallo, R. C. and Fischinger, P. J. (1987). Serological responses in chimpanzees inoculated with human immunodeficiency virus glycoprotein (gp120) subunit vaccine. *Proc. Natl. Acad. Sci., USA*, **84**, 8583–7
61. Allison, A. C. and Byars, N. E. (1986). An adjuvant formulation that selectively elicits the formation of antibodies of protective isotypes and of cell-mediated immunity. *J. Immunol. Methods*, **95**, 157–68
62. Kenney, J. S., Hughes, B. W., Masada, M. P. and Allison, A. C. (1989). Influence of adjuvants on the quantity, affinity isotype and epitope specificity of murine antibodies. *J. Immunol. Methods*, **121**, 157–66
63 Ribi, E. and Cantrell, J. (1985). A new immunomodulator with potential clinical applications: monophosphoryl lipid A, a detoxified endotoxin. *Clin. Immunol. Newsletter*, **6**, 33–6
64. Ribi, E. (1986). Structure-function relationship of bacterial adjuvants. In Nervig, R. M., Gough, P. M., Kaeberle, M. L. and Whetstone, C. A. (eds) *Advances in Carriers and Adjuvants for Veterinary Biologics* (Ames, IA: Iowa State University Press), pp. 35–49
65. Odean, M. J., Franc, C. M., Van der Vieren, M., Tomai, M. A. and Johnson, A. G. (1990). Involvement of gamma interferon in antibody enhancement by adjuvants. *Infect. Immun.* **58**, 427–32
66. Tomai, M. A. and Johnson, A. G. (1989). T cell and interferon gamma involvement in the adjuvant action of a detoxified endotoxin. *J. Biol. Response Mod.*, **8**, 625–43
67. Gregoriadis, G. (1990). Immunological adjuvants: a role for liposomes. *Immunol. Today*, **3**, 89–97
68. Pyle, S. W., Morein, B., Bess, J. W., Akerblom, L., Nara, P. L., Nigida, S. M., Lerche, N. W., Robey, W. G., Fischinger, P. J. and Arthur, L. O. (1989). Immune response to immunostimulatory complexes (ISCOMs) prepared from human immunodeficiency virus type 1 (HIV-1) or the HIV-1 external envelope glycoprotein (gp120). *Vaccine*, **7**, 465–73
69. Kingsman, S. M. and Kingsman, A. J. (1988). Polyvalent recombinant antigens: a new

vaccine strategy. *Vaccine*, **6**, 304.

70. Evans, D. J., McKeating, J., Meredith, J. M., Burke, K. L., Katrak, K., John, A., Ferguson, M., Minor, P. D., Weiss, R. A. and Almond, J. W. (1989). An engineered poliovirus chimaera elicits broadly reactive HIV-1 neutralizing antibodies. *Nature*, **339**, 385–8
71. Michel, M-L., Mancini, M., Riviere, Y., Dormont, D. and Trollais, P. (1990). T- and B-lymphocyte responses to human immunodeficiency virus (HIV) type 1 in macaques immunized with hybrid HIV/hepatitis B surface antigen particles. *J. Virol.*, **64**, 2452–5
72. Arthur, L. O., Bess, J. W. Jr, Waters, D. J., Pyle, S. W., Kelliher, J. C., Nara, P. L., Krohn, K., Robey, W. G., Longlois, A. J., Gallo, R. C. and Fischinger, P. J. (1989). Challenge of chimpanzees (*Pan troglodytes*) immunized with human immunodeficiency virus envelope glycoprotein gp120. *J. Virol.*, **63**, 5046–53
73. Pukonen, P., Thorstensson, R., Albert, J., Hild, K., Norby, E., Biberfeld, P. and Biberfeld, G. (1990). Infection of cynomolgus monkeys with HIV-2 protects against pathogenic consequences of a subsequent simian immunodeficiency virus infection. *AIDS*, **4**, 783–9
74. Kestler, H., Kodama, T., Ringler, D., Marthas, M., Pedersen, N., Lackner, A., Regier, D., Sehgal, P., Daniel, M., King, N. and Desrosiers, R. (1990). Induction of AIDS in Rhesus monkeys by molecularly cloned simian immunodeficiency virus. *Science*, **248**, 1109–12
75. Hoxie, J. A., Haggarty, B. S., Bonser, S. E., Rackowski, J. L., Shan, H. and Kanki, P. J. (1988). Biological characterization of a simian immunodeficiency virus – like retrovirus (HTLV-IV): evidence for CD4-associated molecules required for infection. *J. Virol.*, **62**, 2557–68
76. Sparger, E. E., Luciw, P. A., Elder, J. A., Yamamoto, J. K., Lowensteine, L. J. and Petersen, N. C. (1989). Feline immunodeficiency virus is a lentivirus associated with an AIDS-like disease in cats. *AIDS*, **3** (Suppl. 1), S43–9
77. McCune, J. M., Namikawa, R., Kaneshima, H., Shultz, L. D., Lieberncan, M. and Weissman, I. L. (1988). The SCID-hu mouse: murine model for the analysis of human hematolymphoid differentiation and function. *Science*, **241**, 1632–9
78. McCune, J. M., Kaneshima, H., Lieberman, M., Weissman, I. L. and Namikawa, R. (1989). The SCID-hu mouse: current status and potential applications. In Bosma, M. J., Phillips, R. A. and Schuler, W. (eds.), *Current Topics in the SCID Mouse: Characterization and Potential Uses. Curr. Top. Microbiol. Immunol.*, **152**, 183–93
79. Mosier, D. E., Gulizia, R. J., Baird, S. M. and Wilson, D. B. (1988). Transfer of a functional human immune system to mice with severe combined immunodeficiency. *Nature*, **335**, 256–9
80. Mosier, D. E., Gulizia, R. J., Baird, S. M., Spector, S., Spector, D., Kipps, T. J., Fox, R. I., Carson, D. A., Cooper, N., Richman, D. D. and Wilson, D. B. (1989). Studies of HIV infection and the development of Epstein Barr virus-related B cell lymphomas following transfer of human lymphocytes to mice and severe combined immunodeficiency. In Bosman, M. J., Phillips, R. A. and Schuler, W. (eds), *The SCID Mouse, Characterization and Potential Uses. Curr. Top. Microbiol. Immunol.*, **152**, 175–99
81. Berman, P. W., Gregory, T. J., Riddle, L., Nakamura, G. R., Champe, M. A., Porter, J. P., Wurm, F. M., Hersberg, R. D., Cobb, E. K. and Eichberg, J. W. (1990). Protection of chimpanzees from infection by HIV-1 after vaccination with recombinant glycoprotein gp120 but not gp160. *Nature*, **345**, 622–5
82. Berman, P. W., Groopman, J. E., Gregory, T., Clapham, P. R., Weiss, R. A., Ferriani, R. A., Riddle, L., Shimasaki, C., Lucas, C., Lasky, L. A. and Eichberg, J. W. (1988). Human immunodeficiency virus type 1 challenge of chimpanzees immunized with recombinant envelope glycoprotein gp120. *Proc. Natl. Acad. Sci., USA*, **85**, 5200–4
83. Hu, S. L., Fultz, P. N., McClure, H., Eichberg, J. W., Thomas, E. K., Zarling, J., Singhal, M. C., Kowawski, S. G., Swenson, R. B., Anderson, D. C. and Todaro, G. (1987). Effect of immunization with a vaccinia–HIV env recombinant on HIV infection of chimpanzees. *Nature*, **328**, 721–3
84. Arthur, L. O., Pyle, S. W., Nara, P. L., Bess, J. W. Jr, Gonda, M. A., Kelliher, J. C., Gilden, R. V., Robey, W. G., Bolognesi, D. P., Gallo, R. C. and Fischinger, P. J. (1987). Serological responses in chimpanzees inoculated with human immunodeficiency virus glycoprotein (gp120) subunit vaccine. *Proc. Natl. Acad. Sci., USA*, **84**, 8583–7
85. Girard, M., Kieny, M-P., Pinter, A., Barre-Sinoussi, F., Nara, P., Kolbe, H., Kusumi, K., Chaput, A., Reinhart, T., Muchmore, E., Ronco, J., Kaczorey, M., Gomard, E., Gluckman, J-C. and Fultz, P. N. (1991). Immunisation of chimpanzees confers protection against challenge with human immunodeficiency virus. *Proc. Natl. Acad. Sci. USA*, **88**, 542–6

86. Emini, E. A., Schleif, W. A., Quintero, J. C., Conard, P. G., Eichberg, J. W., Vlasuk, G. P., Lehman, E. D., Polokoff, M. A., Schaeffer, T. F., Schultz, L. D., Hofmann, K. J., Lewis, J. A. and Larson, V. M. (1990). Yeast-expressed p55 precursor core protein of human immunodeficiency virus type 1 does not elicit protective immunity in chimpanzees. *AIDS Res. Hum. Retrovir.*, **6**, 1247–50
87. Desrosiers, R. C., Wyand, M. S., Kodama, T., Ringler, D. J., Arthur, L. O., Sehgal, P. K., Letvin, N. L., King, N. W. and Daniel, M. D. (1989). Vaccine protection against simian immunodeficiency virus infection. *Proc. Natl. Acad. Sci., USA*, **86**, 6353–7
88. Murphey-Corb, M., Martin, L. N., Davison-Fairburn, B., Montelaro, R. C., Miller, M., West, M., Onkawa, S., Baskin, G. B., Zhang, J.-Y., Putney, S. D., Allison, A. C. and Eppstein, D. A. (1989). A formalin-inactivated whole SIV vaccine confers protection in macaques. *Science*, **246**, 1293–7
89. Gardner, M. B. (1990). Vaccination against SIV infection and disease. *AIDS Res. Hum. Retrovir.*, **6**, 835–45
90. Stott, E. J., Chan, W. L., Mills, K. H. G., Page, M., Taffs, F., Cranage, M., Greenway, P. and Kitchin, P. (1990). Preliminary Report: protection of cynomologus macaques against simian immunodeficiency virus by fixed infected-cell vaccine. *Lancet*, **i**, 1538–41
91. Allen, D., Cumano, A., Dildrop, R., Kochs, C., Rajewsky, K., Roes, J., Stablitzky, F. and Siekevitz, M. (1987). Timing, genetic requirements and functional consequences of somative hypermutation during B-cell development. *Immunol. Rev.*, **96**, 5–22
92. Berek, C. and Milstein, C. (1988). The dynamic nature of the antibody repertoire. *Immunol. Rev.*, **105**, 5–26
93. Marthas, M. L., Sutjipto, S., Higgins, J., Lohman, B., Torten, J., Luciw, P. A., Marx, P. A. and Pedersen, N. C. (1990). Immunization with a live, attenuated simian immunodeficiency virus (SIV) prevents early disease but not infection in rhesus macaques challenged with pathogenic SIV. *J. Virol.*, **64**, 3696–700
94. Sutjipto, S., Pederson, N. C., Muller, C. J., Gardner, M. B., Hanson, C. V., Gettie, A., Jennings, M., Higgins, J. and Marx, P. A. (1990). Inactivated simian immunodeficiency virus vaccine failed to protect rhesus macaques from intravenous or genital mucosal infection but delayed disease in intravenously exposed animals. *J. Virol.*, **64**, 2290–7
95. Carlson, J. R., McGraw, T. P., Keddie, E., Yee, O. J. L., Rosenthal, A., Langlois, A. J., Dickover, R., Donovan, R., Luciw, P. A., Jennings, M. B. and Gardner, B. (1990). Vaccine protection of rhesus macaques against simian immunodeficiency virus infection. *AIDS Res. Hum. Retrovir.*, **6**, 1239–46
96. Murphey-Corb, M., Martin, L. N., Davison-Fairburn, B., Ohkawa, S., Baskin, G. B., Zhang, J-Y., Montelaro, R. C., Miller, M., West, M., Allison, A., Eppstein, D. and Putney, S. (1990). Induction of protective immune responses to viral infection by immunization of rhesus monkeys with formalin-inactivated whole SIV and glycoprotein-enriched SIV subunit vaccines. In Brown, F., Chanock, R. M., Ginsberg, H. S. and Lerner, R. A. (eds), *Vaccines 90. Modern Approach to New Vaccines Including Prevention of AIDS* (Coldspring Harbor Laboratory Press), pp. 393–9
97. Koff, W. C. and Fauci, A. S. (1989). Human trials of AIDS vaccines: current status and future directions. *AIDS*, **3**, (Suppl. 1), 5125–9
98. Zagury, D., Leonard, R., Fouchard, M., Reveil, B., Bernard, J., Ittele, D., Cattan, A., Zirimwabagabo, L., Kalumbu, M., Justin, W., Salaun, J-J. and Goussard, B. (1987). Immunization against AIDS in humans. *Nature*, **326**, 249–50
99. Smith, G. and Volvovitz, F. (1990). Vaxsyn HIV-1 (RGP160) vaccine recipients demonstrate functional immune responses classically associated with protective immunity. In VI International Conference on AIDS, San Francisco: Abstract SA75
100. Dolin, R., Graham, B., Greenberg, S., Tachett, C., Belshe, R., Clements, M., Fernie, B., Stablein, D., Smith, G. and Koff, W. (1989). Safety and immunogenecity of HIV-1 recombinant gp160 vaccine candidate in normal volunteers. In V International Conference on AIDS, Montreal: Abstract ThCO33
101. Cooney, F., Zarling, J., Hu, S-L., Watson, A., Corey, L. and Greenberg, P. (1989). T cell responses to HIV in humans immunized with recombinant vaccinia virus containing HIV envelope. In V International Conference on AIDS, Montreal: Abstract, ThCO 34
102. Coles, P. (1988). AIDS vaccine trials to begin in Geneva. *Nature*, **330**, 792
103. Goldstein, A. L., Naylor, P. H., Sarin, P. S., Kirkley, J. E., Stombak, D., Rios, A., Zagury,

D., Achour, A., Gazzard, B. and Youle, M. (1989). Progress in the development of a p17 based HIV vaccine: immunogenecity of HGP-30 in humans. In VI International Conference on AIDS, San Francisco: Abstract SA76

104. Orentas, R. J., Hildreth, J. E. K., Obah, E., Polydefkis, M., Smith, G. E., Clements, M. L. and Siliciano, R. F. (1990). Induction of CD4$^+$ human cytolytic T cells specific for HIV-infected cells by a gp160 subunit vaccine. *Science*, **248**, 1234–7
105. Viscidi, R., Ellerbeck, E., Garrison, L., Midthun, K., Clements, M. L., Clayman, B., Fernie, B., Smith, G. and the NAID vaccine clinical trials network (1990). Characterization of serum antibody responses to recombinant HIV-1 gp160 vaccine by enzyme immunoassay. *AIDS Res. Hum. Retrovir.*, **6**, 1251–6
106. Cooney, E. L., Corey, L., Hu, S. L., Collier, A., Arditti, D., Hoffman, M., Smith, G., Steimer, K. and Greenberg, P. (1990). Enhanced immunogenecity in humans of an HIV subunit vaccine regimen employing priming with a vaccine gp160 recombinant virus (VAC/env) by boosting with recombinant HIV envelope. In VI International Conference on AIDS, San Francisco: Abstract ThA 333
107. Salk, J. (1989). Prospects for the control of AIDS by immunizing seropositive individuals. *Nature*, **327**, 473–6
108. Levine, A., Henderson, B. E., Groshen, S., Burnett, K., Jensen, F., Peters, R., Carlo, D., Gersten, M., Salk, J. *et al.* (1990). Immunization of HIV-infected individuals with inactivated HIV immunogen significance of HIV-specific cell mediated immune response. In VI International Conference on AIDS, San Francisco: Abstract ThA 339
109. Gibbs, C. J., Mora, C., Peters, R., Jensen, F. C., Carlo, D. J. and Salk, J. (1989). HIV immunization and challenge of HIV seropositive and seronegative chimpanzees. In V International Conference on AIDS, Montreal: Abstract ThCO 46
110. Gardner, M. B., Jennings, M., Carlson, J. R., Lerche, N., McGraw, T., Luciw, P., Marx, P. and Pedersen, N. (1989). Postexposure immunotherapy of simian immunodeficiency virus (SIV) infected rhesus with an SIV immunogen. *J. Med. Primatol.*, **18**, 321–8
111. Javaherian, K., Langlois, A. J., LaRosa, G. L., Profy, A. T., Bolognesi, D. P., Herlihy, W. C., Putney, S. D. and Matthews, T. J. (1990). Broadly neutralizing antibodies elicited by the hypervariable neutralizing determinant of HIV-1. *Science*, **250**, 1590–3
112. Palker, T. J., Matthews, T. J., Langlois, A., Tanner, M. E., Martin, M. E., Scearce, R. M., Kim, J. E., Berzofsky, J. A., Bolognesi, D. P. and Haynes, B. F. (1989). Polyvalent human immunodeficiency virus synthetic immunogen comprised of envelope gp120 T helper cell sites and B cell neutralizing epitopes. *J. Immunol.*, **10**, 3612–9
113. Weinhold, K. J., Lyerley, H. K., Stanley, S. D., Austin, A. A., Matthews, T. J. and Bolognesi, D. P. (1989). HIV-1 gp120-mediated immune suppression and lymphocyte destruction in the absence of viral infection. *J. Immunol.*, **142**, 3091–7
114. Wiley, D. C., Wilson, I. A. and Skehel, J. J. (1981). Structural identification of the antibody binding sites of Hong Kong influenza haemagglutinin and their involvement in antigenic variation. *Nature*, **289**, 373–8
115. Mills, K. H. G., Skehel, J. J. and Thomas, D. B. (1986). Extensive diversity in the recognition of influenza virus hemagglutinin by murine T helper clones. *J. Exp. Med.*, **163**, 1477–80
116. Pircher, H., Moskophidis, D., Rohrer, U., Burki, K., Hengartner, H. and Zinkernagel, R. M. (1990). Viral escape by selection of cytotoxic T cell-resistant virus variants *in vivo*. *Nature*, **346**, 629–33
117. Buck, D. W., Schroeder, K., Suni, M., Kelkenberg, J., Estess, P., Healey, D., Sweet, R. and Truneh, A. (1990). Anti-CD4 idiotypes: potential for AIDS vaccination. In VI International Conference on AIDS, San Francisco: Abstract ThA 353
118. Wilhelm, J., Kalyan, N., Chanda, P., Murthy, S., Vernon, S., Molnar-Kimber, K., Mizutani, S., Davis, A., Lee, S. and Hung, P. (1990). Expression and processing of HIV gag proteins with recombinant adenovirus vectors. In VI International Conference on AIDS, San Francisco: Abstract ThA 348
119. Chatfield, S. N., Strugnell, R. A. and Dougan, G. (1989). Live salmonella as vaccines and carriers of foreign antigenic determinants. *Vaccine*, **7**, 495–8
120. Hunter, R. L. and Bennett, B. (1984). The adjuvant activity of nonionic block polymer surfactants. II. Antibody formation and inflammation related to the structure of trublock and octablock copolymers. *J. Immunol.*, **133**, 3167–75
121. Woodard, L. F. and Jasman, R. L. (1985). Stable oil-in-water emulsions: preparation and

use as vaccine vehicles for lipophilic adjuvants. *Vaccine*, **3**, 137–44
122. O'Hagan, D. T., Palin, R., Davis, S. S., Artursson, P. and Sjoholm, I. (1989). Microparticles as potentially orally active immunological adjuvants. *Vaccine*, **7**, 421–4
123. Brynested, K., Babbitt, B., Huang, L. and Rouse, B. T. (1990). Influence of peptide acylation, liposome incorporation, and synthetic immunomodulators on the immunogenecity of a 1–23 peptide of glycoprotein D of herpes simplex virus: implications for subunit vaccines. *J. Virol.*, **64**, 680–5
124. Naylor, P. T., Larsen, H. S., Huang, L. and Rouse, B. T. (1982). *In vivo* induction of anti-herpes simplex virus immune response by type 1 antigens and lipid A incorporated into liposomes. *Infect. Immun.*, **36**, 1209–16
125. Allison, A. C. and Gregoriadis, G. (1990). Vaccines: recent trends and progress. *Immunol. Today*, **11**, 427–9
126. Kawamura, H. and Berzofsky, J. A. (1986). Enhancement of antigenic potency *in vitro* and immunogenecity *in vivo* by coupling the antigen to anti-immunoglobulin. *J. Immunol.*, **136**, 58–65
127. Carayanniotis, G. and Barber, B. H. (1987). Adjuvant-free IgG responses induced with antigen coupled to antibodies against class II MHC. *Nature*, **327**, 59–61
128. Allison, A. C. (1987). Vaccine technology: adjuvants for increased efficacy. *Biotechnology*, **5**, 1041–5
129. Mills, K. H. G., Barnard, A. L., Williams, M., Stott, E. J., Silvera, P., Page, M., Ling, C., Taffs, F., Kingsman, A. S., Adams, S. E., Almond, N., Kitchin, P. A. and Gaisford, W. C. Vaccine-induced $CD4^+$ T cells against the simian immunodeficiency virus gag protein: epitope specificity and relevance to protective immunity. *J. Immunol.* (in press)

Index

MIX
Papier aus verantwortungsvollen Quellen
Paper from responsible sources
FSC® C105338

If you have any concerns about our products,
you can contact us on
ProductSafety@springernature.com

In case Publisher is established outside the EU,
the EU authorized representative is:
Springer Nature Customer Service Center GmbH
Europaplatz 3, 69115 Heidelberg, Germany

Printed by Libri Plureos GmbH
in Hamburg, Germany